T0073639

Vascular
ULTRASOUND
HOW, WHY AND WHEN

Vascular
ULTRASOUND
HOW, WHY AND WHEN

FOURTH EDITION

Abigail Thrush, MSc
Clinical Scientist (retired)
Chesterfield Royal Hospital NHS Trust
Chesterfield
United Kingdom

Timothy Hartshorne, AVS
Clinical Scientist
University Hospitals of Leicester NHS Trust
Leicester
United Kingdom

Colin Deane, PhD
Clinical Scientist
King's College Hospital
London
United Kingdom

ELSEVIER

Notice

Practitioners and researchers must always rely on their own experience and knowledge in evaluating and using any information, methods, compounds or experiments described herein. Because of rapid advances in the medical sciences, in particular, independent verification of diagnoses and drug dosages should be made. To the fullest extent of the law, no responsibility is assumed by Elsevier, authors, editors or contributors for any injury and/or damage to persons or property as a matter of products liability, negligence or otherwise, or from any use or operation of any methods, products, instructions, or ideas contained in the material herein.

ISBN: 978-0-7020-4656-8

Content Strategist: Trinity Hutton
Content Development Specialist: Andrea Akeh
Publishing Services Manager: Shereen Jameel
Project Manager: Nadhiya Sekar
Design: Renee Duenow
Marketing Manager: Kristen Oyirifi

Printed in the United Kingdom

Last digit is the print number: 9 8 7 6 5 4 3 2 1

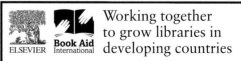

CONTENTS

Introduction

In the 12 years since the last edition of this book, ultrasound has developed considerably. Image quality has improved, automatic optimization of images is now commonplace although not yet perfect, and the proliferation of smaller scanners brings ultrasound to the patient rather than the reverse for selected applications. In vascular ultrasound practice, there have been service developments. Screening for aortic aneurysms is done in the community, vascular surgeons and sonographers use low-cost scanners in clinics. The increase in venous lines has brought a commensurate increase in the number of upper-limb deep venous thrombosis (DVTs). Ultrasound screening for giant cell arteritis is proven, and many centers now run routine transcranial Doppler ultrasound screening for stroke risk in children with sickle cell disease; these last applications are new additions to the book. Vascular ultrasound departments in hospitals are busy as their capabilities and efficacy are increasingly recognized.

The scope of vascular ultrasound brings its own challenges. It is a wide discipline serving a wide range of referring clinicians, not only vascular surgeons, stroke physicians, neurologists, and hematologists but also nephrologists, cardiac physicians and surgeons, pediatricians, ophthalmologists, endocrinologists, and any clinical team for whom investigation of the circulation is part of patient care. The skill required to scan is also varied. The use of small scanners to screen aortic aneurysms in primary care has been shown to be feasible; venous intervention using portable ultrasound in theatre is now routine. However, for many vascular ultrasound applications, high-end scanners are required with staff who are trained to use all aspect of imaging, color flow, and spectral Doppler and who have the understanding to image and measure changes in the circulation to determine the cause and extent of abnormal vascular conditions.

For those of us who practice and enjoy vascular ultrasound, the examination can be like solving a puzzle (Fig. 1.1). A complex scan of the leg arteries might require three different transducers and a large range of measurements to tease out why the flow to the foot looks like it does. The ultrasound practitioner—we have used the word sonographer to include anyone from any profession who is trained to undertake the role—must have the confidence to optimize the B-mode images, the color flow images, and the spectral Doppler measurements to obtain the best information available. They must also have an understanding of normal and abnormal flow to be able to use these findings to report what is occurring in an individual patient. On the occasions when imaging is suboptimal, they must have the confidence and candor to describe the limitations of any scan and to know when the images are inadequate for a full report.

Ultrasound scanning is still very much dependent on the skill and knowledge of the operator. Basic errors such as inadequate image gain setting, or poor spectral Doppler angle correction, can lead to misdiagnosis and potential harm to patients; more subtle errors, for example the wrong transmit frequency or sample volume size, can affect image quality. As always with ultrasound, moving the transducer to image through a better acoustic window or to obtain clearer reflections from an interface or an improved alignment with a vessel to optimize the Doppler trace is an integral part of scanning. The sonographer's proprioception of the scanning hand combines with their understanding of the plane of imaging so that the experienced vascular sonographer will

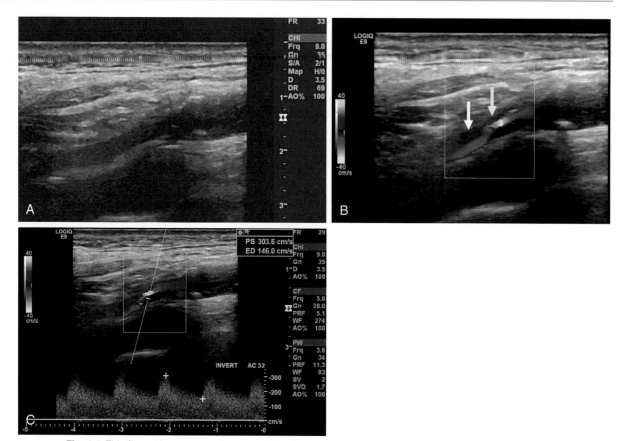

Fig. 1.1 This figure demonstrates how a combination of imaging and Doppler ultrasound can be used identify and grade carotid artery diseases in clinical practice. The artery is seen in image (A), but the lumen is unclear. Color flow imaging (B) shows aliasing *(yellow arrow)* indicating increased velocities with bidirectional flow *(white arrow)* suggesting poststenotic flow. Spectral Doppler (C) records a peak velocity of 304 cm/s indicating a severe stenosis of greater than 70%.

turn the probe to look along and across a vessel, using the image to guide their hand to build up a complete picture of the tissue underneath. This is particularly challenging for vascular sonographers where the image is best shown when interfaces are orthogonal to the beam but when Doppler is best where flow is in line with it.

There is occasional controversy within the medical community related to the professional status and qualification of sonographers and their ability to interpret and report scans. There are often limitations when a person who has not been present during the examination is responsible for issuing a report from static images captured during an examination. There is the potential for detail or information that was evident in real time to be missed. Video recording of images can help a third

party, but the highly trained vascular sonographer has a unique viewpoint from which to understand the full picture.

We have tried to show how ultrasound can be used well for vascular ultrasound applications, when it falls short and how to use it optimally, whether for carotid arteries, DVTs, or the many and increasing applications that continue to be used. The opening chapters review B-mode, color, and spectral Doppler ultrasound, not just from a theoretical aspect but to show how these can be modified and optimized to best display and measure arteries and veins and the flow through them. The chapter on blood flow introduces the physical principles of flow and shows how ultrasound can be used to image this and provide an understanding of specific vascular conditions. Practitioners should be aware of possible errors and the limits of ultrasound; these are reviewed and recommendations and tips for good clinical practice are provided. The following chapters then address each major clinical application, giving the clinical background, scanning techniques, normal appearance, and measurements and changes to these in the presence of disease. Tips as to how to optimize the scan are included for each investigation.

Our perspective is that of vascular sonographers and we do not attempt to tread on the medical and surgical teams' toes; we are there to serve the interests of the patient in providing the best information possible within the larger clinical team. Development of understanding of service needs is best in the context of good communication with the referring clinicians. It is also recognized that vascular ultrasound does not work in isolation; the reader should also obtain an overview of other imaging modalities in order to have an understanding of vascular ultrasound in the context of these other techniques in the care of patients with vascular disorders. They should also take time to study the different radiological, surgical, and medical treatments used to treat peripheral vascular disease.

Ultrasound and B-Mode Imaging

INTRODUCTION

It is important to understand how ultrasound interacts with tissue to be able to interpret ultrasound images and to identify artifacts. Knowledge of how an image is produced allows optimal use of the scanner controls and helps in the understanding of the changes to images seen with manipulation of the transducer. The aim of this and the next few chapters is to give a simple explanation of the process involved in producing images and blood velocity and flow measurements.

NATURE OF ULTRASOUND

Ultrasound, as the name implies, is high-frequency sound. Sound waves travel through a medium by causing local displacement of particles within the medium; however, there is no overall movement of the medium. Unlike light, sound cannot travel through a vacuum, as sound waves need a supporting medium. Consider a piece of string held at both ends; with one end briefly shaken, the vibration caused will travel along the string and in so doing transmit energy from one end of the string to the other. This is known as a transverse wave, as the movement of the string is at right angles to the direction in which the wave has moved. Ultrasound is a longitudinal wave, as the displacement of the particles within the medium is in the same direction as that in which the wave is traveling. Fig. 2.1 shows a medium with particles distributed evenly within it. The position of the particles within the medium will change as a sound wave passes through it, causing local periodic displacement of these particles (see Fig. 2.1B). The size, or amplitude, of these displacements is shown in Fig. 2.1C. As the particles move within the medium, local increases and decreases in pressure are generated (see Fig. 2.1D).

Wavelength and Frequency

Ultrasound is usually described by its frequency, which is related to the length of the wave produced. The wavelength of a sound wave is the distance between consecutive points where the size and direction of the displacement are identical and the direction in which

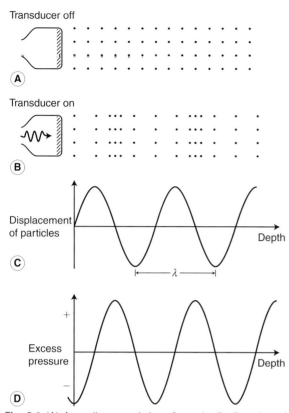

Transducer off

A

Transducer on

B

Displacement of particles

Depth

λ

C

Excess pressure

Depth

+

−

D

Fig. 2.1 (A) A medium consisting of evenly distributed particles. (B) The positions of the particles change (shown here at a given point in time) as the ultrasound wave passes through the medium. (C) The amplitude of the particle displacement. (D) Excess pressure.

TABLE 2.1	Speed of Sound in Different Tissues
Medium	**Speed of Sound (m/s)**
Air	330
Water (20°C)	1480
Fat	1450
Blood	1570
Muscle	1580
Bone	3500
Soft tissue (average)	1540

the tissue (Table 2.1) (e.g., sound travels faster through bone than it does through water). The speed of a sound wave, c, is given by the distance traveled by the disturbance during a given time and is constant in any specific material. The relationship between the speed of sound, its frequency, and wavelength is:

$$c = \lambda f \qquad (2.2)$$

Knowledge of the speed of sound is needed to determine how far an ultrasound wave has traveled. This is required in both imaging and pulsed Doppler (as will be seen later), but ultrasound systems usually make an estimate by assuming that the speed of sound is the same in all tissues: 1540 m/s. This can lead to small errors in the estimated distance traveled because of the variations in the speed of sound in different tissues.

GENERATION OF ULTRASOUND WAVES

The term "transducer" simply means a device that converts one form of energy into another. In the case of an ultrasound transducer, this conversion is from electrical energy to mechanical vibration. The piezoelectric effect is the method by which most medical ultrasound is generated. Piezoelectric materials will vibrate mechanically when a varying voltage is applied across them. The frequency of the voltage applied will affect the frequency with which the material vibrates. The thickness of the piezoelectric element will determine the frequency at which the element will vibrate most efficiently; this is known as the resonant frequency of the transducer. When an appropriate coupling medium is used (e.g., ultrasound gel), this vibration will be transmitted into a surrounding medium, such as the body. The named frequency of a transducer is its resonant frequency. This

the particles are traveling is the same. The wavelength is represented by the symbol λ and is shown in Fig. 2.1C. The time taken for the wave to move forward through the medium by one wavelength is known as the period (τ). The frequency, f, is the number of cycles of displacements passing through a point in the medium during 1 second (s) and is given by:

$$f = 1/\tau \qquad (2.1)$$

The unit of frequency is the hertz (Hz), with 1 Hz being one complete cycle per second. Audible sound waves are in the range of 20 Hz to 20 kHz, whereas medical ultrasound scanners typically use high frequencies of between 1 and 20 MHz (i.e., between 1,000,000 and 20,000,000 Hz).

Speed of Ultrasound

Sound travels through different media at different speeds and is dependent on the stiffness and density of

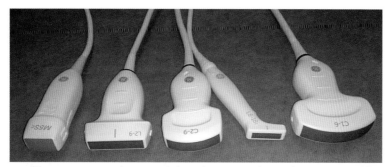

Fig. 2.2 A range of linear array, curved array, and phased array transducers that operate at different frequency ranges. Right to left: curved array (frequency range 1–6 MHz), linear "hockey stick" (8–18 MHz), curved array (2–9 MHz), linear array (2–9 MHz), phased array (1–5 MHz). Between them, these transducer types and frequencies cover most vascular ultrasound applications.

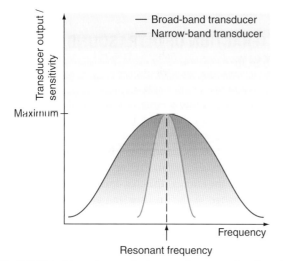

Fig. 2.3 Plot of transducer output versus frequency for a broadband and a narrow-band transducer. A broad-band transducer will be more efficient over a wider range of frequencies than a narrow-band transducer for both transmitting and receiving ultrasound.

is not to say that the transducer will not function at a different frequency, but it will be much less efficient at those frequencies. Most modern imaging transducers are designed as broad-band transducers, meaning that they will function efficiently over a wide range of frequencies, and these are usually labeled with the frequency range over which they operate, for example, 1 to 6 MHz, as seen on the far right in Fig. 2.2. Fig. 2.3 shows how the transducer output of narrow-band and broad-band transducers varies with the frequency of the excitation voltage. A broad-band transducer is more efficient over a wider range of frequencies than a narrow-band transducer. Ultrasound transducers also use the piezoelectric effect to convert the returning ultrasound vibrations back into electrical signals. These signals can then be amplified, analyzed, and displayed to provide anatomical images together with flow information.

Pulsed Ultrasound

Simple Doppler systems (as seen in Fig. 9.6) operate with a continuous single-frequency excitation voltage and are known as continuous-wave (CW) Doppler, but all imaging systems and pulsed Doppler systems use pulsed-wave (PW) excitation signals. If ultrasound is continuously transmitted along a particular path, the energy will also be continuously reflected back from any boundary in the path of the beam, and it will not be possible to predict where the returning echoes have come from. However, when a pulse of ultrasound is transmitted, it is possible to predict the distance (d) of a reflecting surface from the transducer if the time (t) between transmission and reception of the pulse is measured and the velocity (c) of the ultrasound along the path is known, as follows:

$$d = \frac{tc}{2}$$

(2.3)

The factor 2 arises from the fact that the pulse travels along the path twice, once on transmission and once on its return. This pulse echo relationship can be used to determine where returning echoes have originated from within the body.

Frequency Content of Pulses

Typically, the pulses used in imaging ultrasound are very short and will only contain one to three cycles in order that reflections from boundaries that are close together

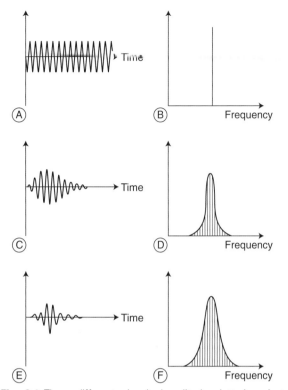

Fig. 2.4 Three different signals (amplitude plotted against time) and their corresponding frequency spectra (power plotted against frequency). (A, B) For a continuous single frequency. (C, D) A long pulse. (E, F) A short pulse. The shorter the pulse, the greater the range of frequencies within the pulse.

can be easily separated. Pulsed Doppler signals are longer and contain several cycles. In fact, a pulse is made up not of a single frequency but of a range of frequencies of different amplitudes. Different-shaped pulses will have different frequency contents. The frequency content of a signal can be displayed on a graph, such as those shown in Fig. 2.4 (right panels). This is known as a frequency spectrum and displays the frequencies present within the signal against the relative amplitudes of these frequencies. Fig. 2.4A provides an example of a continuous signal consisting of a single frequency. As only one frequency is present in the signal, the frequency spectrum displays a single line at that frequency (Fig. 2.4B). Figs. 2.4C and E give examples of two differently shaped pulses along with their frequency spectra (Fig. 2.4D and F), showing the range of frequencies present in each of the different pulses. The shorter pulse in Fig. 2.4E contains a wide range of frequencies (Fig. 2.4F). As ultrasound imaging uses pulsed ultrasound, the transducer is not transmitting

a single frequency but a range of frequencies. A broadband transducer can produce a shorter pulse, which enables better visualization of structures that are close together, giving better resolution.

Beam Shape

The shape of the ultrasound beam produced by a transducer will depend on the shape, number of the element(s), the transmitted frequency, and whether the beam is focused. The shape of the beam will affect the region of tissue that will be insonated and the region from which returning echoes will be received. Array transducers, used in ultrasound imaging, use several elements to produce the beam, as discussed later in this chapter.

INTERACTION OF ULTRASOUND WITH TISSUE

The creation of an ultrasound image depends on the way in which ultrasound energy interacts with the tissue as it passes through the body. When an ultrasound wave meets a large smooth interface between two different media, some of the energy will be reflected back, and this is known as specular reflection. The relative proportions of the energy reflected and transmitted depend on the change in the acoustic impedance between the two materials (see Fig. 2.5). The acoustic impedance of a medium is the impedance (similar to resistance) the material offers against the passage of the sound wave through it and depends on the density and compressibility of the medium. The greater the change in the acoustic impedance across a boundary, the greater the proportion of the ultrasound that is reflected. There is, for example, a large difference in acoustic impedance between soft tissue and bone, or between soft tissue and air, and such interfaces will produce large reflections. This is the reason why ultrasound cannot be used to image beyond lung or bone, except in limited situations, as only a small proportion of the ultrasound is transmitted. It is also the reason for the loss of both imaging and Doppler information beyond calcified arterial walls (see Fig. 8.17B and D), bone, and bowel gas, leading to an acoustic shadow beyond. Table 2.2 shows the ratio of the reflected to incident wave amplitude for a range of reflecting interfaces.

The path along which the reflected ultrasound travels will also affect the amplitude of the signal detected by the

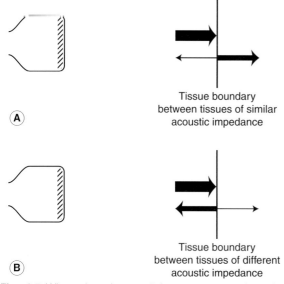

(A)

Tissue boundary
between tissues of similar
acoustic impedance

(B)

Tissue boundary
between tissues of different
acoustic impedance

Fig. 2.5 When the ultrasound beam meets a boundary between two media, some of the ultrasound will be transmitted and some will be reflected. (A) When the two media have similar acoustic impedances, the majority of the ultrasound will be transmitted across the boundary. (B) When the two media have markedly different acoustic impedances, most of the ultrasound will be reflected.

TABLE 2.2 The Ratio of Reflected to Incident Wave Amplitude for an Ultrasound Beam Perpendicular to Different Reflecting Interfaces	
Reflecting Interface	**Ratio of Reflected to Incident Wave Amplitude**
Muscle/blood	0.03
Soft tissue/water	0.05
Fat/muscle	0.10
Bone/muscle	0.64
Soft tissue/air	0.9995

After McDicken 1981, with permission.

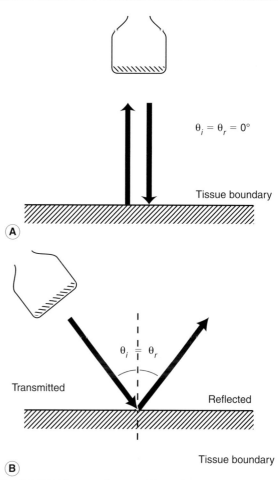

$\theta_i = \theta_r = 0°$

Tissue boundary

(A)

$\theta_i = \theta_r$

Transmitted

Reflected

Tissue boundary

(B)

Fig. 2.6 (A) When an ultrasound beam is perpendicular to an interface, the reflected ultrasound will return by the same path. (B) If the interface is not perpendicular to the beam, then the reflected ultrasound will travel along a different path. The angle of incidence of the beam (θ_i) is equal to the angle of reflection (θ_r).

transducer. If the beam is perpendicular to the interface, the reflected ultrasound will travel back along the same path to the transducer. If, however, the beam intercepts the interface at an angle of less than 90°, then the beam will be reflected along a different path. Fig. 2.6 shows that the angle of incidence (θ_i) is the same as the angle of reflection (θ_r) measured from a line perpendicular (orthogonal) to the interface. This means that when the beam is at 90° to the interface, all the reflected ultrasound will travel back toward the transducer, but when the beam is no longer perpendicular to the interface, the ultrasound beam will be reflected away from the transducer, leading to little or no echoes returning to the transducer. The best image of an interface will be obtained when the interface is at right angles to the beam, and likewise the poorest image will be obtained when the interface is parallel to the beam. Fig. 2.7 shows an ultrasound image of a catheter in a vein. Being a smooth reflective surface, the beam is reflected by the catheter. In Fig. 2.7A the ultrasound beam *(yellow arrows)* is at right angles to the catheter *(yellow*

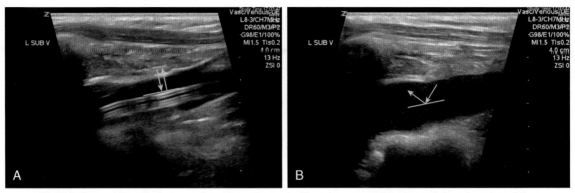

Fig. 2.7 Steered B-mode images of a catheter in a vein. The ultrasound beam is parallel to the edge of the field of view. (A) The ultrasound beam *(yellow arrows)* is at right angles to the catheter *(yellow line)*, so the beam is reflected back to the transducer and the catheter is seen on the image as a bright white structure. (B) The beam is steered in a different direction and is no longer at right angle to the catheter *(arrows)*, so the beam is reflected away from the transducer and the catheter is not detected or displayed.

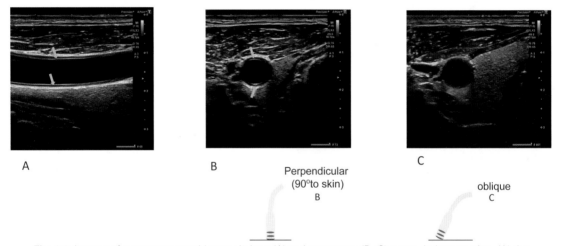

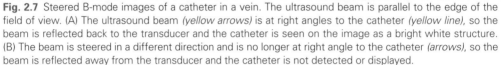

Fig. 2.8 Images of a common carotid artery in long (A) and transverse (B, C) scans. In long section, (A) the intima-media layer is seen on the superficial and deep walls *(arrows)*. In the transverse scans (B, C), the effect of angle dependence is seen where the intima-media layer *(arrows)* is only seen clearly along the beam direction where the specular reflections are reflected back toward the transducer (B) and not along the lateral walls where the reflections are in other directions. In image (C) the transducer is tilted relative to the vessel, so the beam is no longer perpendicular (90°) to vessel wall leading to a loss of clarity and contrast, and the intima-media layer is no longer seen.

line), so the beam is reflected back to the transducer, and the catheter is seen on the image as a bright white structure. In Fig. 2.7B the beam is steered in a different direction and is no longer at right angle to the catheter, so the beam is reflected away from the transducer and is therefore not detected. This results in the catheter not being displayed on the image. In Fig. 2.8 the effect of angle dependence is apparent in the detail seen of the common carotid artery wall in a longitudinal and transverse

scan where the intima-media layer (described in Ch. 5 and Ch.8) is only seen clearly along the beam direction where the specular reflections are directed back toward the transducer and not along the lateral walls where the reflections are in other directions (Fig. 2.8). The effects can also be seen when scanning an artery in transverse when the transducer is tilted relative to the vessel (Fig. 2.8C) so the beam is no longer perpendicular (90°) to the vessel wall. The clarity and contrast of the image of the vessel depends on the angulation of the probe to the vessel; it is optimal at 90°, and the contrast deteriorates as the angle decreases.

If the ultrasound beam is not perpendicular to the interface and there is a change in the speed of sound in the media on either side of the interface, the path of the beam will deviate. This is known as refraction and is illustrated in Fig. 2.9. Refraction causes the beam to change its direction of travel and can lead to artifacts whereby the signal detected by the transducer has

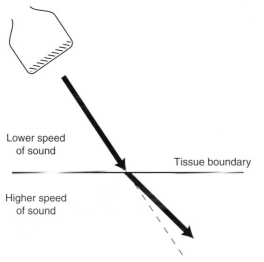

Fig. 2.9 Refraction. When a beam is transmitted through an interface between two media in which the sound travels at different speeds and the beam is not perpendicular to the interface, the path of the beam will be bent.

originated from a different point in the tissue than that displayed on the image. This is most important where there are large changes in the velocity of sound between media. In vascular imaging this can lead to duplicated images of the aorta (Fig. 2.10) and cerebral arteries, when using transcranial Doppler, and can contribute to edge shadowing from artery walls seen in transverse scans (Fig. 2.11).

Although specular reflection occurs at large, smooth boundaries, the majority of signals returning from tissue are made up of ultrasound energy that has been back-scattered from rough surfaces or small structures within the tissue. When the ultrasound beam interacts with a rough surface or small structure, it will be scattered in all directions rather than reflected back along one path. Fig. 2.12 shows the difference between specular reflection and scattering from rough surfaces and small structures. Scattering occurs when the small structures are of a similar size to or smaller than the wavelength of the ultrasound and will result in less of the ultrasound returning to the transducer along the original beam path. The amount of energy lost from the beam by scattering is highly dependent on the frequency (proportional to the fourth power of the frequency [i.e., f^4] for structures that are much smaller than the wavelength of the ultrasound). In the case of peripheral vascular ultrasound, specular reflection will occur at the vessel walls, which are often perpendicular to the beam in longitudinal section, leading to large reflected signals (see Fig. 2.8A). However, ultrasound will be scattered

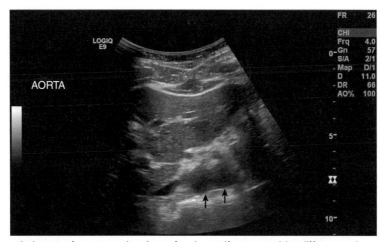

Fig. 2.10 B-mode image of an aorta showing refraction artifact caused by differences in speed of sound between muscle and fat in the abdominal wall, leading to two aortas *(arrows)* being incorrectly displayed.

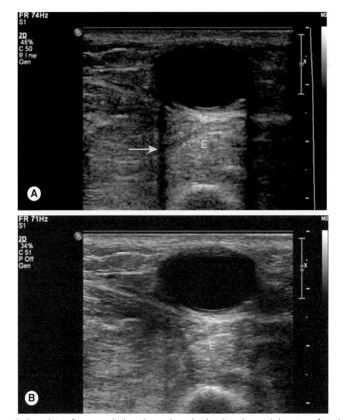

Fig. 2.11 (A) B-mode imaging of a vessel showing edge shadowing *(arrow)* due to refraction. (B) The effect of this refraction artifact can be reduced by the use of compound imaging. Enhancement, *E*, of the echoes beneath a structure of low attenuation.

by groups of red blood cells within the lumen, leading to much smaller returning signals, which will not normally be visible on an image (within the carotid lumen in Fig. 2.8). When blood is moving quickly as in normal arterial and typical venous flow, low-level back-scatter is generated. However, when blood cells move very slowly or even become temporarily stationary, the blood cells aggregate and produce a larger back-scatter signal that can be seen on B-mode imaging. Fig. 2.13 shows images of gastrocnemius veins. In Fig. 2.13A the blood in the veins is moving slowly, and low-level echoes can be seen within the veins. In Fig. 2.13B, where the flow is traveling more quickly following calf compression, the low-level echoes are no longer present, and the lumen now appears black. This static flow can have the misleading appearance of deep vein thrombosis (DVT).

When looking closely at an ultrasound image, it is possible to see a speckle pattern within different organs or tissues, for example, in the thyroid (right of the carotid artery in Fig. 2.8C), the liver, or venous thrombus. Echoes back-scattered from the small structures within the tissue interfere with each other, and the random spacing and back-scatter strength of the echoes of any scatterers within the beam will contribute to the speckle pattern produced at a given depth, giving a grainy appearance on the image. These speckle patterns do not represent true individual structures within the organ but are considered a source of noise within the image. There are various techniques available, discussed later in the chapter, that are used to reduce the impact of speckle on image contrast and spatial resolution.

LOSS OF ULTRASOUND ENERGY IN TISSUE

Attenuation is the loss of energy from the ultrasound beam as it passes through tissue. The more the ultrasound energy is attenuated by the tissue, the less energy will be available to return to the transducer or to penetrate deeper into the tissue. Attenuation is caused by several different processes. These include absorption, scattering, reflection, and beam divergence. Absorption causes ultrasound energy to be converted into heat as the beam passes through the tissue. The rate of absorption

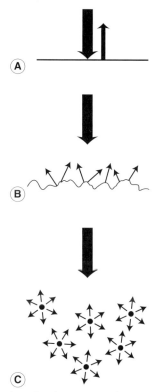

Fig. 2.12 Specular reflections occur at large smooth interfaces (A), whereas ultrasound is scattered by rough surfaces (B) and small structures (C).

varies in different types of tissue. Ultrasound energy can also be lost by scattering from small structures within the tissue or reflection from large boundaries that are not perpendicular to the beam, preventing the ultrasound from returning to the transducer. The attenuation coefficients of various tissues are presented in Table 2.3, from which it can be seen there is a greater attenuation through muscle than through fat. The units of the coefficient of attenuation are in dB MHz^{-1}cm^{-1}, showing that the rate of attenuation depends on frequency of ultrasound, with higher frequencies being attenuated more quickly than lower frequencies. This is why higher ultrasound frequencies penetrate tissue less effectively than lower ultrasound frequencies and can only be used for imaging superficial structures. This is similar to the situation in which you can hear your neighbor's hi-fi bass through the partition wall more than the treble.

PRODUCING AN ULTRASOUND IMAGE

Ultrasound imaging uses information contained in reflected and scattered signals received by the transducer. If it is assumed that the speed of the ultrasound through the tissue is constant, it is possible to predict the distance from a reflective boundary or scattering structure to the transducer. When an ultrasound pulse returns to the transducer, it will cause the transducer to vibrate, and this will generate a voltage across the piezoelectric element. The amplitude of the returning pulse will depend on the proportion of the ultrasound reflected or back-scattered to the transducer and the

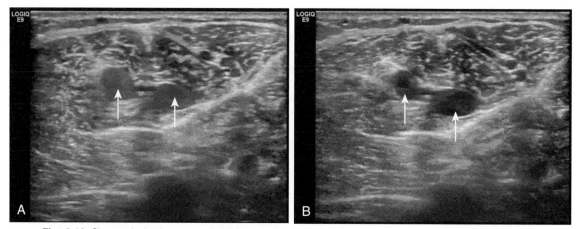

Fig. 2.13 Change in back-scatter signal from blood due to movement. In the two gastrocnemius veins (*arrows*) the image (A) shows increased echoes from stationary blood as it starts to form larger groups of scatterers. (B) If flow is increased, for example following a calf compression image, there is less scattering from flowing blood and the veins appear darker.

amount by which the signal has been attenuated along its path. The amplitude of the pulse received back at the transducer can be displayed against time. This display can be calibrated such that the time delay of the returning pulse represents the distance of the boundary from the transducer, thus showing the depth of the boundary in the tissue. The varying amplitude of the signal can be displayed as a spot of varying brightness that travels down the display with time. This type of display is known as a B-mode (brightness) scan. If the group of transducer elements used to form the beam is moved

slightly so that the beam now passes through the tissue along a path that is adjacent to the first, and the returning signal is displayed next to that from the first pulse, a B-mode image can be produced, as shown diagrammatically in Fig. 2.14A. In this display the distance traveled by the pulse is shown along the vertical axis and the distance between adjacent pulses is shown along the horizontal axis, with the amplitude of the received signal represented by the brightness on the screen. An example of a B-mode image showing a bifurcating artery is presented in Fig. 2.14B.

Ultrasound scanners use electronic multielement array transducers that typically comprise 128 or more piezoelectric elements, capable of producing many adjacent beams or scan lines. The quality of the image depends on the distance between adjacent beam paths, known as the scan line density. The more closely the scan lines are arranged, the more time it will take to produce an image of a given size, which will affect the rate at which the image is updated. This would not be important if a stationary object was being imaged, but most structures in the body are in motion due to cardiac

TABLE 2.3 **Values of Attenuation for Some Tissues**	
Medium	Attenuation (dB cm^{-1} Mhz^{-1})
Water	0.02
Blood	0.15
Muscle	0.57
Bone	22

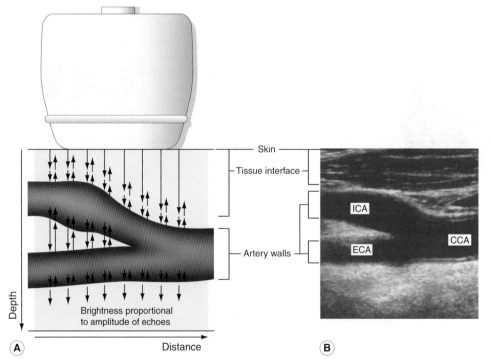

Fig. 2.14 If consecutive ultrasound pulses are transmitted along adjacent paths (A) and displayed in brightness mode in adjacent scan lines, a B-mode image (B) is produced. *CCA,* Common carotid artery; *ECA,* external carotid artery; *ICA,* internal carotid artery.

and respiratory movements. The rate at which complete images are produced per second is known as the frame rate and is affected by the number of scan lines and by the width and depth of the region of tissue being imaged. The deeper the tissue being interrogated, the longer it will take for the returning signal to reach the transducer before the next pulse can be transmitted. In B-mode imaging, it is rarely a problem to produce images with a high enough line density and frame rate.

AMPLIFICATION OF RECEIVED ULTRASOUND ECHOES

There are two methods of increasing the amplitude of the returning signal: increasing the output power and increasing the receiver gain. Increasing the voltage of the excitation pulse across the transducer will cause the transducer to transmit a larger-amplitude ultrasound pulse, thus increasing the amplitude of reflections. However, increasing the output power causes the patient to be exposed to more ultrasound energy, although this is

not usually a cause for concern in vascular imaging with the exception of transorbital imaging. The alternative is to amplify the received signal, but there is a limit at which the amplitude of the received signal is no greater than the background noise, and at which no amount of amplification will assist in differentiating the signal from the noise. Fig. 2.15 shows an image of a thrombus with different gain settings. With the gain set too low (Fig. 2.15A), the thrombus is difficult to visualize. With the gain set high (Fig. 2.15C), the image starts to become saturated to bright white, and image detail is lost. For a given frequency of transducer, the depth at which the reflected or back-scattered signals are no longer greater than the noise is known as the penetration depth.

Increasing the overall gain of the received signal will increase both the high-amplitude signals detected near the transducer and the lower-amplitude signals detected from deeper in the tissue, which have been attenuated to a greater extent. Ideally, reflections from similar boundaries at different depths should be displayed at a similar brightness level on the image. Fig. 2.16A and B show a

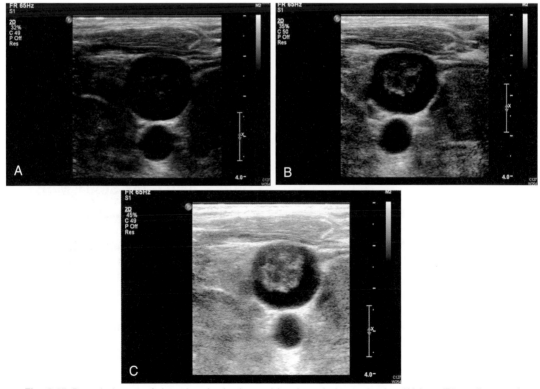

Fig. 2.15 B-mode image of thrombus in the internal jugular vein imaged using (A) low, (B) medium, and (C) high gain.

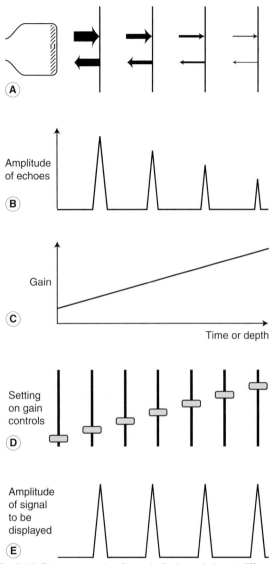

Fig. 2.16 Echoes returning from similar boundaries at different depths (A) will be of different amplitudes (B) due to attenuation. The receiver gain of the scanner can be increased during the time that the echoes are received (C) using the gain controls (D) to produce signals of similar amplitude (E).

diagram of signals returning from four identical boundaries at different depths in an attenuating medium. It can be seen that the echoes received from the deeper boundaries have been attenuated more than those from the shallower boundaries. If the gain of the receiver amplifier is increased over the time during which the pulse is returning to the transducer (Fig. 2.16C and D), it is possible to use greater amplification for the signal received from the deeper boundaries. By changing the gain over time, the returning echoes from the four boundaries can now be displayed at a similar brightness (Fig. 2.16E). When the next pulse is transmitted, the gain would return to the baseline value and increase with time as before. This method of varying gain over time is known as time gain compensation (TGC). The ultrasound scanner makes automatic gain compensations based on assumptions of attenuation in soft tissue, but the sonographer can adjust the TGC, for example, if intervening tissue is highly attenuating, by a set of sliding knobs or paddles to allow different gains to be set for signals returning from different depths, as shown in Fig. 2.16D. Fig. 2.17 shows an abdominal image where ascites, excess fluid in the abdominal cavity, is leading to low attenuation of ultrasound in the near field. The TGC can be adjusted to overcome this change in attenuation rate compared to that which is typical in soft tissue, enabling an optimized view of the deeper tissue.

It is important to select gain levels appropriate to the examination and to be prepared to adjust it during the scan. Some plaques and thrombus can have weak scattering that do not have high contrast with the surrounding blood (which is why compression ultrasound for leg DVTs is used). While increasing gain may produce a saturated and unpleasant looking image, weak echoes may be amplified to display thrombus and plaque where necessary (Fig. 2.18). Different manufacturers describe gain values differently; operators should be aware of the range of gain levels in the scanners they use and the typical values for a particular application.

DYNAMIC RANGE, COMPRESSION CURVES, AND GRAY-SCALE MAPS

The range of echoes received by the transducer—the dynamic range—is enormous; the highest amplitudes are of an order of 100,000 times that of the smallest signal detected. This large range of signal amplitudes can best be described using the decibel scale (see Appendix A) as 100 dB. The range of signals that can be displayed by different gray levels is much less than 100 dB, typically 20 dB, and therefore the range of signal amplitudes needs to be reduced in order to be displayed best to suit the type of scan. For example, the transducer detects strong echoes from tissue-air or tissue-bone and weak echoes from blood, yet we might want to see differences in the gray scale between plaque and thrombus

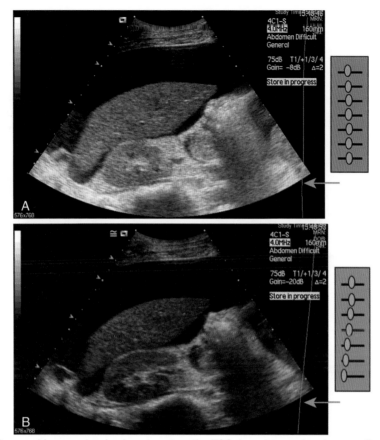

Fig. 2.17 Ultrasound images showing how to set up the TGC *(arrow)* to produce image uniformity. Ascites, excess fluid in the abdominal cavity, leads to low attenuation of ultrasound in the near field resulting in liver and kidney being insonated at greater power (A) than normal at this depth and echoes are bright. TGC can be adjusted to produce a more uniform image by reducing gain for deeper echoes (B). *TGC,* Time gain compensation.

where the differences in echoes are subtle. This can be achieved by restricting the dynamic range of echoes for the gray scale used, for example, choosing white for all echoes above a certain level and black for all echoes below it, and also by compressing the signal where more gain is applied to lower-amplitude signals than higher-amplitude signals, so reducing the dynamic range of the signal to be displayed.

Fig. 2.19A gives an example of a compression curve, showing how the amplitude of the signal to be displayed relates to the amplitude of the input signal. The input signal is the received signal, which has already been amplified by the TGC. This compression curve accentuates the differences in lower- to mid-range amplitude signals. The choice of compression curve used depends on what aspect of the image is important in a given application, for example, the fine detail of back-scatter

from tissue or the presence of large boundaries, such as vessel walls. There are usually a range of compression curves available on modern scanners, which are often selected automatically by the system, depending on the application preset used (e.g., vascular or abdominal). Alternatively there may be a control called the dynamic range which enables the degree of compression used to be altered directly by the sonographer. Figs. 2.19B and C show the aorta and liver imaged using two different dynamic range settings, (B) being a low dynamic range and (C) a high dynamic range. Fig. 2.18 shows the interaction of altering both the gain and dynamic range on the appearance of a carotid plaque.

Finally, the scanner uses a gray-scale map to assign a level of gray dependent on the amplitude of the amplified signal, to produce the gray-scale image. Some systems have a choice of gray-scale maps, used in different

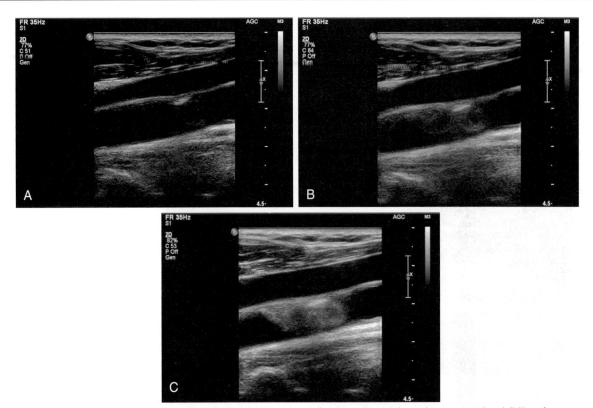

Fig. 2.18 B-mode images showing the interaction when adjusting gain and dynamic range on the visibility of a carotid plaque. (A) Gain 77%, dynamic range 51; (B) gain 77%, dynamic range 64; (C) gain 82%, dynamic range 63. (With permission from Allan et al., Churchill Livingstone.)

applications, and these will affect the appearance of the image. Many systems also offer maps with a different hue (for example, red or blue tints), which may help in the perception of images. Once again, different manufacturers have a range of values and descriptors of dynamic range, and it is worthwhile learning the options available and to explore the effect of the compression curves and gray-scale maps used on the image obtained.

TRANSDUCER DESIGNS AND BEAM-FORMING

To produce an image, the transducer has to send ultrasound into the area of tissue to be examined and will then receive echoes from the insonated tissue. This is done by array transducers containing many elements arranged in a row. Fig. 2.20 shows a schematic diagram of a range of different-shaped transducers (linear array, curved array, and phased array and a linear in trapezoidal mode), producing a range of field of views (region

scanner by the transducer). This schematic diagram also gives an indication of how the scan lines are arranged to cover the field of view. To form an individual scan line or beam, a group of elements are all excited simultaneously (see Fig. 2.21A), and the wavelets will interfere to produce a beam that is perpendicular to the transducer face. The groups of elements within the array that are excited can be varied to produce ultrasound beams that follow adjacent paths (see Fig. 2.21B). For example, elements 1–5 produce the first beam, 2–6 the second, 3–7 the third, and so on until all the tissue under investigation is insonated. Using several elements to form the ultrasound beam enables the beam shape to be manipulated. If the elements used to form the beam are excited at slightly different times, the wavefronts produced by the elements will interfere differently than they would if they were all excited at the same time. For example, if the element on the far right in the array (Fig. 2.22A) is excited first, with the next element excited after a very short delay, and so forth, the wavefronts produced will

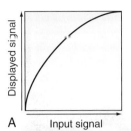

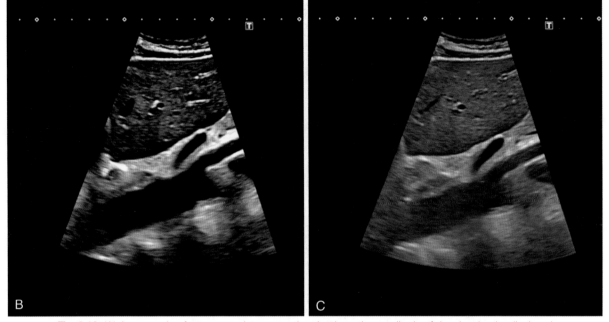

Fig. 2.19 (A) An example of a compression curve, showing how the amplitude of the signal to be displayed relates to the amplitude of the input signal. (B,C) Aorta and liver imaged using two different dynamic range settings, (B) low dynamic range and (C) high dynamic range.

interfere in such a way that the beam is no longer perpendicular to the front of the transducer. The angle at which the beam is produced will depend on the delay between the excitation pulses of the different elements. By changing the delay between each set of excitation pulses, it is possible to steer the beam through a range of angles from left to right. This is used for compound imaging (discussed later in the chapter) and for steering color flow imaging and spectral Doppler beams in linear arrays. In phased array sector transducers, beam steering is used to sweep the beam though the field of view.

Alterations in the timing of elements are also used to produce focused transmit beams. Fig. 2.22B shows how, if the elements at each end of the group of active elements are excited first, with the next two elements being excited after a short delay, and so forth, the wavelets will interfere to produce a concave wavefront causing the

beam to converge at the focal point. The distance of the focal point from the front of the transducer is governed by the length of the time delays, with longer delays producing a shorter focal length.

A wide range of transducers are available on most scanners all serving different functions. Each transducer is optimized, for example, by transmit frequency, footprint (size of the transducer face in contact with the skin), and elevation width (slice thickness) for a range of applications and imaging formats at depths appropriate to the application. For a comprehensive vascular ultrasound service, up to five or six transducers might be needed depending on the versatility of individual transducers (see Fig. 2.2).

Transducer types used are:

Linear arrays give a rectangular image (for example, Fig. 2.8), although many offer a trapezoid option in

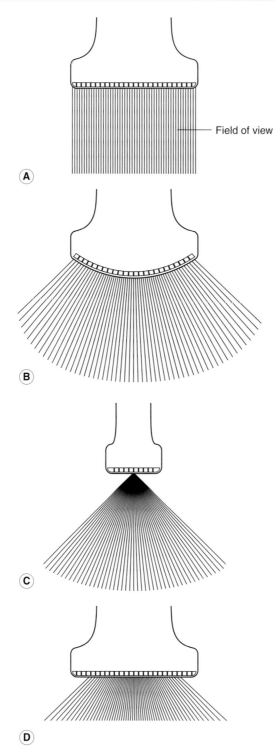

Field of view

Fig. 2.20 (A) Linear array transducer. This is typically made up of 128 elements in a row and produces a rectangular field of view. (B) Curved array transducer. This produces a sector image, with a field of view that diverges with depth. (C) Phased array transducer. This uses a narrower array of 128 elements using all the element simultaneously to electronically steer the beam to produce a sector image. (D) Some linear array transducers can steer the beam at both ends of the transducer to produce a trapezoidal shape field of view.

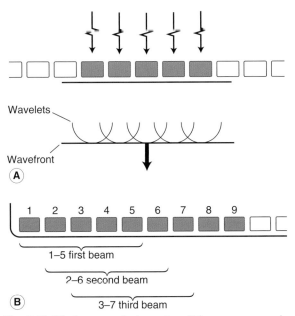

Fig. 2.21 (A) A group of elements within an array can be excited simultaneously, and the resulting wavelets will interfere to produce a wavefront perpendicular to the transducer face. (B) The group of elements excited within an array can be varied to produce beams following parallel adjacent paths.

B-mode (see Fig. 8.5). These are usually higher-frequency probes and are used for carotid arteries, peripheral arteries, DVTs in the leg and arm, and for varicose veins. They come in a range of frequencies, but probes of approximately 3 to 12 MHz are suitable for carotid, DVT, and the thigh and calf; higher-frequency probes may be beneficial for varicose veins and vessels in the arm and foot. "Hockey stick" high-frequency linear arrays give excellent images of the first 2 cm of tissue (Fig. 2.2) and are useful for pedal arteries, temporal arteries, the veins and arteries in the forearm, and in young children.

Curvilinear arrays produce an image that fans out from the curved surface, enabling a wider region of tissue to be imaged in the field of view. They are used for abdominal scanning and in vascular imaging for imaging the aorta (Fig. 2.10), the iliac arteries and veins, and the abdominal vessels. The frequency range is typically 1 to 5 MHz, and the design is optimized for tissue deeper than 4 cm. They can be useful in the assessment of femoral vessels in large patients. They can be useful to examine the patency and to exclude gross disease of carotid arteries in patients with thick necks, although the resolution is significantly inferior to higher-frequency linear arrays. Higher-frequency curvilinear arrays are designed

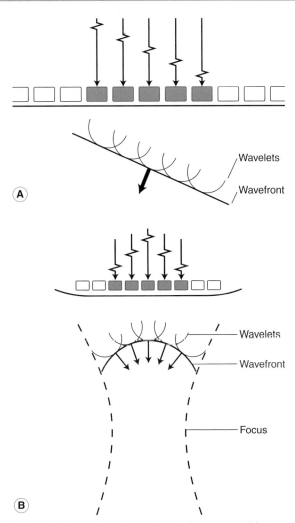

Fig. 2.22 (A) Introducing a time delay between exciting consecutive elements within the array causes the wavelets to interfere in such a way that the beam is steered away from the path perpendicular to the transducer face (e.g., steered left or right). (B) Delays between excitation of the elements in the array can be used to focus the beam.

to image more superficially and can be useful in subclavian and brachiocephalic vessels, and in the thigh and popliteal fossa where the wider field of view helps the practitioner to assess occlusions and collaterals.

Phased array transducers produce a "sector" image from a small flat surface. Designed for cardiac applications where their small footprint allows for imaging from small "acoustic windows" (for example, intercostally), the image quality is inferior to curvilinear probes because of the reduced aperture for focusing.

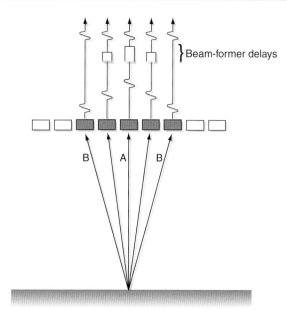

Fig. 2.23 Introducing delays before summing the signals received at different elements allows dynamic focusing of the received beam. In this case, dynamic focusing allows the signals that have traveled farther along path *B* to be added to the signal that has traveled along path *A* by delaying the signal received by the middle element before summing it with the signals received by the outer elements.

Nevertheless, low-frequency (2–3 MHz) phased arrays have good color and Doppler sensitivity and are useful as a backup for imaging renal arteries. They are also used for transcranial Doppler imaging (see Fig. 17.7).

FOCUSING THE BEAM

The ultrasound beam can be focused in transmission to improve the image quality within the focal zone as described earlier. Many scanners enable the use of multiple zone focusing whereby the image will be created in zones, using different focal lengths for different depths. The advantage is that image quality is improved throughout the image; however, the disadvantage is that the frame rate (number of new images a second) is reduced by a factor of 1/(number of focal zones).

The focus of the beam is also altered during reception. This is known as dynamic focusing. In this case, delays are introduced between consecutive elements on reception, rather than transmission, before the received signals are summed together. This is illustrated in Fig. 2.23; dynamic focusing allows the signals that have traveled farther along path B to reach the target to be added to the signal that has traveled along path A by delaying the signal received by the middle element before summing it with the signals received by the outer elements. The focal point of the received signal again depends on the lengths of the delays introduced and is automatically adjusted during the time the pulse is received to optimize for the depth of returning pulse. The receive focus can utilize small apertures for early returned signals for superficial tissue and can introduce a wider aperture for deeper echoes. The effective beam is where the transmit and receive beams overlap and is the area of the tissue from which echoes will be used to form the image.

Beam focusing in transmit and receive assumes a consistent and known speed of sound in the tissue through which the ultrasound passes. This is a major limitation of ultrasound, since variations or in homogeneities of tissue in the field of view may cause beam aberration whereby the beam becomes defocused, for example, if there are areas of fat in the field of view where the speed of sound is reduced. Manufacturers are introducing speed-of-sound corrections and optimization to improve compensation of these variations and produce improved images, but this still plays a significant part in the quality of ultrasound imaging. Experienced ultrasound practitioners know that by moving a transducer to look through an improved "acoustic window" the spatial and contrast resolution is improved as the ultrasound to and from the target passes through tissue with more consistent acoustic properties. Each application has particular scanning approaches that may lend themselves to better imaging; an example of this is shown in Fig. 2.24. It is good practice not to fixate on the first images obtained but to move the transducer and optimize the controls to see if better images are achievable.

A technique known as parallel beam-forming may be used to improve the frame rate (number of images produced per second). This uses a wide, weakly focused transmitted beam. The received signal produced from this transmitted beam can then be processed using different sets of delays in order to form two or more different received beams, simultaneously, as shown in Fig. 2.25 (Whittingham and Martin 2019). This allows two or more received beams, producing two or more scan lines, for each transmitted pulse, thus enabling higher frame rates. Some modern scanners form the image

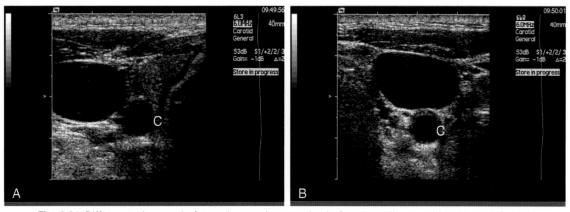

Fig. 2.24 Differences in speed of sound cause inaccuracies in focusing. Ultrasound has to pass through tissue to the target (transmit) and back through tissue to the transducer (receive). (A) An image of the carotid artery *(C)* is unclear because of the variation in tissues superficial to the artery. (B) The jugular vein acts as an acoustic window leading to improved image quality from better beam-forming and reduced attenuation.

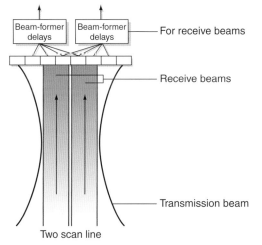

Fig. 2.25 Parallel beam-forming of two or more received beams from a single wide transmitted beam permits improvements in imaging frame rate. (With permission, Hoskins et al. 2019).

using very wide transmit beams and multiple receive beams, which enables high frame rates. These scanners may not have the facility for the sonographer to control the transmit focus.

IMAGE RESOLUTION

The resolution of a system is defined as its ability to distinguish between two adjacent closely placed objects. Figs. 2.26A and B demonstrate how the echoes from two reflecting surfaces can be resolved, seen as separate boundaries, and that they can no longer be distinguished

from each other if the two objects are closer together (Fig. 2.26C and D). The resolution of an ultrasound image can be described in three planes: axial (along the beam), lateral (across the image), and slice thickness (elevation plane)—as shown in Fig. 2.27. Axial resolution depends on the length of the excitation pulse, which in turn depends on the transmit frequency of the transducer. The higher the frequency, the better the axial resolution. There is, however, a compromise, as the higher the frequency, the greater the attenuation and therefore the poorer the penetration. This can be seen when comparing images from two different frequency transducers in Fig. 2.28. Choosing the frequency of transducer to use for a given examination depends on a compromise between the depth of the region to be imaged and the axial resolution that can be obtained. It is preferable to select the highest-frequency transducer that will provide adequate penetration.

Lateral resolution depends on the focusing of the beam (Fig. 2.29) and the density of the scan lines. The focus is in turn dependent on the aperture available and the consistency of the tissue through which the beam is focused. Image quality can be improved by having a higher line density or using multiple focal zones; however, these will lead to lower frame rates with reduced temporal resolution. The sonographer can decide whether a particular application requires an improved static image or a faster updated image (higher frame rate). Lateral resolution is generally poorer than axial resolution and may vary with depth and lateral position in the image. In those scanners that still have a

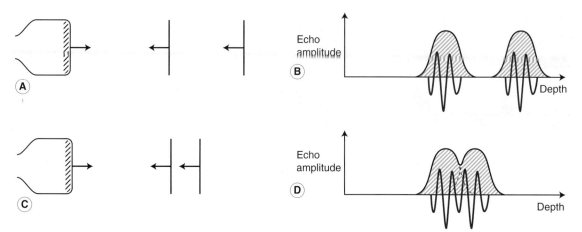

Fig. 2.26 Echoes returning from two boundaries (A) can be resolved (B). However, if the boundaries are close together (C), they can no longer be seen as different echoes (D).

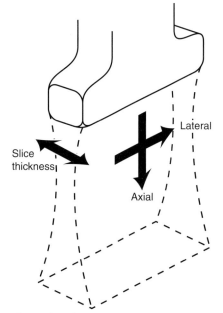

Fig. 2.27 Resolution of a transducer can be described in different planes—axial and lateral. The slice thickness of the beam relates to the width of the beam in the nonimaging (elevation) plane and governs the thickness of the slice of tissue being imaged.

transmit focus, the focus should be set at the depth of the region of most interest to improve spatial and contrast resolution. It is also important to set the depth of imaging to just cover the depth of imaging required and not to display unnecessary depth as this will reduce frame rate and can impact on spatial resolution. If a detailed image of a smaller structure at depth is required, zoom controls are available to facilitate this.

The thickness in the elevation plane (slice thickness) should be thin as possible over a wide range of depths to maintain image quality. Focusing is conventionally done using a fixed lens on the front of the transducer, although more recently there is increased use of matrix arrays where a grid of elements allows focusing in both the imaging plane and the plane at right angles to the image, the elevation plane.

TISSUE HARMONIC IMAGING

Tissue harmonic imaging (THI) can improve the image quality by reducing noise. THI utilizes the fact that high-amplitude ultrasound pulses undergo nonlinear propagation, whereby the pulse becomes progressively distorted as it passes through tissue (Fig. 2.30; Whittingham 1999). This distortion of the pulse results in the frequency content of the returning pulse being significantly different from that of the transmitted pulse. Fig. 2.30D shows how the energy spectrum of the distorted pulse will contain harmonic frequencies ($2f$, $3f$, etc.) that are multiples of the original transmitted frequency, f. These harmonic frequencies can be extracted and used to form the B-image.

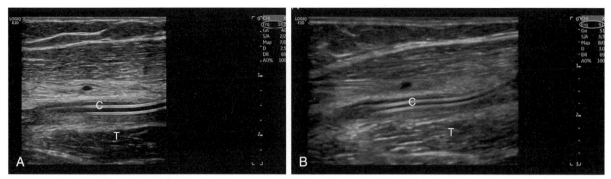

Fig. 2.28 Frequency *(circled)*, resolution, and penetration. The images are of a catheter in a subclavian vein. With a high-frequency transducer, 18 MHz (A) the outer and inner surfaces of the catheter *(C)* are separated (the edge of the catheter is a smooth surface and the thickness of the line from the specular reflection in the image is dependent on the pulse length). With a lower-frequency transducer, 9 MHz (B) the pulse echoes from the surface of the catheter are longer and the outer and inner surfaces are not seen as separated. However, the lower-frequency probe has better penetration to the deeper tissue *(T)*.

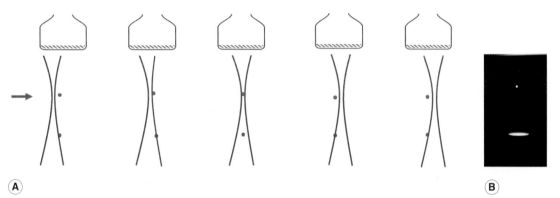

Fig. 2.29 Schematic diagram showing the effect of the beam width on the appearance of a small structure on the image. (A) Shows consecutive scan lines with a focus beam (focal point shown by *arrow*) as it images two small structures *(dots)*. (B) Shows that where the beam is narrow, at the focal point, the object is shown as a narrow point on the image, but where the beam is wider and has intercepted the beam on several scan lines, the image of the structure appears wider.

The stated benefits of harmonic imaging are that the harmonic beam is concentrated in the center of the original beam and that this confers advantages with improved lateral and slice thickness resolution, due to a reduction in the beam width (Fig. 2.31B). The harmonic image also contains fewer artifacts from the tissue just underneath the transducer, since tissue harmonics develop as the pulse becomes deeper so that there is a reduction in noise from reverberations, grating lobes, and side lobes that result from high intensities of the fundamental frequency in the near field. The implementation of harmonic imaging is complex and may combine elements of the fundamental and harmonic signals. Most scanners now used THI as a default image setting although non-THI imaging (fundamental imaging) is usually still an option and produces different, sometimes better, images; the sonographer should experiment with the THI settings available in their particular scanner.

SPATIAL COMPOUND IMAGING

In spatial compound imaging, the B-mode image is formed by obtaining multiple images with the beam steered at several slightly different angles (Fig. 2.32). The returning echoes from these beams, steered at

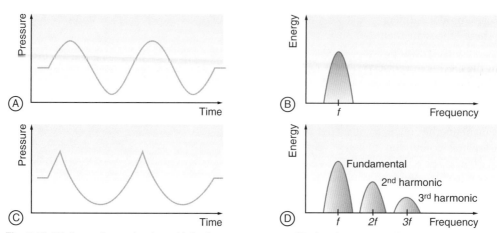

Fig. 2.30 (A) An undistorted pulse with its frequency spectra (B) showing a center frequency *f*. (C) Large-amplitude signals become progressively distorted as they pass through tissue. (D) The distorted pulse contains harmonics (2*f*, 3*f*, etc.) of the fundamental frequency *f*. (From Whittingham, T. A. (1999). Tissue harmonic imaging. *European Radiology*, 9 (Suppl. 3): S323–S326. With kind permission from Springer Science + Business Media.)

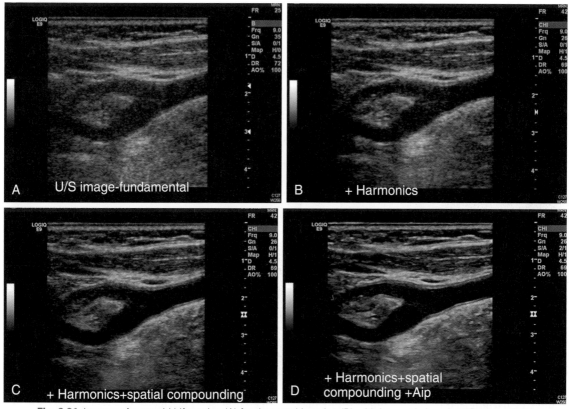

Fig. 2.31 Images of a carotid bifurcation (A) fundamental imaging (B) with harmonic imaging (C) plus spatial compound imaging (D) plus adaptive image processing.

different angles, produce different speckle patterns at each point. These echoes are then combined to produce a single image, and the speckle patterns are averaged out, thus reducing the speckle and noise within the image. This technique also gives improved imaging of interfaces that are not parallel to the transducer face, for example, curved boundaries such as vessel walls. Fig. 2.31C shows the improvement in the image that can be provided when using spatial compound imaging. Compound imaging also reduces the effect of shadowing for highly reflective structures. In practice, there are occasions when this shadow artifact is useful; Fig. 2.33 shows an

example where scanning without spatial compounding helps locate a catheter in the ultrasound image.

ADAPTIVE IMAGE PROCESSING

Ultrasound scanners have image-processing techniques to help enhance the image. For example, edge enhancement can be used to accentuate edges or boundaries; however, this may be at the expense of increasing the impact of noise or speckle on the image. Image-smoothing techniques can reduce the impact of noise on the image but can reduce the sharpness of edges. With adaptive image processing, a scanner analyzes the content of the image at each point on the image and applies the appropriate image-processing technique to optimize edges while reducing noise and speckle. The techniques and their names vary between ultrasound manufacturers, and the sonographer may need to consult the scanner manual (or on-board help function) to identify this facility, which is usually automatically applied to all imaging. Fig. 2.31D shows the change to an image when adaptive processing is added, along with other image optimization techniques.

Harmonic imaging, spatial compounding, and adaptive processing give the operator several combinations of options to optimize images (see Fig. 2.31). The advent of these technologies, with improvements in penetration from higher frequencies, better beamforming, and better control of the slice thickness, has led to significant improvements to ultrasound imaging performance.

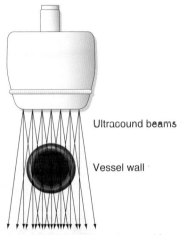

Fig. 2.32 Compound scanning sums several images obtained with the ultrasound beam steered at slightly different angles, to improve imaging of boundaries that are perpendicular to the transducer face and to reduce noise and speckle.

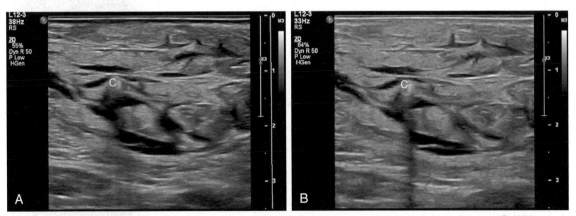

Fig. 2.33 Disadvantages of compound imaging. The catheter is seen as a bright echo in the images *(C)*. With compound imaging, there is weak shadowing seen in several directions (A). By turning the compounding off (B) there is strong single shadow that makes the location of the catheter easier to determine during the procedure.

CONTRAST AGENTS AND B-MODE IMAGING

Contrast agents have been developed to enhance the visualization of blood flow and perfusion. Ultrasound contrast agents are gas-filled bubbles with a thin outer shell, injected in solution via a vein, which are comparable in size to red blood cells and thus able to pass through the circulation. The presence of the contrast agent can be viewed using ultrasound as they travel through both large vessels and perfuse smaller vessels within organs such as the liver.

There are several ways in which microbubbles interact with ultrasound. First, the compressibility of the bubble makes it a strong scatter of ultrasound. However, when the microbubbles are diluted in the blood flow, this effect is limited. Second, when a gas bubble is insonated by an ultrasound pulse, the changing pressure generated by the pulse will cause the bubbles to oscillate. During the positive pressure (compression) part of the oscillation the bubble will contract, and during the negative pressure (rarefaction) the bubble will expand. The bubbles oscillate most effectively at their resonant frequency, which is within the range of frequencies used in diagnostic ultrasound. This can be detected and displayed by the ultrasound scanner. The

way the microbubbles react will also depend on the acoustic pressure of the pulse (often indicated by the Mechanical Index, MI, discussed in Ch. 7). As shown in Fig. 2.34, at low acoustic pressure the bubbles will oscillate symmetrically; however, at higher acoustic pressures the bubbles are unable to contract as much as they can expand, so the oscillations are asymmetric (nonlinear), and this will result in the scattered signal containing not only the incident frequencies but also the second harmonic. These harmonic frequencies can be extracted and displayed to enable better detection of the presence of contrast. At even higher acoustic pressures, the bubbles will burst and then can no longer be seen. This makes it possible to use a brief high-amplitude pulse to burst the contrast agent bubbles then, using a low MI imaging to visualize the reperfusion of the tissue. Therefore, there are different contrast imaging techniques that rely on different values of MI. In contrast imaging mode, the standard B-mode images are often displayed side by side with the contrast-enhanced image (see Fig. 11.22). In vascular ultrasound, contrast-enhanced ultrasound imaging (CEUS) has been used in imaging endovascular aortic repair grafts for detection of endoleaks, which may result in low flow into the aneurysm sac, which is difficult to detect on color flow imaging.

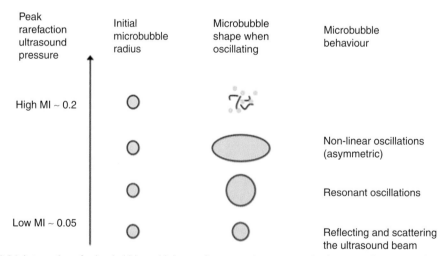

Fig. 2.34 Interaction of microbubbles with increasing acoustic pressure. As the acoustic pressure increases, the microbubbles oscillate nonlinearly and eventually collapse, releasing free gas bubbles. (From Moran, C., & Butler, M. (2019). Contrast agents. In Hoskins et al (with permission).

B-MODE IMAGING ARTIFACTS

An imaging artifact is a feature on the image that does not relate exactly to a structure within the tissue being investigated. This can be due to a feature being misplaced on the image, a feature appearing on the image that is not present within the tissue, or an existing structure that is absent from the image. The creation of an image relies on the assumption that the ultrasound beam travels in a straight path between the transducer and the structures within the tissue and returns along the same path once reflected. It is also assumed that the speed of sound and the attenuation of tissues in the path of the pulse are constant. Any process that alters this situation can lead to the misplacement or absence of information or the presence of image features not present in the tissue. This can be caused by the following:

- Multiple reflections can lead to reverberation artifacts, seen as several equidistant echoes that reduce in brightness with depth. This is due to multiple reflections, along the same path, between the transducer and a strongly reflecting boundary (Fig. 2.35A) or between two parallel, strongly reflecting surfaces (Fig. 2.35B). If the multiple reflections do not return along the same path, the structure may be misplaced on the image (Fig. 2.35C), as the scanner assumes the pulse has traveled in a straight line to the target and back and positions the echo at a depth dependent on the time taken for the pulse to return.

- A mirror image of a structure can be produced in the presence of a strongly reflecting surface. Fig. 2.35D shows how the true position of a structure, that scatters the ultrasound, is displayed, with a second ghost

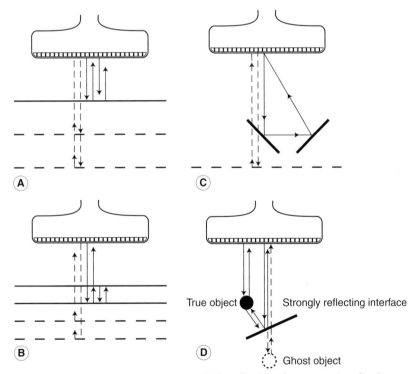

Fig. 2.35 Imaging artifacts can be produced by multiple reflections from strongly reflecting surfaces. The *solid line* shows the true path of the ultrasound beam. The *dashed lines* show the path of the beam assumed by the ultrasound scanner and the assumed interfaces displayed on the ultrasound images. (A) Multiple reflections between the transducer and a strongly reflecting boundary. (B) Multiple reflections between two parallel, strongly reflecting surfaces. (C) Multiple reflections not returning along the same path. (D) Mirror image produced in the presence of a strongly reflecting surface.

image also displayed. The ghost image has been created by an ultrasound beam that has undergone multiple reflections from the strongly reflecting surface.

- Structures can also be absent from the image if their interface with the beam is not perpendicular or near perpendicular to the beam, as the echo will be reflected away from the transducer (Fig. 2.6) and not detected and displayed as seen in Fig. 2.7.
- Refraction can lead to bending of the path of the ultrasound when the beam passes through an interface between two media in which the speed of sound is different (see Fig. 2.9). An example of an imaging artifact that occurs due to refraction is shown in Fig. 2.10 with two images of the aorta, rather than the true single aorta, seen. Another refection artifact is edge shadowing (Fig. 2.11A).
- Echoes can be displaced on the image if the tissue which the pulse passes through has a different speed of sound than is assumed for soft tissue, for example, a region of fat. This can lead to distortion of boundaries.
- Grating lobes are areas of lower-intensity ultrasound outside the main beam and are produced as a function of the multielement structure of array transducers. These grating lobes can lead to strongly reflecting surfaces outside the main beam

being displayed in the image. These artifacts may be reduced by THI.

- If there is a significant difference in the attenuation seen by different scan lines, the tissue at depth may appear as different levels of gray, despite having similar back-scatter properties (see Fig. 2.36). The tissue beneath a low-attenuation, anechoic region such as a vessel may appear brighter than adjacent areas (see E in Fig. 2.11A). Highly attenuating tissue, however, such as calcified plaque, can cause loss of ultrasound information beneath the calcification, leading to a shadow (see Fig. 8.36 and Fig. 8.17B).

The image in Fig. 2.37 shows how an artifact, created by multiple reflections from a strongly reflecting surface such as the vein wall or a muscle boundary, can give the appearance of a dissection, or tear, of the carotid artery wall. If an artifact is suspected, the vessel should be imaged in different planes or from different angles by tilting the transducer. The artifact may then appear in a different position relative to the vessel or may not appear at all, confirming that it is not a true structure that has been visualized. Slight changes in probe pressure can help demonstrate reverberation artifacts as the artifact will move the position within the image. It is usually easier to identify artifacts in real-time imaging than on a frozen image.

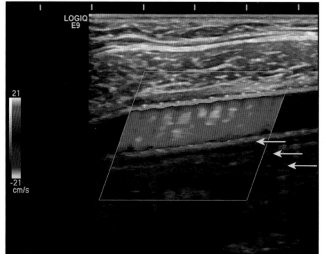

Fig. 2.36 Differences in attenuation can be observed in this image of a synthetic bypass graft. The graft has spaced external supporting rings that are causing increased attenuation in the tissue lying below the rings *(arrows)*. This effect can be seen on both the B-mode and color flow imaging.

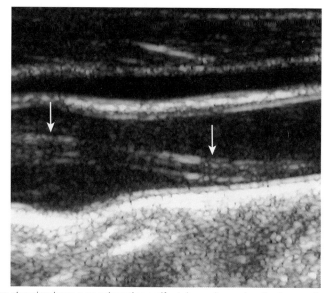

Fig. 2.37 An image showing how a reverberation artifact *(arrow)* can give the impression of a dissection, or tear, of the carotid artery wall.

Doppler Ultrasound

THE DOPPLER EFFECT

The Doppler effect enables ultrasound to be used to detect blood flow and to quantify vascular disease. The Doppler effect is the change in the observed frequency due to the relative motion of the source and the observer. This effect can be heard when the pitch of a police car's siren changes as the car travels toward you and then away from you. Fig. 3.1 helps to explain the effect in more detail. In Fig. 3.1A the source of the sound and the observer are both stationary, so the observed sound has the same frequency as the transmitted sound. In Fig. 3.1B the source is stationary and the observer is moving toward it, causing the observer to cross the wavefronts of the emitted wave more quickly than when stationary, so that the observer witnesses a higher-frequency wave than that emitted. If, however, the observer is moving away from the source (Fig. 3.1C), the wavefronts will be crossed less often, and the frequency witnessed will be lower than that emitted. Fig. 3.1D shows the opposite case, in which the source is moving toward a stationary observer. The source will move a short distance toward the observer between the emission of each wave, resulting in a shorter wavelength and the observer witnessing a higher frequency. Similarly, if the source is moving away from the observer, the wavelength is increased,

leading to observation of a lower frequency (Fig. 3.1E). The resulting change in the observed frequency is known as the Doppler shift, and the magnitude of the Doppler shift frequency is proportional to the relative velocity of the source and the observer.

History Behind the Discovery of the Doppler Effect

This effect was first described by an Austrian physicist named Christian Doppler in 1842. He used the Doppler effect to explain the "color of double stars." A rival Dutch scientist working at the same time tried to prove Doppler's theory wrong by hiring a train and two trumpeters. One trumpeter stood on the train while the other stood by the track, and an observer compared the pitch of the trumpeter who passed by on the train with that of the stationary trumpeter. This experiment verified Doppler's theory, although Doppler's use of this effect to explain the "color of double stars" was in fact incorrect.

DOPPLER EFFECT APPLIED TO VASCULAR ULTRASOUND

In the case of vascular ultrasound, the Doppler effect is used to study blood flow. The ultrasound transducer will transmit a pulse, separate from that used to form the B-mode image, and receive the returning echoes

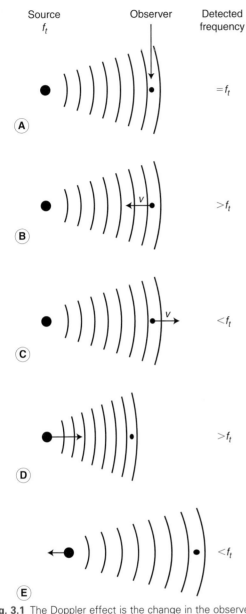

Source f_t	Observer	Detected frequency

(A) $= f_t$

(B) $> f_t$

(C) $< f_t$

(D) $> f_t$

(E) $< f_t$

Fig. 3.1 The Doppler effect is the change in the observed frequency due to motion between the source and the observer. (A) The source of the sound and the observer are both stationary, so the observed sound has the same frequency as that transmitted. (B) The source is stationary and the observer is moving toward the source (with velocity v), so that the observer witnesses a higher frequency than that emitted. (C) The observer is moving away from the source, so the frequency detected is lower than that emitted. (D) The source is moving toward a stationary observer, so the detected frequency is increased. (E) The source is moving away from the observer, thus decreasing the frequency observed.

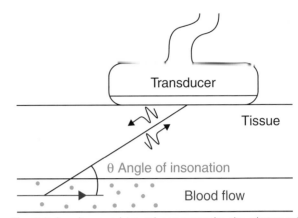

Fig. 3.2 An ultrasound transducer transmits the ultrasound beam into the tissue and the returning echoes are back-scattered from the moving blood cells. The frequency of the Doppler signal detected depends on the angle between the beam and the path of the blood flow, the angle of insonation θ.

back-scattered from the moving blood cells (Fig. 3.2, the solid line shows the path of the transmitted and received Doppler beam). In this situation, the Doppler effect occurs twice. First, the transducer is a stationary source while the blood cells are moving receivers of the ultrasound waves (see Fig. 3.1B). The ultrasound is then back-scattered from the blood cells, which now act as a moving source, with the transducer acting as a stationary observer (see Fig. 3.1D). The Doppler shift observed depends on the frequency of the ultrasound originally transmitted by the transducer and the velocity of the blood cells from which the ultrasound is back-scattered. The observed frequency also depends on the angle from which the movement of the blood is observed (i.e., the angle between the ultrasound beam and the direction of the blood flow). The Doppler shift frequency, f_d (i.e., the difference between the transmitted frequency, f_t, and received frequency, f_r) is given by:

$$f_d = f_r - f_t = \frac{2vf_t\cos\theta}{c} \tag{3.1}$$

where v is the velocity of the blood, θ is the angle between the ultrasound beam and the direction of blood flow, known as the angle of insonation, and c is the speed of sound in tissue. The factor of 2 is present in the Doppler equation as the Doppler effect has occurred twice, as explained above.

Consider, for example, a 5 MHz transducer used to interrogate a blood vessel with a flow velocity of 50 cm/s

BOX 3.1   Another Way of Writing the Doppler Equation

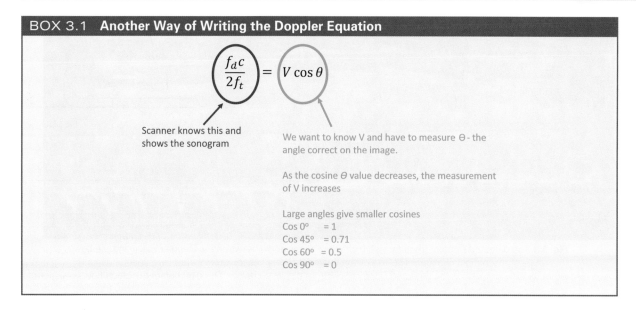

$$\left(\frac{f_d c}{2 f_t} \right) = \left(V \cos \theta \right)$$

Scanner knows this and shows the sonogram

We want to know V and have to measure Θ - the angle correct on the image.

As the cosine Θ value decreases, the measurement of V increases

Large angles give smaller cosines
Cos 0°   = 1
Cos 45° = 0.71
Cos 60° = 0.5
Cos 90° = 0

using an angle of insonation of 60°. Taking the speed of sound in tissue to be 1540 m/s, the Doppler equation can be used to estimate that the Doppler shift frequency will be 1.6 kHz. In fact, it is a useful coincidence that the typical values of blood velocity found in the body and the transmitted frequencies used in medical ultrasound result in Doppler shift frequencies that are in the human audible range (from 20 Hz to 20 kHz). The simplest Doppler systems can extract the Doppler shift frequency and output it to a loudspeaker, enabling the operator to listen to the Doppler shifts produced from the blood flow.

The Doppler equation shows that the detected Doppler shift depends on the angle of insonation, θ, through the term cosθ. Box 3.1 shows how the cosθ term varies between 0 and 1 as the angle changes from 0° to 90°. When the angle of insonation is 90°, the cosθ term is 0, so virtually no Doppler shift is detected. When the angle of insonation is 0° (i.e., the Doppler beam is parallel to the direction of flow), the cosθ term is 1, giving the maximum detectable Doppler shift frequency for a given velocity of blood and transmitted frequency. Fig. 3.3 shows how the detected Doppler waveform changes as the Doppler angle changes. When the angle of insonation is 60° a good spectral Doppler waveform is obtained; however, a poorer waveform is obtained at 70° and very poor waveform seen at 90°. Whether the waveform is above or below the

baseline will depend on the direction of the flow relative to the Doppler beam, i.e., toward or away from the transducer and this is shown as positive and negative numbers either side of the baseline on the velocity scale. This can be inverted by the sonographer, therefore it is important to be able to interpret this, so the direction of the flow can be understood.

Back-Scatter From Blood

Blood is made up of red blood cells (erythrocytes), white blood cells (leukocytes), and platelets suspended in plasma. Red blood cells occupy between 36% and 54% of the total blood volume. They have a biconcave disc shape and a diameter of 7 μm, which is much smaller than the wavelength of ultrasound used to study blood flow. This means that groups of red blood cells act as scatterers of the ultrasound (see Fig. 2.12).

The back-scattered signal from blood received at the transducer is small, partly due to the back-scattered energy being radiated in all directions, unlike specular reflections, and partly because the effective cross-section of the blood cells is small compared with the width of the beam. The back-scattered power is proportional to the fourth power of the frequency (i.e., f^4), and therefore as the transmitted frequency selected to detect flow is increased, there is an increase in back-scattered power. However, this is offset by the increase

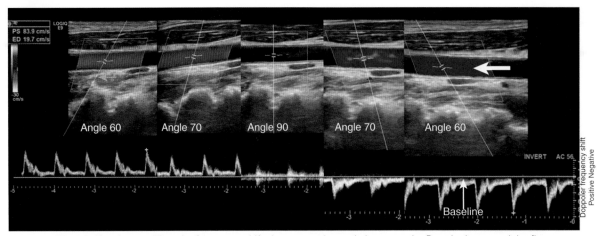

Fig. 3.3 The detected Doppler frequency shift changes as the angle between the Doppler beam and the flow (the angle of insonation) changes. The top of the image shows a vessel interrogated by a spectral Doppler beam *(orange arrow)* with the detected Doppler spectrum displayed below. The direction of the blood flow is shown by the *white arrow*. On the left side of the figure, the angle of insonation is 60° with the flow traveling away from the transducer (spectral Doppler negative value on the scale). In the center of the figure the angle of insonation changes to an angle of 90° giving a poor spectral waveform. On the right side of the screen the flow is now toward the transducer and the spectrum is now shown below the baseline *(vertical arrow)* as positive values. The spectral Doppler waveforms obtained at 60° (far left and far right) are superior to those obtained at 70° and a very poor signal is obtained at 90°. It is possible to invert the spectrum, so flow toward the transducer is above the baseline and flow away below.

in attenuation of the overlying tissue with the increase in frequency. Ultrasound systems will often use a lower transmitted frequency for Doppler recordings than for B-mode imaging. The imaging and Doppler transmitted frequencies are usually indicated on the image and are often under the control of the sonographer. In situations in which blood velocity is low or blood cells are stationary, such as aneurysms or venous flow, the cells may aggregate into clumps that can sometimes produce sufficiently high-amplitude back-scattered echoes to be displayed on the B-mode image (see Fig. 2.13). Similarly, slower venous flow can produce higher amplitude color flow and spectral Doppler signal strength than that from fast-moving arterial blood.

EXTRACTING THE DOPPLER SIGNAL

The simplest Doppler systems, such as handheld Doppler systems used to detect pulses at the ankle (see Fig. 9.6), consist of a transducer with two piezoelectric elements (Fig. 3.4A), one continuously transmitting ultrasound and the other continuously receiving back-scattered signals both from stationary tissue and flowing blood. This is known as continuous-wave (CW)

Doppler. This received signal therefore consists of the transmitted frequency reflected by stationary objects and the Doppler-shifted frequencies back-scattered from moving blood cells. As the returning echoes are of low amplitude, first they must be amplified. The Doppler shift frequency can then be extracted from the received signal, amplified, and the output sent to a loudspeaker (giving the sound we hear when using the Doppler) or investigated using a spectrum analyzer. With experience, it is possible for the operator to recognize the different sounds produced by normal and diseased vessels.

Information about the direction of flow relative to the transducer is available in the returning signal, as objects moving toward the transducer will produce an increase in the detected frequency, while those moving away will produce a decrease in the detected frequency. When the flow directions have been separated, stereo loudspeakers can be used with one channel for forward flow and the other for reverse.

Once the Doppler signal has been analyzed (discussed later), it is preferable to display both the forward and reverse Doppler signals simultaneously on the same spectrum. This is done by displaying the signals

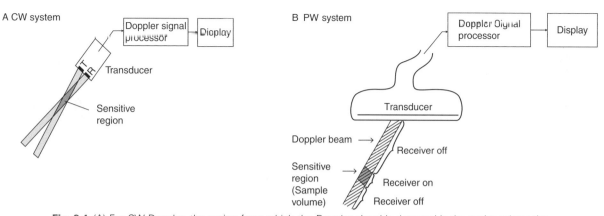

Fig. 3.4 (A) For CW Doppler, the region from which the Doppler signal is detected is the region where the transmit beam and receive beam overlap and this cannot be controlled by the sonographer. (B) For PW Doppler, the sensitive region, sample volume, is governed by the time the receiver is switched on to obtain the signal and is controlled by the sonographer. The sample volume can be positioned anywhere along the path of the beam. *CW*, Continuous-wave; *PW*, pulsed-wave.

on either side of a baseline, with flow toward the transducer displayed above the baseline and flow away from the transducer displayed below, although this can be inverted by the sonographer. Fig. 3.5A shows the flow in the vertebral artery and vein displayed in different directions on the spectrum. The fact that the display is inverted is usually indicated on the screen (Fig. 3.5B) and shows the negative values above the baseline and positive values below. The baseline can also be shifted up and down to make maximum use of the spectral display (Fig. 3.5C).

As well as obtaining Doppler shift frequencies from the flowing blood, the slow-moving vessel walls act as large reflective surfaces, producing large-amplitude, low-frequency Doppler shift signals along with the low-amplitude high frequencies obtained from blood. These signals are known as wall thump, due to their audible sound, and are removed by high-pass filters, which will remove any signals with a frequency below the cut-off frequency of the filter. This can be controlled by the sonographer; if it is set too low, the wall thump signal (Fig. 3.6A) will not be removed, whereas if it is set too high, important Doppler information will be removed, possibly altering the waveform shape (Fig. 3.6C) (e.g., by suggesting the absence of diastolic flow). The ideal filter setting (Fig. 3.6B) should remove unwanted signals such as wall thump without removing important blood flow information.

ANALYSIS OF THE DOPPLER SIGNAL

The Doppler signal can be investigated using spectral analysis, allowing waveforms to be displayed (as seen in Fig. 3.5) and enabling blood velocity to be measured. The blood cells flowing through a vessel will be moving at different velocities within the vessel; for example, cells near the vessel wall will be moving more slowly than those in the center (see Ch. 5). The velocity of the blood cells will vary with time, owing to the pulsatile nature of arterial blood flow. This means that the Doppler shift signal obtained from flowing blood will contain a range of frequencies, due to the range of velocities present, and the frequency content will vary with time. Spectral analysis can be used to break down the Doppler signal into its component frequencies (an analogy would be a prism splitting white light into the colors of the rainbow). These component frequencies can be displayed to show how the blood velocities vary with time. Fig. 3.7 shows how a spectrum is displayed, with time along the horizontal axis and the Doppler shift frequencies (or calculated velocities) along the vertical axis. The third axis, the brightness of the display, relates to the backscattered power of the signal at each frequency (i.e., the proportion of the blood cells moving at a particular velocity). Spectral analysis is carried out using mathematical techniques such as the fast Fourier transform (FFT). Fig. 3.5C shows a typical spectral display produced by a Doppler system. In this case, each vertical

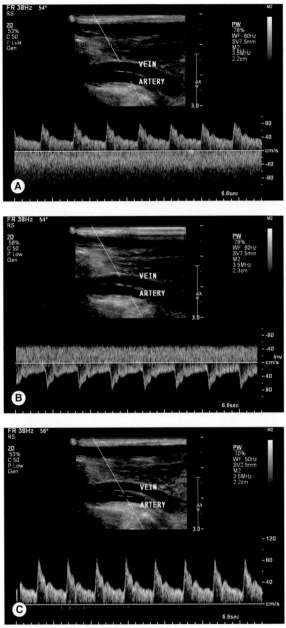

Fig. 3.5 The use of an offset, or baseline, allows both forward and reverse flows to be displayed on the same spectrum (A) with the sample volume covering both the artery and vein. This can be inverted if required (B), shown by negative values of the velocity being displayed above the spectral Doppler baseline (labeled *inv*). The baseline can be altered to make maximum use of the spectral display (C). The sample volume size is reduced compared to (A) and (B) to select a signal that only arises from the artery.

line of data on the spectral display is produced every 5 to 10 ms (i.e., 100–200 lines of data per second).

Continuous Wave Doppler

CW Doppler continuously emits a single frequency while the receiving element continuously detects any echoes from the sensitive region of the beam (i.e., where transmitted and received beams overlap) (shaded region in Fig. 3.4A). This region usually covers a depth of a few centimeters, and any flow within this area will be detected. This means that CW Doppler is unable to provide information about the depth from which the Doppler signal is returning and therefore has poor range resolution. Veins often lie adjacent to arteries and so, in some situation, the CW Doppler will simultaneously detect arterial and venous flow as the operator is unable to select the depth at which the signal is detected.

Pulsed-Wave Doppler

The poor range resolution of CW Doppler can be overcome by using an ultrasound pulse, known as pulsed-wave (PW) Doppler, enabling the use of the pulse echo effect (as used in B-mode imaging) to determine the depth from which a signal has returned. The scanner can select and analyze the returning signal from a specific time after the pulse has been transmitted. Thus, by knowing the speed of sound in tissue, the depth from which the signal has returned can be calculated, in the same way as described for B-mode pulsed echo imaging (Eq. 2.3), enabling the signal to only be acquired from the desired depth. As the piezoelectric element is only emitting ultrasound for a short period of time, it is possible to use the same element, or group of elements, to transmit and to receive the returning signal. Fig. 3.8 shows how the pulse of ultrasound is transmitted and how the receiver then waits a given time before acquiring the signal over a short period of time. Although the system acquires no further signals, it must wait for the echoes from greater depths to return before sending the next pulse. The time during which the received signal is acquired is known as the sample volume or range gate. The time the receiver is on for will govern the size of the sample volume, and this can be altered by the operator in order to determine the region within the tissue from which the Doppler signal is obtained (see Fig. 3.4B). The sample volume size depends not only on the size of the range gate (time the receiver is on) but

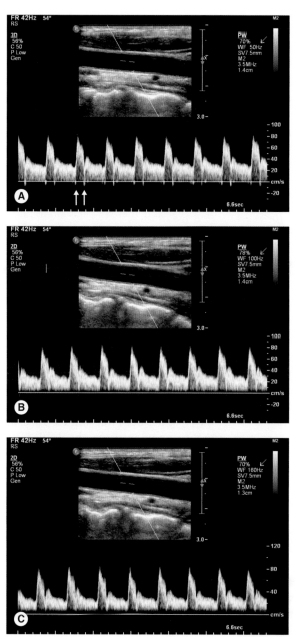

Fig. 3.6 (A) Arterial wall motion gives a low-frequency, high-amplitude signal, wall thump *(large arrows)*. (B) A filter can be used to remove wall thump from the Doppler signal, but if the filter cut-off frequency is set too high (as in C), this can alter the appearance of the waveform. *Small arrows* show wall filter setting in A: 50 Hz, B: 100 Hz, and C: 160 Hz.

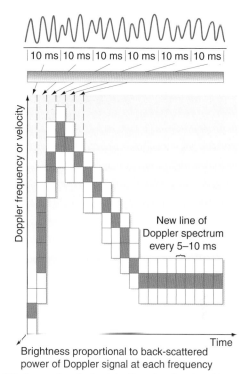

Fig. 3.7 Spectral analysis of the Doppler signal enables the frequencies present within the signal to be displayed as consecutive spectra. This produces a display of the changes in blood velocity over time.

also on the shape and length of the transmitted pulse and the shape of the ultrasound beam. The path of the Doppler beam is typically displayed on an ultrasound image as a solid or dotted white line (Fig. 3.9), and the sample volume is typically displayed as two parallel lines perpendicular to the line showing the path of the beam. The combination of the B-mode image and superimposed PW Doppler beam and sample volume markers enables the operator to select the location of the sample volume so that it is within the desired anatomical area as displayed on the B-mode image. The size of the sample volume has a significant effect on the Doppler spectrum produced. For example, in Fig. 3.5A,B the sample volume is set to encompass both the artery and the vein so both the arterial and venous signal is displayed. In Fig. 3.5C a smaller sample volume is placed only over the artery, enabling only the arterial signal to be displayed. A large sample volume is required if the operator wishes to record both the fast-moving blood in the center of the vessel and the slower-moving blood near the walls. This is discussed further in Chapter 6.

In order to measure the frequencies present in the blood flow, thousands of pulses are sent along the beam path per second. The frequency at which these pulses are

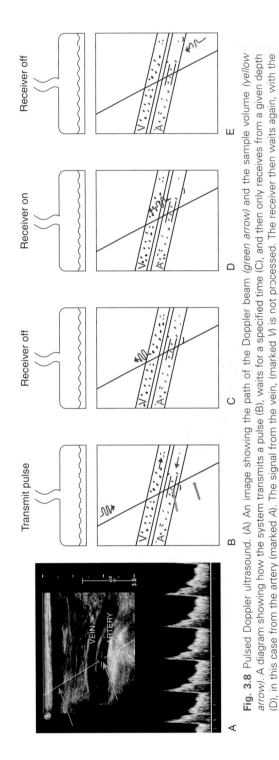

Fig. 3.8 Pulsed Doppler ultrasound. (A) An image showing the path of the Doppler beam *(green arrow)* and the sample volume *(yellow arrow)*. A diagram showing how the system transmits a pulse (B), waits for a specified time (C), and then only receives from a given depth (D), in this case from the artery (marked A). The signal from the vein, (marked V) is not processed. The receiver then waits again, with the receiver off (E), for all the echoes to return from greater depths before transmitting the next pulse.

sent is known as the pulse repetition frequency (PRF) and is in the kHz range. The PRF can be adjusted by the sonographer by using a control typically called "Scale." The upper limit of the PRF is given by the constraint that the system has to wait for all the echoes from the last pulse to return before transmitting the next pulse. In fact, the pulsed Doppler method, unlike CW systems, does not actually measure the Doppler shift, but rather measures the phase change in echoes from consecutive pulses. However, the final output of the detected signal is similar to the Doppler shift that would be obtained from a CW system, so it can be described by the Doppler equation and is typically referred to as the Doppler signal. The ultrasound pulses enable the changing velocity of the blood to be sampled, and the resulting signal can be analyzed to obtain a frequency spectrum using an FFT.

The values of the PRF (Scale), sample volume size, and depth are usually displayed at the side of the image. Pulsed Doppler is able to provide good depth information, but the disadvantage is that pulsed Doppler suffers

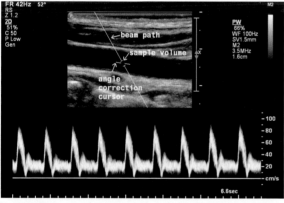

Fig. 3.9 The path of the Doppler ultrasound beam, sample volume size, and position are displayed on the image.

from an artifact known as aliasing, that puts an upper limit on the maximum frequency that can be detected.

Aliasing

Aliasing is an effect that results in the incorrect estimation of the Doppler shift frequency of a signal due to insufficient sampling of the signal. Imagine that you have a clock with only a minute hand and you wish to estimate the speed at which the hand is moving. If you look at the face every 45 minutes (Fig. 3.10), starting on the hour, first the hand would point at 12, then, 45 minutes later, it would point at 9, then at 6, at 3, and at 12 again. This would give the impression that the hand was traveling slowly anticlockwise. The speed of the hand would appear to be one complete revolution every 3 hours rather than, as expected, once an hour. In order to estimate the speed of the hand correctly, the clock would have to be viewed at least twice in a complete cycle (i.e., at least twice an hour).

Fig. 3.11 shows how the frequency of a simple sine wave, indicated by the solid line, can be underestimated when the signal is sampled less than twice in a complete cycle. If the dots represent the points at which the signal is sampled, then the lowest-frequency sine wave that would fit the sampled data is that shown by the dashed line. If, instead, the signal is sampled at least twice in a complete cycle, shown by the crosses, it is no longer possible to fit a lower-frequency sine wave to the sampled data and the correct frequency is measured. Aliasing occurs when the sampling frequency is less than twice the frequency to be estimated, a limit known as the Nyquist frequency.

An example of aliasing of a Doppler signal can be seen in Fig. 3.12A, where the frequency or velocity detected at peak systole is underestimated and displayed below the baseline of the spectrum. Aliasing can be overcome

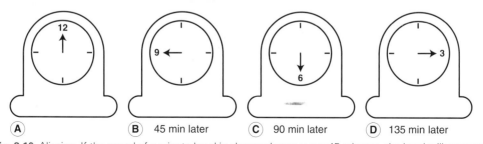

Fig. 3.10 Aliasing. If the speed of a minute hand is observed once every 45 minutes, the hand will appear to be moving slowly anticlockwise due to not being observed frequently enough.

by increasing the sampling rate (i.e., increasing the PRF or scale). There is, however, an upper limit to the PRF that can be used, as the system has to wait for each pulse to return before the next pulse can be transmitted, in order to prevent confusion as to where a returning signal has originated. Therefore, there is also a limit to the maximum Doppler shift frequency that can be detected. This limits the maximum detectable Doppler frequency (f_{dmax}) and velocity (V_{max}) as follows:

$$f_{dmax} = \frac{PRF_{max}}{2} = \frac{2V_{max}f_t\cos\theta}{c} \qquad (3.2)$$

This can be rewritten as:

$$V_{max} = \frac{PRF_{max}c}{4f_t\cos\theta} \qquad (3.3)$$

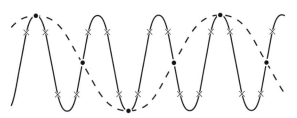

Fig. 3.11 Aliasing. The frequency of a simple sine wave *(solid line)* can be underestimated *(dashed line)* when the signal is sampled *(dots)* less than twice in a complete cycle. If sampled more than twice a cycle *(crosses)*, the correct frequency is obtained.

For a depth of interest, d, and speed of sound, c,

$$PRF_{max} = \frac{c}{2d} \qquad (3.4)$$

The 2 in the equation above arises from the fact that the pulse has to go to and return from the target. This gives:

$$V_{max} = \frac{c^2}{8df_t\cos\theta} \qquad (3.5)$$

The maximum velocity that can be detected without aliasing therefore depends on the depth of the vessel. When measuring very high blood flow velocities at depth, some scanners will allow a "high PRF" mode to be selected. This allows more than one pulse to be in flight at a given time. The higher PRF allows higher velocities to be measured, but it also introduces range ambiguity (i.e., a loss of certainty as to the origin of the Doppler signal). In this mode, the scanner will typically show more than one sample volume displayed on the scan line (Fig. 3.13). Using a lower transmitted frequency delays the appearance of this effect, since lower transmit frequencies result in lower Doppler frequencies that do not require such high PRFs. However, in practice, this is a limitation when imaging renal artery stenosis and in some cases of transcranial Doppler (TCD) imaging. Using a lower transmit frequency can also be useful when assessing high volume flow as seen in fistulae, due to a reduction in aliasing.

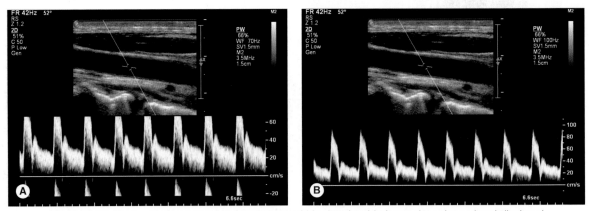

Fig. 3.12 (A) Aliasing leads to the high frequencies within the signal being underestimated and displayed below the baseline of the spectrum. (B) Aliasing can be overcome by increasing the pulse repetition frequency (shown as an increase in the upper limit of the velocity displayed on the velocity scale from 60 cm/s in A to100 cm/s in B).

Limitations of CW Versus PW Doppler

CW Doppler and PW Doppler have different limitations. There is no upper limit to the velocity of blood that can be detected by CW Doppler, but no information is available regarding the depth of the origin of the signal, and it is not always possible to detect arterial flow without the venous flow from a nearby vein also being detected. CW is most commonly used in simple handheld systems to listen to blood flow, enabling ankle blood pressures to be measured (see Ch. 9). It can also be used in cardiology to allow high velocities to be measured through the heart valves. PW Doppler provides information regarding the origin of the signal, enabling detailed studies of a specific vessel; however, this restricts the maximum velocity that can be detected. PW methods are used in duplex systems both for spectral Doppler and color flow imaging.

DUPLEX ULTRASOUND

Combining the pulse echo imaging with Doppler ultrasound allows interrogation of a vessel in a known location and permits close investigation of the hemodynamics around areas of atheroma visualized on the image. Ideally, to produce a good image of a vessel wall, the vessel should be at right angles to the ultrasound beam. This is the case in the majority of peripheral vessels, as they mainly lie parallel to the skin. However, the Doppler equation shows that no Doppler signal will be obtained when the angle of insonation is at right angles to the direction of flow (as cosθ = 0). The greatest Doppler shift is detected when the beam is parallel to the direction of flow (angle of insonation of zero). Therefore, there is a conflict between the ideal angle of the beam used for imaging and that used for Doppler recordings. Linear array transducers are able to produce Doppler beams that can be steered left or right to the

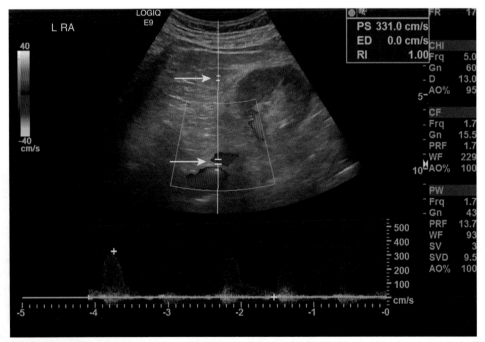

Fig. 3.13 High pulse repetition frequency (PRF) used to measure high velocities in a renal artery stenosis. The high velocities at the renal artery origin (sample volume indicated by the lower *yellow arrow*) coming directly toward the beam require a high scale. This produces PRFs that result in a second pulse being sent out before the first arrives back to the transducer. This leads to a received signal from a second, more superficial sample volume (*upper yellow arrow*), which, with less attenuation, is stronger than that from the deeper sample volume in the stenosis. Despite this, the peak systolic velocity can be measured.

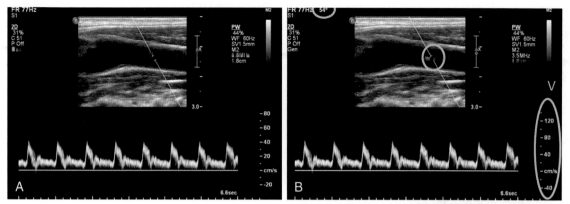

Fig. 3.14 (A) and (B) The image and sonogram are identical. The sonogram shows the range of Doppler frequencies f_d changing with time. The velocity scale displayed will change as the operator changes the angle correction cursor (*ringed*). In (A), no angle correction is made. $\Theta = 0$ so cos $\Theta = 1$. In (B), an angle correction of 54° is made, estimating the true angle of insonation. Cos 54° = 0.59 so the velocity scale now is 70% higher and displays an accurate estimation of the velocity. As the cosine Θ value decreases, the velocity scale V increases to compensate.

central axis of the probe, as described in Chapter 2 (see Fig. 2.22A, and seen in Fig. 3.3). The transducer elements are most sensitive to the returning signals that are at right angles to the front face of the element. This means that, as the beam is steered, the sensitivity of the Doppler transducer will fall to some extent, and therefore the Doppler beam can only be steered by about 20° to 30° left and right of center. There is thus a compromise between the choice of Doppler angle and sensitivity.

Velocity Measurements Using Duplex Ultrasound

An important consequence of duplex ultrasound is that it allows the image of the vessel to be used to estimate the angle of insonation between the Doppler beam and the vessel. This enables the detected Doppler frequency to be converted into a velocity measurement using the Doppler equation (Eq. 3.1) and is fundamental to measure velocities accurately. PW Doppler extracts the Doppler shift from the velocity *component* in the direction of the beam. This may be understood by writing the Doppler equation in a different way:

$$\frac{f_d c}{2 f_t} = V \cos \theta$$

$$(3.6)$$

The scanner extracts the Doppler frequency and knows the speed of sound and the transmit frequency. The operator then has to measure the angle of insonation, Θ, the angle between the beam and flow, by adjusting the angle correction cursor control, for the scanner to calculate and display the correct velocity scale and allow accurate measurement of V. For a given Doppler frequency, if the cosine Θ value is large, then the calculated V will be small, if the cosine Θ value is small, then calculated V will be larger. Fig. 3.14 shows what happens when no angle correction is made and when the operator sets it to line up with the flow.

It can be difficult to align the angle correction with the true direction of flow, and the use of high angles can lead to errors. Fig. 3.15A demonstrates how the image of a vessel can be used to enable the angle of insonation to be measured by lining up an angle correction cursor with the vessel wall, the expected path of the flow. In Fig. 3.15B the angle correction cursor has been lined up correctly with the cursor parallel to the vessel wall, but the angle of insonation is 70°, which is too large to make accurate measurements (see Ch. 6). The peak velocities seen in Fig. 3.15B are higher than those seen in Fig. 3.15A. The angle of insonation should be 60° or less to make velocity measurements, with smaller angles leading to a smaller potential for measurement errors. In Fig. 3.15C the angle has been set to read an angle of insonation of 60°, but the angle correction cursor has not been aligned parallel to the vessel walls, therefore giving an incorrect angle of insonation, leading to incorrect velocity measurements. Very large errors in velocity measurement can be generated by incorrect alignment of the angle correction cursor.

Although there are many potential sources of errors when using Doppler ultrasound to calculate blood flow velocity (see Ch. 6), it is a powerful technique for detecting and quantifying the degree of disease present in a vessel.

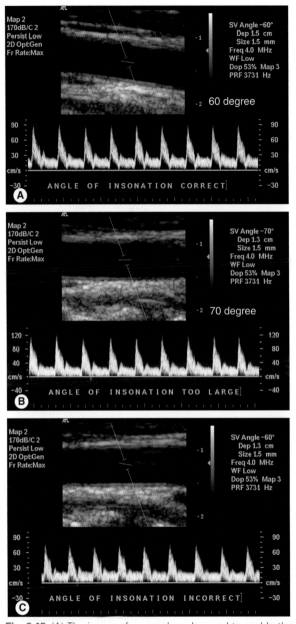

Fig. 3.15 (A) The image of a vessel can be used to enable the angle of insonation to be measured by lining up an angle correction cursor with the vessel wall. (B) The angle correction cursor has been lined up correctly with the cursor parallel to the vessel wall, but the angle of insonation is 70°, which is too large to make accurate measurements. (C) The angle has been set to read an angle of insonation of 60°, but the angle correction cursor has not been aligned with flow, assumed to be parallel to the vessel walls, therefore giving an incorrect angle of insonation, leading to incorrect velocity measurements. The correct value of the velocity is that obtained in (A).

Color Flow Imaging

INTRODUCTION

Vascular ultrasound was revolutionized in the late 1980s when color flow imaging (CFI) was introduced. By mapping images of moving blood in color over the two-dimensional (2D) gray-scale images of tissue, flow within arteries and veins was displayed in a different way. CFI showed vessels invisible to B-mode and displayed particular flow characteristics, for example, locally increased velocities at sites of stenosis, to aid in imaging and guide spectral Doppler measurement of blood velocity. B-mode, CFI, and spectral Doppler are complementary; they show different information and each works and is optimized in a different way. Good vascular ultrasound practice requires an understanding of each and an appreciation of how they are used together for optimum imaging, measurement, and diagnostic efficacy.

BASIC PRINCIPLES

CFI is essentially a dynamic measurement of movement within an area of the image selected by the sonographer. The scanner detects movement along multiple beams transmitted in a region of interest (ROI) within the area scanned by the B-mode image (see Fig. 4.1). For each beam the depth is divided into closely spaced sample volumes along the beam, each sample being at a different time delay after the transmitted pulse corresponding to slightly different depths in the tissue. CFI uses specific pulses, separate from those used for B-mode, and several pulses must be transmitted and received along the scan line for the movement of the blood to be detected. Once sufficient samples have been detected from each sample volume in a beam, pulses are then directed along a second scan line adjacent to the first followed by further scans lines until the whole of the ROI is examined for flow.

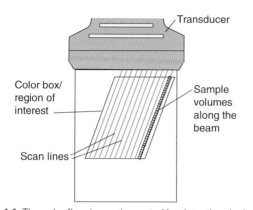

Fig. 4.1 The color flow image is created by detecting the back-scattered ultrasound from hundreds of sample volumes along over a hundred different scan lines.

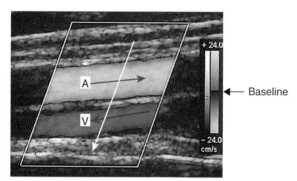

Fig. 4.2 The color flow displays the mean velocity of flow relative to the ultrasound beam detected within each sample volume. This image of an artery *(A)* overlying a vein *(V)* demonstrates the difference in the velocity and direction of the blood flow in the two vessels. The direction of the blood flow is shown as *red arrows* and the beam direction in *white*. The top half of the color scale, in this case colors from red to yellow, shows flow toward the beam. In this image, flow in the artery is toward the beam and is displayed as red, whereas flow in the vein is away from the transducer and is displayed as blue.

The estimated mean relative velocity (equivalent to the Doppler frequency) from each sample volume within the tissue is displayed in color, as shown in Fig. 4.2. In this image of an artery lying next to a vein, the flow toward the transmitted beam is displayed by the red scale, and flow away from the beam is displayed by the blue scale. The higher relative velocities are shown as yellow and light blue, whereas the lower relative velocities are displayed as deep red and deep blue.

The need for separate pulses for CFI and for several pulses along each beam to detect flow puts more constraints on the time available to produce images. Color flow images showing movement in an area are typically updated between 6 and 30 times a second. By comparison, the spectral display in a Doppler sonogram shows the distribution of changing flow over 100 times a second in a single sample volume location. Later on in this chapter we will see that the sonographer can make changes that affect how quickly the flow information is updated and what the effects are on the sensitivity of the color flow image and its spatial resolution and that of the B-mode image.

METHODS OF ESTIMATING THE VELOCITY OF BLOOD

Spectral Doppler ultrasound uses fast Fourier transform (FFT) to provide detailed information on the frequency content of the Doppler signal from the velocity distribution within a specific sample volume. For CFI, mapping flow over a 2D area, the requirements are different. CFI measures the movement of blood by sending short series of pulses to track the characteristic echo pattern from groups of red blood cells as they move through the beam.

The echoes from stationary tissue are subtracted leaving echoes from moving blood, which are time shifted from each transmitted pulse. By measuring the movement between pulses and knowing the interval between pulses, the velocity component in the direction of the beam is measured. The movement is calculated by measuring the change in phase of the returning echoes (Fig. 4.3) using correlation techniques. Autocorrelation compares two consecutive pulses returning from a given sample volume to produce an output that is dependent on the phase shift. The phase shifts between four or more pulses are used to estimate the mean velocity (the velocity of the group of cells does not change significantly during the short time over which the blood flow velocity is estimated). The more pulses used, the more accurate is the result as long as the time taken is not so great that the velocity of the blood cells has changed. This relatively small number of pulses required for each beam means that the image itself, built from measurements from several beams, can be updated many times a second.

ELEMENTS OF A COLOR FLOW SCANNER

Fig. 4.4 shows the basic elements of a color flow scanner. Before any analysis of the returning echoes is carried out, the signal is filtered by the clutter filter to remove the high-amplitude signals returning from the surrounding stationary tissue and the slow-moving vessel walls, while preserving the low-amplitude signals from the blood. The filtered signal is analyzed to obtain an estimate of the mean velocity relative to the path of the beam in each sample volume. Postprocessing is then used to smooth the data in order to produce a less noisy color image. This can be done by combining the data obtained from consecutive images, known as frame-averaging. As each point on the image can only be assigned either a

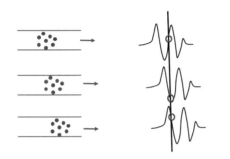

Blood cell scatterers   Echo from scatterers

Fig. 4.3 Phase change in echoes from moving blood. The diagram shows a group of blood cells moving along a vessel. If ultrasound pulses are sent in the direction of movement, then the returning echoes from each will have a slight time shift. This can be measured by examining the phase change in the echo between pulses. The vertical line represents a specific time from transmit to reception. The phase *(red circles)* of the echo is different as the blood moves.

specific color or level of gray, a decision has to be made as to whether to display the B-mode pulse echo information or any flow information detected. This involves the process known as blood–tissue discrimination.

Blood–Tissue Discrimination

Generally, the returning pulse echo signals from blood have very low amplitude compared with those from the vessel walls and surrounding tissue. In addition, rapidly moving blood leads to higher velocities in comparison to the lower velocities obtained from the slow-moving vessel walls. Ultrasound systems are designed with an adjustable setting that discriminates between high amplitude, low velocity, or static echoes, where the gray scale is shown and low-amplitude, higher-velocity echoes where the scanner assumes that this is from blood and color is displayed. This color write priority can be set in the presets so that, for example, for superficial low flow tissues, more emphasis can be given to flow displays whereas for applications where more tissue motion is expected, the color display may be more suppressed. In many scanners this can be altered by a "priority" control, choosing to emphasize the gray scale or color according to the flow conditions, although it is rarely altered during an examination.

Most systems also have a flash filter. This is designed to remove color flashes, known as flash artifacts, that are generated by rapid movement between the transducer and tissue, such as when the sonographer moves the transducer during scanning.

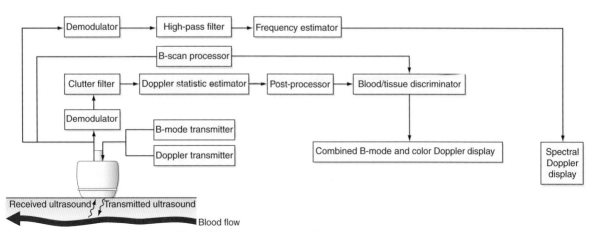

Fig. 4.4 The basic elements of a color flow scanner.

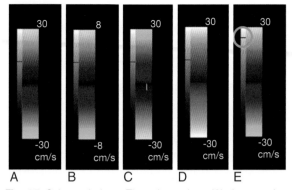

Fig. 4.5 Color scale bars. The color scale at (A) shows red as flow toward the transducer and blue away from it. The numbers, 30 and −30, represent the velocity in cm/s of blood flowing directly toward the beam that would be shown as the yellow and light blue hues at the top and bottom of the bar. Higher scales indicated that higher pulse repetition frequencies (PRFs) are being used. This scale might be used for arterial flow. In scale (B) the color scale number is 8 and −8. This is a result of lowering the scale which reduces PRF producing greater sensitivity to low flows but with increased risk of aliasing. This scale would be more appropriate for slow-moving venous flow. Scale (C) shows an inverted scale with flow toward the transducer as blue. Scale (D) shows a different color map with higher velocities as lighter reds and blues. In scale (E) the indicator on the adjacent gray bar *(ringed)* shows that there is more emphasis of the color overwriting strong gray levels (compared with A–D) by changing the color write priority setting.

Color-Coding the Flow Information

Having obtained values of the mean velocity along the beam in the multiple sample volumes, these data now have to be displayed on the image. This is done by color-coding the velocity information. The color on the screen has three attributes: luminosity, hue, and saturation. Luminosity is the degree of brightness or shade of the displayed color; hue is the wavelength (the actual color displayed, from violet through red), and saturation is the degree to which the color is mixed with white light (e.g., from red through light pink, producing up to 20 identifiable tints). These three attributes can be used to produce a variety of color scales, as shown in Fig. 4.5, which can be displayed as a bar at the side of the image. The scale usually consists of a different color representing different flow directions, with red often used to show flow toward the transducer and blue depicting flow away from the transducer. The color scale can be inverted to display flow toward the transducer as blue and flow away as red; this is indicated by the reversed color scale

displayed at the side of the image (see Fig. 4.5C). It is essential for the sonographer to be aware of which colors represent which directions of flow within the image, otherwise serious diagnostic errors can occur. Ultrasound scanners provide a range of color scales, and certain scales may be more appropriate in particular imaging situations. The various color scales may be selected to accentuate the different parts of the range of detected relative velocities seen in different clinical situations. For example, in an arterial scan, the color scale may accentuate the differences in the upper portion to highlight velocity changes in the higher range of velocities.

Another form of color display uses increasing luminosity of orange to display the increasing back-scattered power detected. This is known as power Doppler and is discussed later in this chapter.

EFFECT OF ANGLE OF BEAM TO FLOW ON THE COLOR FLOW IMAGE

CFI works by measuring the movement of blood in the direction of the ultrasound beam between pulses and calculating the velocity component along it. Like other Doppler-based techniques, this is larger if blood flow is aligned to the beam and is lower as the angle between blood and the beam increases (see Fig. 4.6). In theory, if the flow is at 90° to the beam there is no movement in the direction of the beam and there will be no signal. This has profound implications for using CFI in vascular imaging and for the images that CFI produces.

Many peripheral arteries run parallel, or close to parallel, with the skin surface. While this is optimal for B-mode imaging of vessels, CFI requires the sonographer to move the transducer or steer the CFI beams to obtain consistent color images of flow. Fig. 4.7 shows the effect in a transverse scan of a carotid artery. Using a linear array and with beams transmitted vertically from the transducer face, the color image produced is confusing when the probe is at 90° to the skin and vessel. The main direction of flow is through the plane of the image; the color image shows the slight change of velocities across the artery caused by corkscrewing of blood as it flows up the artery. By tilting the probe in a cephalad direction the angle between the beam and the main direction of flow is less, and there is a consistent movement through the beam as blood flows away from the beam direction. The sonographer cannot use this plane of image to measure velocities; the angle correction between the

Angle dependence of Doppler ultrasound

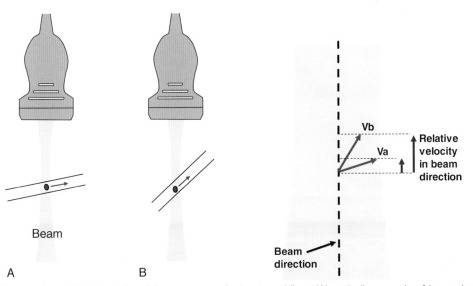

Fig. 4.6 The diagram shows blood velocity of the same magnitude at an oblique (A) angle (large angle of insonation) and angled more toward the beam (B) (small angle of insonation). The scanner measures the movement between pulses in the direction of the beam *(dashed line)* and calculates the velocity component in the direction of the beam. The velocity from the flow more aligned to the beam gives a larger velocity component than that at higher angles.

direction of the beam and flow is unknown, but they can use CFI to determine the presence of flow and its direction in this plane. For this examination it is invaluable to show filling of the lumen as an indication of any narrowing. Since B-mode images are optimal around 90°, the sonographer will constantly adjust the angle of the probe depending on the anatomy underneath the probe and the direction of flow to obtain the required images.

For longitudinal imaging of peripheral arteries with linear arrays, angling of the beam can be achieved by steering the beam so that the direction of the beam is no longer vertical but angled obliquely to the left or right, typically from 20° to 30° to the vertical (see Fig. 4.8). By using the appearance of the vessel in the image to guide the steering, the angle between the direction of flow and the beam can be reduced so that there is a consistent velocity component toward or away from the beam and a consistent flow direction, red or blue shown on the image. The sonographer uses probe positioning and orientation, beam steering, and awareness of the color scale to confirm the direction of the flow in arteries and veins. This is a crucial skill; if sonographers encounter flow in an unexpected direction, confidence in the displayed image is essential to understand the scan. The color scale

can be inverted from red for flow toward the beam to blue. The effect is shown in two images in Fig. 4.9 where arterial flow can be shown as red or blue depending on the color scale assignment.

During an examination, the sonographer may alter beam steering to the left or right depending on the orientation of the artery or vein under investigation (see Fig. 4.10). This is particularly relevant when scanning curved or tortuous vessels when the velocity component measured in the direction of the beam will change, causing a change in color hue even though the true blood velocity is the same (see Fig. 4.11).

Curvilinear and phased array transducers produce scan lines that fan out (diverge) in the image. This leads to more complex changes of angle between the beams and the vessels. For example, in a straight vessel parallel to the skin, the different beam/vessel angles produce a range of hues as the flow direction relative to the beam is altered (see Fig. 4.12). In images where there are vessels with different flow paths and even flow direction within them, an understanding of the beam direction, expected flow, and color scale allows accurate interpretation of the arterial and venous anatomy and the flow within them (see Fig. 4.13).

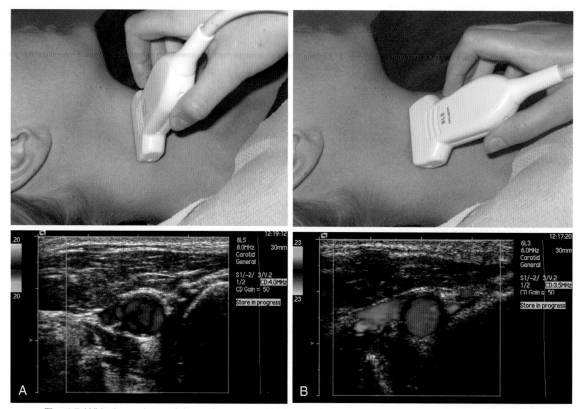

Fig. 4.7 With the probe at right angles to the skin (and vessel) the color flow image is ambiguous, since the main direction of flow is perpendicular to the image plane and beam direction (A). With the probe more aligned to the vessels, color flow is improved (B); note that the color scale has been inverted to show flow away from the probe as red.

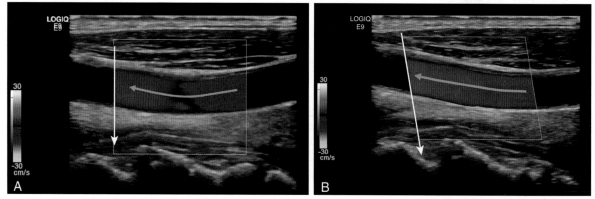

Fig. 4.8 Longitudinal imaging of flow in an artery. Flow is from right to left, the flow direction is highlighted by the *red arrow*. The beam direction is parallel to the sides of the color flow box *(white arrow)*. (A) The ultrasound beams are steered vertically and detect the small flow component away or toward the beam as the artery becomes slightly deeper and then superficial. This leads to blue-coded flow as the artery becomes deeper (right side of the image) and red-coded flow as the artery becomes more superficial (left side of the image) with no flow signal as it turns through 90° to the beam in the center. (B) The beam is electronically steered so that there is a consistent flow direction toward the beam resulting in a consistent red-coded flow.

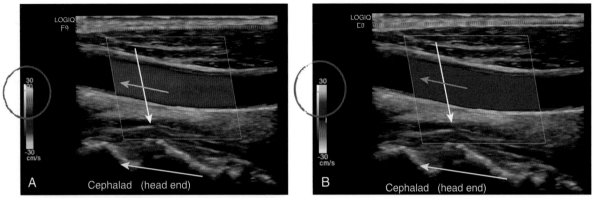

Fig. 4.9 The relationship between direction of flow, color scale direction, and color appearance. Two images of flow in the common carotid artery (CCA). The sonographer has aligned the transducer in the axis of the artery with the left of the image in the headwise (cephalad) direction. The beam is steered to the right *(white arrows)* with the direction of flow toward the beam. (A) The color scale is set with red as flow toward the beam *(ringed)* and since the headwise flow in the CCA is from right to left in the image, it is shown as red. (B) If the color scale is inverted, flow toward the beam is now shown as blue. As arterial flow is toward the beam, it is also now shown as blue.

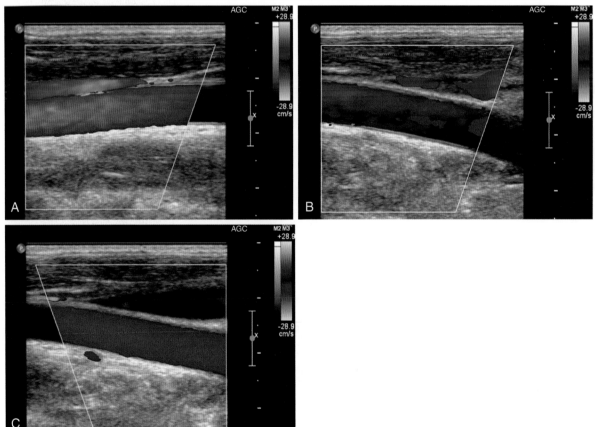

Fig. 4.10 Beam steering to optimize color flow imaging. In image (A) of the mid common carotid artery (CCA), the color box is steered to the left as the artery becomes deeper from right to left in the image so the beam direction is well aligned to the flow. In image (B), the proximal CCA rises from right to left in the image and the beam/flow angles are large. By steering the beam to the right (C), there is better alignment of beam and flow, and the image is clear and unambiguous. Note that the color scale has inverted so that flow away from the beam (images A and B) is displayed as red, but as the beam direction is changed (image C), flow toward the beam is now displayed as red. This is normally done automatically by the scanner as the beam transitions through steering between left and right.

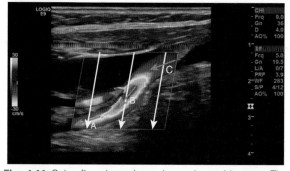

Fig. 4.11 Color flow hues in an internal carotid artery. The beam direction is shown as *white arrows*, the velocity direction is in *red arrows*. At *(B)*, the beam/flow angle is markedly less than at *(A)* and *(C)*. The better alignment leads to a higher velocity component in the beam direction with hues that are higher on the velocity scale and demonstrate aliasing. It is important to appreciate that the true velocity may not be different; the change in flow direction relative to the beam causes changes in the color appearance.

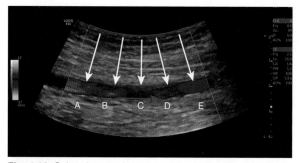

Fig. 4.12 Color changes in an artery imaged with a curvilinear array. The *white arrows* show the direction of the beams. Flow in the artery is from left to right in the image *(red arrow)*. At *(A)* and *(E)* the beam/flow angle is small enough that consistent color flow with lighter red and blue hues is displayed toward *(A)* and away *(E)* from the beam. At *(B)* and *(D)*, the beam/flow angle approaches 90°, color filling of the lumen is less consistent, and the red and blue hues are darker. At *(C)*, the beam/flow angle is 90° and there is no color flow for a short length.

COLOR FLOW IMAGING CONTROLS, THEIR FUNCTION, AND USE

PRF/Scale, Aliasing, and Sensitivity

The range of velocities displayed by the color scale (Fig. 4.5) is governed by the pulse repetition frequency (PRF). Generally, imaging arterial flow with high velocities usually requires a high scale/PRF; the low velocities in venous flow require low scales/PRFs, but it is a control

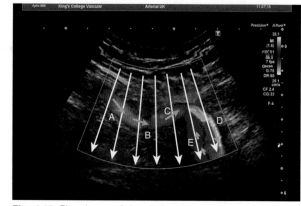

Fig. 4.13 Flow in a graft imaged with a curvilinear transducer. Flow is from left to right and the flow direction is shown by the pink arrows. The color assignment is red for flow away from the beam *(white arrows)*, blue toward the beam. At the left of the image *(A)*, flow is away from the beam. At *(B)*, flow is at 90° to the beam so there is no color. At *(C)*, flow is toward the beam and is coded blue. At the right of the image there is an area of dilatation in the graft with flow both away and toward the beam. The flow at *(D)* is closely aligned to the beam direction and so there is aliasing, the change in color arises from the smaller beam/flow angle, not higher velocities. At *(E)* the low reverse velocities in the dilated region are coded blue.

that sonographers will often change during an examination. By increasing or decreasing the scale, the PRF is increased or decreased to investigate the flow conditions in the vessels under examination.

The maximum velocity that can be detected with CFI is limited by the sampling frequency (PRF) in the same way as described for spectral Doppler (see Ch. 3). If the PRF is too low, then aliasing occurs and velocities will be displayed in the opposite flow direction colors (examples are seen in Figs. 4.11 and 4.13). As will be seen in the clinical chapters, aliasing is enormously useful to identify areas in an artery where velocities increase, especially in stenoses (Fig. 4.14).

One potential problem is differentiating aliasing from true flow reversal. True flow reversal, shown as a change in color within a vessel (i.e., from red to blue), can be seen where there is both forward and reverse flow present within a vessel due to a hemodynamic effect. Flow reversal is often seen in a normal carotid artery bulb, as described in Chapters 5 and 8. Apparent flow reversal can be due to an artifact, aliasing and can occur when a vessel changes direction relative to the CFI ultrasound beam (Fig. 4.11), although flow within the vessel has not changed direction. It is possible to distinguish between

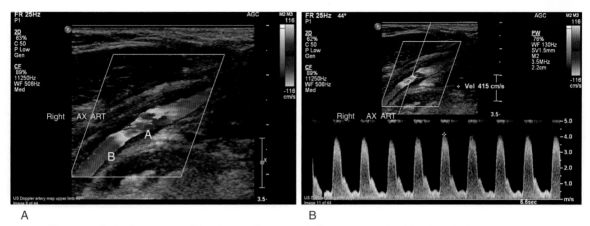

A   B

Fig. 4.14 Aliasing in an image of flow in an axillary artery indicates a stenosis. (A) In the color image there is an area of aliasing at *A* that is not due to change in direction relative to the beam. The lumen size does not look very different at *B*, but there is narrowing in the elevation plane causing an eccentric stenosis. Doppler measurement (B) shows a velocity of over 4 m/s, confirming a severe stenosis. Note that the color scale is high (± 115 cm/s). The sonographer should choose a scale that shows normal velocities as clear unambiguous hues, with aliasing then an indication of a change, either due to direction (Figs. 4.11 and 4.13) or increased velocities.

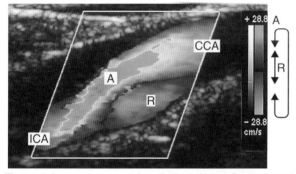

Fig. 4.15 Image demonstrating aliasing *(A)* and flow reversal *(R)* in an internal carotid artery *(ICA)*. Aliasing can be recognized as a color change that wraps around from the top to the bottom of the color scale, or vice versa. A change in color due to a relative change in the direction of flow can be recognized as a change in color across the baseline, at the center of the color scale, passing through black (see color scale on right of image). *CCA*, Common carotid artery.

aliasing and changes in the direction of flow relative to the transducer by the fact that the color transition seen in aliasing wraps around the farthest ends of the color scale (the color scale is shown as forward and reverse bars; in fact, it would be more accurate to show it as a color wheel with the highest forward hues transitioning to the highest reverse hues). In contrast, the colors displayed when the flow changes direction are near the baseline and pass through black at the point where no or low flow has been detected. Fig. 4.15 shows an image of a carotid artery that demonstrates both flow reversal and aliasing. The transitions in the colors displayed in both cases are shown as annotations to the right of the color scale.

High scales will be less sensitive to venous flow. When imaging low-velocity flow, the scale is reduced so that the low PRF is better able to detect the slow movement between pulses. Arterial settings have a PRF typically three to four times that for venous flow.

System presets choose PRFs that are appropriate for the specific application. Ideally, a PRF should be selected that displays the highest normal velocities present with the colors near the top of the scale. Fig. 4.16 shows two images of an artery overlying a vein. In Fig. 4.16A the PRF is set high and no aliasing is seen within the artery; however, no flow is detected in the vein, as the scale has been set too high to detect the lower venous flow. In Fig. 4.16B the PRF has been set lower and now flow is detected in the vein but aliasing is seen in the artery.

Color Box Size, Sensitivity, Frame Rate, and Spatial Resolution

As described earlier, CFI requires several pulses along each beam to measure the movement of blood in the direction of the beam to construct the CFI image. These pulses are in addition to those for the B-mode image. CFI requires more time to complete each image and there are compromises that are made between the need

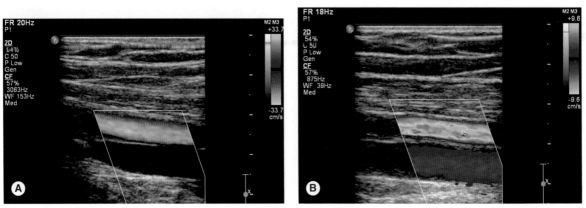

Fig. 4.16 Images of an artery overlying a vein. (A) The pulse repetition frequency (PRF) is set relatively high (3063 Hz) and no aliasing is seen within the artery; however, no flow is detected in the vein, as the scale has been set too high to detect the lower venous flow. (B) The PRF has been set lower (875 Hz), and now flow is detected in the vein but aliasing is seen in the artery. It is important that the appropriate PRF is selected depending on whether low- or high-velocity flow is being imaged to enable flow to be detected but without undesirable aliasing

for accurate sensitivity to flow, good spatial resolution and detail, and an adequate frame rate (number of images per second).

The interaction of these requirements is dependent on:

- The width and depth of the CFI region. If the entire area of the image is assessed for CFI, then more scan lines are required than if a small region of the image is to be investigated.
- The ensemble length. This is a technical term for the number of pulses sent along each beam to measure flow, typically from 4 to 12. More pulses will lead to increased sensitivity to flow and greater accuracy but will require more time.
- The line density. A high line density leads to finer lateral resolution in the color image, but the need for more scan lines will use more time.

The resulting frame rate will depend on the number of pulses sent and how they are used to produce the images. If large areas of CFI are chosen with high line density and high ensemble length, the time to complete each frame is longer than if less demanding parameters are selected. On some scanners the sonographer can alter all these factors independently, but the manufacturers' engineers also set up interaction of parameters so that, for example, if a wide CFI image is chosen, line density will often decrease to maintain an acceptable frame rate. The compromises made will be more visible in abdominal imaging where PRF is already constrained by the time needed for pulses to insonate deep tissue. In superficial applications, the constraints are not as severe. Generally, line density and ensemble length (sometimes described as color quality) are set up for each application preset and are rarely changed during an examination. However, color box size, or ROI, is routinely altered during an examination and, for example, to optimize investigation of a renal artery at depth, the sonographer is wise to reduce the area of color investigation to a minimum to improve the sensitivity to flow and the resolution of the color images of the vessels (see Fig. 4.17).

Transmit Frequency

Wideband transducers allow changes in transmit frequency. Just as in B-mode, lower frequencies give greater penetration, but higher frequencies are more sensitive to weak flow signal from small vessels, since scattering increases at higher frequencies. The effect of change in frequency is demonstrated in Fig. 4.18 where flow in the internal carotid artery is depicted more completely with a lower transmit frequency. Low frequencies also confer another advantage. Because the CFI signals are derived from phase changes and the interaction with PRF, lower transmit frequencies are able to image higher velocities without aliasing (see Eq. 3.5). This is also important in high flows in superficial vessels, particularly those seen in dialysis access where there is a compromise to be made between high frequencies for imaging and low frequencies to image flow with less risk of aliasing and ambiguity.

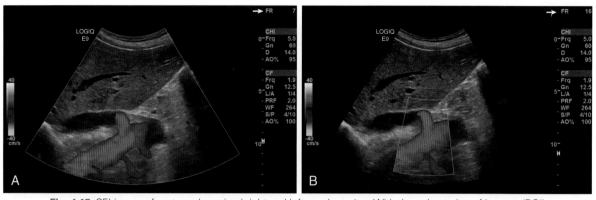

Fig. 4.17 CFI image of aorta and proximal right and left renal arteries. With the color region of interest (ROI) set over the entire image (A), the color resolution is slightly poorer and the frame rate is 7 frame/s *(arrow)*. By concentrating the ROI at the renal artery origins (B) the color image resolution is improved and the frame rate is now increased to 16 frames/s *(arrow)*. *CFI*, Color flow imaging.

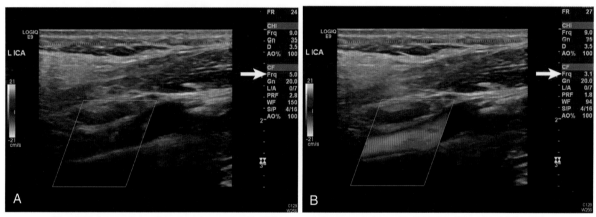

Fig. 4.18 Internal carotid artery imaged with CFI transmit frequency *(arrow)* of 5 MHz (A) and 3.1 MHz (B). The lower frequency provides improved penetration and better sensitivity to flow. *CFI*, Color flow imaging.

Scanners describe change in frequency either in values of MHz or in resolution/penetration options. This is a control that is optimized by experienced sonographers during a scan.

Focus

For those scanners that have a transmit focus control, setting the focus at the area of color flow interest improves sensitivity to flow and spatial resolution at the required depth. By moving a color ROI/box, focusing is often automatically altered, although the sonographer can also optimize this. An example of the improvement in image quality is shown in Fig. 4.19.

Gain

As for other modes, increasing gain boosts the signal, in this case increasing the color in the image. Used judiciously, it can enhance color flow sensitivity if images are unclear. Too much gain leads to color "bleed" into surrounding tissue, too little can lead to absence of flow images where they should be seen.

Filter

Filters are used to remove unwanted low-frequency CFI signals, particularly those from tissue movement. The high-pass filter will only allow frequencies greater than the cut-off frequency to be displayed; if this is set too

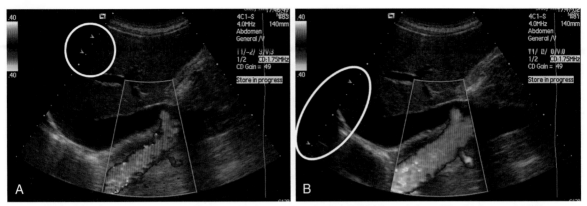

Fig. 4.19 Aorta and renal artery origins with focus, circled, superficial (A), and deep (B) with improved CFI imaging quality when focus is set at the region of interest. *CFI,* Color flow imaging.

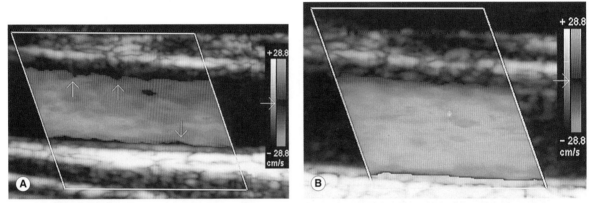

Fig. 4.20 Effect of using the filter. (A) The filter is set too high, removing the low-velocity flow near the vessel walls *(vertical arrows).* (B) The filter setting is reduced to display the low frequencies detected near the vessel walls. The filter setting may be indicated on the color scale *(horizontal arrows).*

high, velocities detected from the lower-velocity blood flow will not be displayed. The level of the high-pass filter is usually displayed on the color scale (Fig. 4.20). Using the wrong filter setting has led to removal of the low velocities at the vessel walls or of low flow during diastole. Filter settings are chosen for specific presets, for example, there is less tissue movement in peripheral veins and a lower filter setting can be chosen when compared with abdominal vascular imaging.

Frame Averaging

For weak flow signals, frame averaging can be used to enhance the color flow image by accumulating signals from several frames to show the presence of flow where sensitivity is inconsistent. This will be at the expense of dynamic display of flow. Typically, settings for venous flow will have greater frame averaging than those for arterial flow where the dynamic of flow is more important and changes occur more rapidly.

Color Map

A variety of color maps are available to suit the sonographer. These are a matter of personal preference, and various maps are shown in the following chapters.

The major controls affecting CFI imaging are summarized in Appendix C.

SPATIAL RESOLUTION OF COLOR FLOW IMAGING

CFI uses longer pulses than B-mode and typically has a lower line density. Because of this, conventional CFI has a lower spatial resolution than B-mode. When

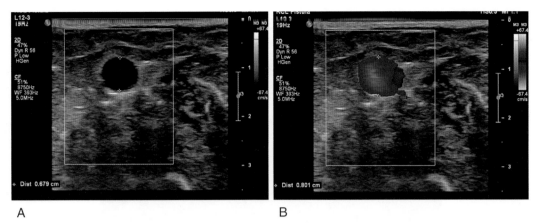

Fig. 4.21 (A) B-mode and (B) CFI transverse images of a fistula vein. The diameter measured on B-mode is approximately 6.8 mm and in CFI is 8.0 mm. The poorer resolution of CFI leads to overestimation of the true diameter. *CFI*, Color flow imaging.

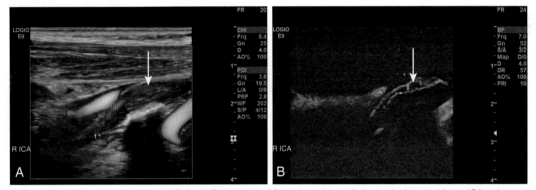

Fig. 4.22 Power Doppler (A) and B-flow (B) images of flow though small channels *(arrows)* in an ICA subocclusion. The high resolution of B-flow shows greater spatial resolution of the narrow lumens. *ICA*, Internal carotid artery.

measuring vessel dimensions, it is prudent to turn off CFI and use the B-mode image, especially when measuring plaque dimensions or the vessel diameter. The effect of CFI on apparent vessel diameter is shown in Fig. 4.21.

POWER DOPPLER IMAGING

So far, this chapter has described how the estimated velocity of blood can be displayed as a color map superimposed on to the gray-scale image. However, instead of displaying the detected velocity with respect to the beam, it is possible to display the back-scattered power of the correlation signal. The color scale used in power Doppler imaging shows increased luminosity with increased back-scattered power. This allows the scanner to display the presence of moving blood and, since the

amount of back-scattering varies less than its velocity, averaging techniques can be used to enhance the flow signal and reduce noise, leading to greater sensitivity of low flows. Initial implementations of power Doppler were nondirectional but there are an increasing number of combinations of directional and nondirectional power Doppler to improve sensitivity to flow. An example of nondirectional power Doppler is shown in Fig. 4.22A.

NEW DEVELOPMENTS IN COLOR FLOW IMAGING

Several manufacturers have introduced color flow modes for enhanced sensitivity to low flows in small vessels. Advanced filtering techniques have been employed to reduce clutter and emphasize blood flow. For superficial peripheral vessels, the improved sensitivity to flow

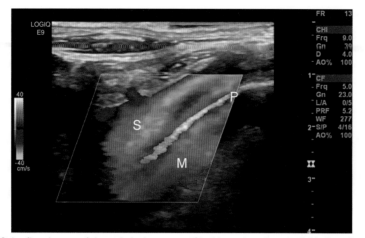

Fig. 4.23 Color flow image of the subclavian artery *(S)* with a mirror image *(M)* below the pleura *(P)*.

reveals a profusion of small arteries and veins and offers the prospect to image and make measurements in vessels significantly smaller than has hitherto been possible.

B-FLOW IMAGING

B-flow imaging is a technique for displaying the presence of blood flow that relies on B-mode type pulses. As seen in Chapter 2, the back-scatter from blood is small and blood is usually displayed as black on B-mode images. However, improvements in sensitivity of ultrasound to blood offer the possibility of imaging moving blood directly. This is done by sending pairs of pulses, then subtracting the returning echoes. If the signal is detected from a stationary structure, such as tissue, the pulses will cancel out and no movement will be displayed. If there is movement, such as blood flow, the two back-scattered signals will differ and will not cancel out. The difference in the signal can be amplified and displayed to give a real-time image of areas of movement. Because it relies on pairs of B-mode pulses, the frame rate is higher than CFI and the resolution is improved, leading to greater clarity of stenoses, ulcerations, and images of small vessels (see Fig. 4.22B)

COLOR FLOW IMAGING ARTIFACTS

CFI is prone to imaging artifacts in a similar way to B-mode imaging (see end of Ch. 2), where assumptions made in forming the image are not correct, or poor

control optimization. This can lead to the absence of flow being displayed or flow being displayed where it is not present.

A common artifact seen in CFI is the absence of flow being displayed resulting from an increased attenuation, due to calcified plaque (Fig. 8.36) or bone, such as the clavicle overlying the subclavian artery (Fig. 10.5), preventing penetration of the CFI and spectral Doppler beam. As discussed earlier, poor angle between the CFI beam and flow (Fig. 4.10B) or inappropriate selection of scale/PRF (Fig. 4.16) can also result in an absence of flow being displayed.

Flow may be displayed in the incorrect location when the CFI pulse undergoes multiple reflections, as the scanner assumes the pulse has traveled in a straight line to the blood flow and back. Fig. 4.23 shows a mirror image of the subclavian artery produced by reflections from the pleura overlying the lung, a highly reflective air–tissue interface, of the back-scattered signal from the blood. A second artifactual image of the subclavian artery has been incorrectly displayed beneath the pleura. The path of the reflected ultrasound has undergone multiple reflections and is different from that of the ultrasound back-scattered directly from the blood to the transducer. Therefore, the detected velocity displayed for the mirror image may not be the same as for the vessel itself. The artifactual flow displayed on the color image can also be detected with spectral Doppler, if the sample volume is placed over the mirror image. Mirror image artifacts may occur from the tibial vessels or bypass grafts when these vessels are overlying bone. Another example of this occurring is shown in Fig. 12.9 with aortic flow incorrectly superimposed on the spine.

Color can also be introduced into the CFI where flow is not present if the color gain is set too high, giving the appearance of the color "bleeding" out of the vessel. Anechoic areas on B-mode can be filled with speckled color due to noise if the gain is set high or if there is low-velocity tissue motion present (e.g., due to respiration). Tissue bruits, for example, near a stenosis may result in color appearing outside the vessel wall (Fig. 16.24) due to tissue vibration being detected.

A bright B-mode imaging artifact (such as seen in Fig. 2.37) may be displayed in preference to the color flow information, and this may give the appearance of a structure within the vessel lumen, around which the flow is displayed. If the color write priority is set too low in the presence of a noisy B-mode image, flow detected may not be displayed due to the lack of a clear vessel lumen. Giving priority to the CFI means that the B-mode image can be reasonably bright without losing color information on the screen.

The CFI may not give a true representation of the relative blood velocities within the vessel (as discussed earlier). Changes in the angle between the flow and beam can lead to color imaging artifacts, giving the false impression of changes in blood velocity (see Fig. 4.12). Aliasing artifacts will also change the appearance of the color image (see Fig. 4.15).

Blood Flow and Its Appearance on Color Flow Imaging

INTRODUCTION

Interpretation of Doppler images and measurements of flow in arteries and veins require an understanding of the hemodynamics, the dynamics of blood flow. Arterial blood flow is complex and consists of pulsatile flow of an inhomogeneous fluid through viscoelastic arteries that branch, curve, and taper. However, a useful understanding of hemodynamics can be gained by first considering simple models and concepts, such as steady flow in a rigid tube. In this chapter, factors that affect arterial and also venous flow will be discussed with a particular emphasis on how these are displayed by color flow and spectral Doppler ultrasound and how the user interprets these to image and measure flow in normal and diseased vessels. It is also important to remember that ultrasound controls and parameters themselves contribute to the images and can alter their appearance. Artifactual effects also have to be considered carefully before drawing conclusions about the blood flow.

STRUCTURE OF VESSEL WALLS

The arterial and venous systems are often thought of as a series of tubes that transport blood to and from organs and tissues. In reality, blood vessels are highly complex structures that respond to nervous stimulation and interact with chemicals in the blood stream to regulate the flow of blood throughout the body. Changes in cardiac output and the tone of the smooth-muscle cells in the arterial walls are crucial factors that affect blood flow. The structure of a blood vessel wall varies considerably depending on its position within the vascular system.

Arteries and veins are composed of three layers of tissue, with veins having thinner walls than arteries. The outer layer is called the adventitia and is predominantly composed of connective tissue with collagen and elastin. The middle layer, the media, is the thickest layer and is composed of smooth-muscle fibers and elastic tissue. The intima is the inner layer and consists of a thin layer of endothelium overlying an elastic membrane. The capillaries, by contrast, consist of a single layer of endothelium, which allows for the exchange of molecules through the capillary wall. It is possible to image the structure of larger vessel walls using ultrasound and to identify the early stages of arterial disease, such as intimal thickening.

The arterial tree consists of elastic arteries, muscular arteries, and arterioles. The aorta and subclavian arteries are examples of elastic or conducting arteries and contain elastic fibers and a large amount of collagen fibers to limit the degree of stretch. Elastic arteries function as a pressure reservoir, as the elastic tissue in the vessel wall is able to absorb a proportion of the large amount of energy generated by the heart during systole. This maintains the end-diastolic pressure and decreases the load on the left side of the heart. Muscular or distributing arteries, such as the radial artery, contain a large proportion of smooth-muscle cells in the media. These arteries are innervated by nerves and can dilate or constrict. The muscular arteries are responsible for regional distribution of blood flow. Arterioles are the smallest arteries, and their media is composed almost entirely of smooth-muscle cells. Arterioles have an important role in controlling blood pressure and flow, and they can constrict or dilate after sympathetic nerve or chemical stimulation. The arterioles distribute blood to specific capillary beds and can dilate or constrict selectively around the body depending on the requirements of organs or tissues.

WHY DOES BLOOD FLOW?

Energy created by the contraction of the heart forces blood around the body. Blood flow in the arteries depends on two factors: (1) the energy available to drive the blood flow, and (2) the resistance to flow presented by the vascular system.

Energy in blood

A scientist named Daniel Bernoulli (1700–1782) showed that the total fluid energy, which gives rise to the flow, is made up of three parts:
- Pressure energy (p)—this is the pressure in the fluid, which, in the case of blood flow, varies due to the contraction of the heart and the distension of the aorta.
- Kinetic energy (KE)—this is due to the fact that the fluid is a moving mass. KE is dependent on the density (ρ) and velocity (V) of the fluid:

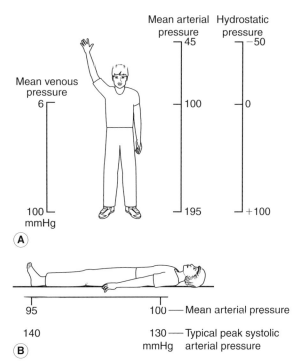

Fig. 5.1 Schematic diagram showing typical pressures in arteries and veins with the subject standing (A) and lying (B). The component due to hydrostatic pressure when the subject is vertical is shown alongside (A).

$$KE = \frac{1}{2}\rho V^2 \qquad (5.1)$$

- Gravitational potential energy—this is the ability of a volume of blood to do work due to the effect of gravity (g) on the column of fluid with density (ρ) because of its height (h) above a reference point, typically the heart.

Gravitational potential energy (ρgh) is equivalent to hydrostatic pressure but has an opposite sign (i.e., $-\rho gh$). For example, when a person is standing, there is a column of blood—the height of the heart above the feet—resting on the blood in the vessels in the foot (Fig. 5.1A) causing a higher pressure, due to the hydrostatic pressure, than that seen when the person is lying down (Fig. 5.1B). As the heart is taken as the reference point, and the feet are below the heart, the hydrostatic pressure is positive. If the arm is raised so that it is above the heart, the hydrostatic pressure is negative, causing the veins to collapse and the pressure in the arteries in the arm to be lower than the pressure at the level of the heart. The total fluid energy is given by:

Total fluid energy = pressure energy +
gravitational energy +
kinetic energy

$$E_{tot} = p + (-\rho gh) + \frac{1}{2}\rho V^2 \qquad (5.2)$$

RESISTANCE TO FLOW

In 1840, a physician named Poiseuille established a relationship between flow, the pressure gradient along a tube, and the dimensions of a tube. The relationship can simply be understood as:

$$\text{Pressure drop} = \text{flow} \times \text{resistance} \qquad (5.3)$$

For constant flow in a rigid tube of uniform diameter, the resistance to flow R is given by:

$$R = \frac{\text{viscosity} \times \text{length} \times 8}{\pi \times r^4} \qquad (5.4)$$

where r is the radius.

Viscosity causes friction between the moving layers of the fluid. Treacle, for example, is a highly viscous fluid, whereas water has a low viscosity and therefore offers less resistance to flow when traveling through a tube. Poiseuille's law shows that the resistance to flow is highly dependent on changes in the radius (r^4). In the normal circulation, the greatest proportion of the resistance occurs at the arteriole level. Tissue perfusion is controlled by changes in the diameter of the arterioles. The presence of arterial disease in the arteries, such as stenoses or occlusions, can significantly alter the resistance to flow, with the reduction in vessel diameter having a major effect on the change in resistance seen. In severe disease, the arterioles distal to the disease may become maximally dilated in order to reduce the peripheral resistance, thus increasing blood flow in an attempt to maintain tissue perfusion. Poiseuille's experiments described nonpulsatile flow in a straight rigid tube, so his equation does not completely represent arterial blood flow; however, it gave him and gives us some understanding of the relationship between pressure drop, resistance, and flow.

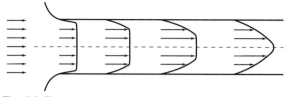

Fig. 5.2 The change in velocity profile with distance along a vessel from a blunt to a parabolic. (After Caro et al. 1978, with permission.)

FLOW PROFILES IN NORMAL ARTERIES

There are two types of flow observed in arteries:
1. laminar
2. turbulent

The term *laminar flow* refers to the fact that the blood cells move in layers, one layer sliding over another, with the different layers being able to move at different velocities. In laminar flow, the blood cells remain in their layers. Turbulent flow occurs when laminar flow breaks down, local inertial forces overcome viscous forces creating random velocity variations in many directions. This is unusual in normal healthy arteries but can be seen in the presence of high-velocity flow caused by stenoses, as discussed later in this chapter. Turbulent flow has greater resistance than laminar flow and so requires a larger pressure drop to drive blood though the artery (Eq. 5.3).

Fig. 5.2 is a schematic diagram showing how the flow profile is expected to change as fluid enters a vessel. When flow enters a vessel from a reservoir (in the case of blood flow, this is the heart), all the fluid is moving at the same velocity, producing a flat velocity profile. This means that the velocity of the fluid close to the vessel wall is similar to that at the center of the vessel. As the fluid flows along the vessel, viscous drag exerted by the walls causes the fluid at the vessel wall to remain motionless, producing a gradient between the velocity in the center of the vessel and that at the walls. As the total flow has to remain constant (as there are no branches in our imaginary tube), the velocity at the center of the vessel will increase to compensate for the low velocity at the vessel wall. This leads to a change in the velocity profile from the initial blunt flow profile to a parabolic flow profile. This is often known as an entrance effect. The distance required for the flow profile to develop from the blunt to the parabolic profile depends on vessel diameter and velocity, but it is usually several times the

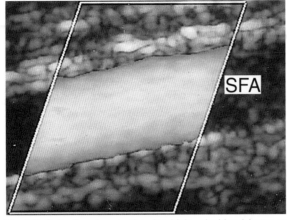

Fig. 5.3 Color flow image showing high velocities (shown as *yellow*) in the center of a normal superficial femoral artery, with lower velocities (shown as *red*) nearer the vessel wall.

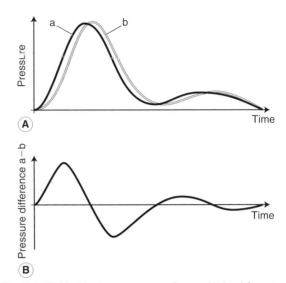

Fig. 5.4 (A) Idealized pressure waveforms obtained from two sites (*a* and *b*) along the femoral artery. (B) The direction of blood flow between *a* and *b* will be governed by the pressure difference, given by *a* − *b*. (From Nichols & O'Rourke, 1990, with permission)

vessel diameter. With blood flow, the velocity profiles are complicated by the pulsatile nature of the flow.

A color flow image obtained from the superficial femoral artery, during systole, is shown in Fig. 5.3. This image shows high velocities in the center of the mid superficial femoral artery and lower velocities near the artery wall.

Pulsatile Flow

The flow profiles considered in Fig. 5.2 describe steady flow, but clearly arterial flow is pulsatile. So how will this affect the velocity profile across the vessel? The mean velocity profile of the pulsatile flow will develop as described for steady-state flow but will have a pulsatile component superimposed upon it. The flow direction and velocity are governed by the pressure gradient along the vessel. The pressure pulse generated by the heart is transmitted down the arterial tree and is altered by pressure waves reflected from the distal vascular bed. Fig. 5.4A shows the pressure waveforms, typical of those seen in the femoral arteries, from two different points along the vessel, "a" and "b." The pressure difference between these two points is given by a − b, as shown in Fig. 5.4B, such that a negative pressure gradient is produced at periods during the cardiac cycle. This leads to periods of reverse flow, as seen in a typical Doppler waveform obtained from a normal superficial femoral artery (Fig. 5.5). If we consider a slowly oscillating pressure gradient applied to the flow, this will slow down, stop, and then reverse the direction of flow. If this oscillation is gradual,

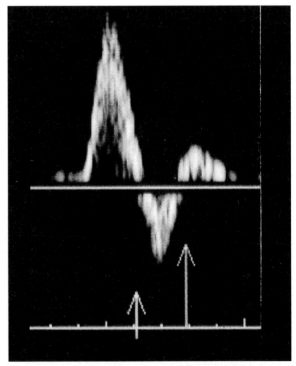

Fig. 5.5 Velocity waveform in a normal superficial femoral artery. The *arrows* represent points in the cardiac cycle where both forward and reverse flows are seen simultaneously.

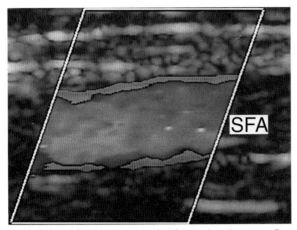

Fig. 5.6 Color flow image showing forward and reverse flow simultaneously in a normal superficial femoral artery *(SFA)*. The red represents forward flow near the vessel wall whereas the blue represents reverse flow in the center of the vessel.

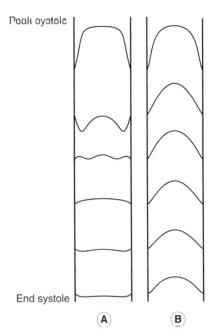

Fig. 5.7 Velocity profiles from a common femoral artery (A) and a common carotid artery (B), calculated from the mean velocity waveforms. (After Evans & McDicken 1999, with permission.)

the near parabolic velocity profile will be maintained, but if the pressure gradient is cycled more frequently, the velocity profile will become increasingly complex.

As the laminae of flowing blood near the vessel wall tend to have a lower velocity (due to the effect of viscosity), and hence lower momentum, they will reverse more easily when the pressure gradient along the vessel reverses. This can lead to a situation in which flow near the vessel wall is in a different direction to flow at the center of the vessel. Fig. 5.6 shows a color image obtained from a normal superficial femoral artery during diastole. The image shows forward flow near the vessel wall, while flow in the center of the vessel is reversed. This would occur at the point in the cardiac cycle marked by the long arrow in Fig. 5.5. The short arrow shows another point at which both forward and reverse flow may occur simultaneously. Fig. 5.7 shows velocity profiles, as they vary over the cardiac cycle, for the common femoral artery (Fig. 5.7A) and the common carotid artery (Fig. 5.7B) that have been calculated from mean velocity waveforms. They show that reversal of flow is seen in the common femoral artery, but that, although the flow is pulsatile, reverse flow is not seen in the normal common carotid artery. Reversal of flow will only be seen if the reverse pulsatile flow component is greater than the steady flow component upon which it is superimposed. This greatly depends on the distal vascular bed. Total reversal of flow is rarely seen in normal renal or internal carotid arteries, both of which

supply highly vascular beds with low resistance. However, there are hemodynamic effects at bifurcations and branches that may cause areas of localized flow reversal. There is a different appearance between waveform shapes obtained from vessels supplying a low-resistance vascular bed (i.e., organs such as the brain and kidney) and those obtained from peripheral vessels in the arms and legs, which supply high-resistance vascular beds.

Changes in peripheral resistance will change the flow pattern. For example, the waveform in the dorsalis pedis artery in the foot changes from bi-directional flow at rest (Fig. 5.8A) to hyperemic multiphasic unidirectional flow (i.e., flow that is always in the same direction; Fig. 5.8B) following exercise. Hyperemic flow can also be induced by temporary occlusion of the calf arteries using a blood pressure cuff. The lack of blood flow during the arterial occlusion with the cuff, or the increase in demand during exercise, causes the distal vessels to dilate in order to reduce peripheral resistance and maximize blood flow, and this is reflected in the change in shape of the waveform seen directly after cuff release. The hyperemic flow soon returns to bi-directional flow once adequate perfusion has occurred. This change in shape can also be seen when hyperemic flow is induced

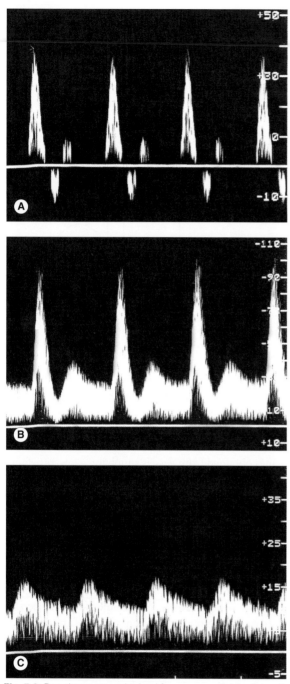

Fig. 5.8 Doppler spectra obtained from a normal dorsalis pedis artery in the foot showing bi-directional flow at rest (A) and uni-directional multiphasic hyperemic flow following exercise (B). Low-volume monophasic flow is seen in the foot distal to an occlusion (C).

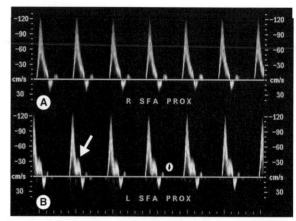

Fig. 5.9 Doppler spectrum obtained from a superficial femoral artery *(SFA)* (A) proximal to normal popliteal artery and (B) proximal to an occluded popliteal artery. The ledge seen *(arrow)* on the downward slope of the systolic peak is an indication of the distal disease.

by infection. Monophasic flow is seen in the lower limb, distal to severe stenoses, or occlusions (Fig. 5.8C). This waveform shape is also due to distal vasodilatation, in an attempt to maximize flow distal to the diseased vessel in response to the reduced pressure pulse. However, this can usually be distinguished from hyperemic flow, as the velocity of the flow is low, and the systolic rise time—the time between the beginning of systole and peak systole—may be longer, and there is less distinction between the systolic and diastolic flow phases.

An occlusion or severe stenosis distal to the site at which a Doppler waveform has been obtained may also cause a change in the waveform shape due to an increase in the resistance to flow. Fig. 5.9A shows a Doppler spectrum obtained from a superficial femoral artery proximal to a normal popliteal artery and demonstrates a normal triphasic waveform shape. Fig. 5.9B shows the Doppler spectrum obtained from the superficial femoral artery in the other leg of the same individual but this time the popliteal artery is occluded. Although the waveform shape in Fig. 5.9B still appears triphasic, a ledge can be seen on the downward slope of the systolic peak, which is caused by the presence of the distal occlusion. This change in appearance of the waveform shape is due to changes in the reflected pressure wave (Fig. 5.4) and can be used as an indication that there may be significant disease distal to the site of measurement that would require further investigation.

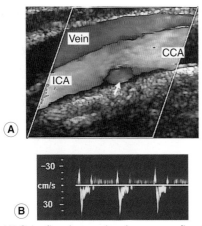

Fig. 5.10 (A) Color flow image showing reverse flow in the origin of a normal internal carotid artery *(ICA)*. (B) Spectral Doppler waveform obtained from the area of flow separation shown by the *arrow* in (A). *CCA,* Common carotid artery.

Flow at Bifurcations and Branches

The arterial tree divides many times, and each branch will affect the velocity profiles seen. The hemodynamics of the carotid bifurcation has been extensively investigated using multigate pulsed Doppler systems and color Doppler systems, and these investigations show that localized reversed flow is seen at the carotid bifurcation in normal subjects. Fig. 5.10A shows reversal of flow, due to flow separation, at the origin of a healthy internal carotid artery. Fig. 5.11 indicates how the asymmetric flow profile in a normal proximal internal carotid artery develops, with the high-velocity flow occurring toward the flow divider and the reverse flow occurring near the wall away from the origin of the external carotid artery. The effect is primarily due to a combination of the pulsatile flow, the relative dimensions of the vessels, the angle of the bifurcation, and the curvature of the vessel walls, making it difficult to predict these profiles. Fig. 5.10B is a spectral Doppler signal obtained from the area of flow separation shown by an arrow in Fig. 5.10A, illustrating reverse flow during systole in that part of the vessel. This normal finding could potentially be misleading if the whole bifurcation is not observed and, typically, spectral Doppler recordings are made beyond the bifurcation unless the presence of disease indicates otherwise (see Ch. 8).

Flow reversal can also occur when a daughter vessel branches at right angles from the parent vessel. Fig. 5.12

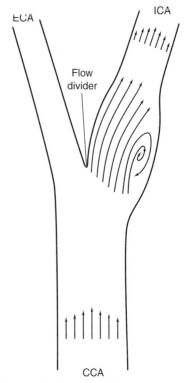

Fig. 5.11 Schematic diagram of the velocity patterns commonly observed in the normal carotid bifurcation. The velocity profile is flat and symmetric in the common carotid artery *(CCA)* and flat but slightly asymmetric in the internal carotid artery *(ICA)*. In the carotid bulb the velocities are highest near the flow divider. Flow separation with flow reversal is observed on the opposite side to the flow divider. *ECA,* External carotid artery. (From Reneman et al. 1985, with permission.)

is a schematic diagram of the results obtained with dye in steadily flowing water in a tube with a right-angled branch and shows how the flow is divided between the main vessel and its branch. The flow is seen to separate from the inner wall of the junction and a region of reverse flow develops, primarily due to the sharp bend.

Flow Around Curves in a Vessel

Curvature of vessels can also have an effect on the velocity profile. When a fluid flows along a curved tube, it experiences a centrifugal force, as well as the viscous forces at the vessel wall, and the combination of these forces results in secondary flow, in the form of two helical vortices (Oates 2008). In the case of parabolic flow, the fluid in the center of the vessel has the

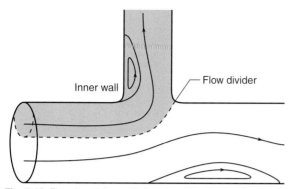

Fig. 5.12 Flow in a right-angle junction. The *dashed line* shows the surface that divides fluid flowing into the side branch from that continuing down the parent vessel. (After Caro et al. 1978, with permission.)

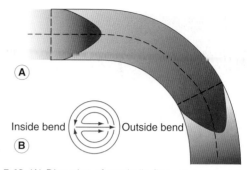

Fig. 5.13 (A) Distortion of parabolic flow caused by tube curvature. (B) Secondary flow, in the form of two helical vortices. (After Caro et al. 1978, with permission.)

highest velocity and will thus experience the greatest force. These vortices will cause the high-velocity flow to move toward the outside wall of the vessel, as seen in Fig. 5.13. Fig. 5.14 shows a color flow image obtained from a tortuous internal carotid artery, with flow going from right to left. The image shows the highest velocities beyond the bend (left), represented in orange due to aliasing, skewed toward the outside of the bend. This is confirmed by spectral Doppler recordings showing that the peak velocity recorded on the outside of the bend (Fig. 5.14B) measures 70 cm/s compared to the peak velocity on the inside of the bend (Fig. 5.14C), which measures 55 cm/s. If the flow profile is blunt when it enters a bend in the vessel (as seen in the ascending aorta), the profile becomes skewed in the opposite direction (i.e., toward the inner wall of the curve). Secondary helical flow also occurs at bifurcations, as the daughter vessels bend away from the path of the parent vessel, leading to skewed velocity profiles in the daughter vessels (Fig. 5.11).

FLOW THROUGH STENOSES

Flow changes in stenoses (narrowings) are fundamental to vascular ultrasound applications. Clinically, stenoses cause alterations to flow that can lead to ischemia or embolic events. Because Doppler ultrasound is a measure of velocity, the changes in velocity through a stenosis mean that it has a unique role not only in identifying the presence and severity of disease, but also providing an assessment of the hemodynamic impact of the stenosis depending on the arteries under investigation.

VELOCITY CHANGES WITHIN STENOSES

The volume flow in a blood vessel is given by:

$$\text{Flow} = \text{mean velocity} \times \text{cross-sectional area}$$
$$Q = V \times A \tag{5.5}$$

where V is the mean velocity across the whole of the vessel, averaged over time, and A is the cross-sectional area of the vessel. This has important ramifications for vascular ultrasound practitioners. For example, with a patient standing at rest, lower-limb veins are distended with large area. Flow is low, so velocities too are low, and augmentation may be required to image the flow. Another practical consequence is pressing too hard on an artery, reducing its cross-sectional area and increasing velocities through it. The most important consequence is the change in velocity through stenoses.

If the vessel has no outlets or branches through which fluid can be lost, the flow along the vessel remains constant. This means that if there are changes in the cross-sectional area of the vessel, there will be changes to velocity, since the velocity at any point along the vessel depends on its cross-sectional area. Fig. 5.15 shows a vessel of changing cross-sectional area (A_1, A_2). Since the flow (Q) along the tube is constant:

$$Q = V_1 \times A_1 = V_2 \times A_2 \tag{5.6}$$

This equation can be rearranged to show that the change in the velocities is related to the change in the cross-sectional area, as follows:

$$\frac{V_2}{V_1} = \frac{A_1}{A_2} \tag{5.7}$$

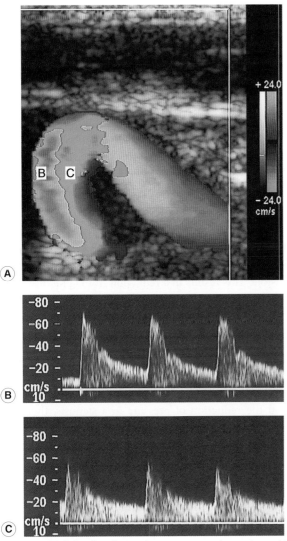

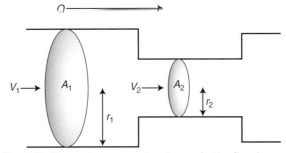

Fig. 5.15 Change in cross-sectional area. As the flow is constant through the tube, the velocity of the fluid increases from V_1 to V_2 as the cross-sectional area decreases from A_1 to A_2.

the mean velocity will change across a stenosis in an artery.

In Doppler ultrasound, measurements of peak systolic velocity are most commonly used to assess the presence and severity of stenosis. This produces an added complexity; the relationship between mean and peak velocity changes depending on the flow profile which in turn is influenced by the flow waveform. For example, a peak velocity increase of × 2 is used to describe a 50% stenosis in the femoral artery where there is pulsatile flow with a blunt flow profile, but the values for internal carotid or renal artery might be different where there is a less pulsatile flow waveform, and here measures of absolute peak velocity are used, alongside ratios. In practice, the geometry of stenoses is very variable. Narrowings are often not symmetrical, sometimes producing eccentric jets, so it is impossible to predict the typical velocity profiles.

ENERGY CHANGES THROUGH A STENOSIS—EFFECTS ON THE CIRCULATION

As well as being useful for diagnosis, the change in velocity through a stenosis is also indicative of changes in pressure as the faster moving blood now has more KE. Fig. 5.16 gives a graphical display of how the KE and pressure alter with continuous flow through an idealized narrowing (it ignores any changes in gravitational potential energy). Usually the KE component of the total energy is small compared with the pressure energy. When fluid flows through a tube with a narrowing, the fluid travels faster as it passes through the narrowed section. As the velocity of the fluid increases in a narrowed portion of the vessel, the KE increases and the pressure energy falls (this is known as the Venturi effect). The

Fig. 5.14 (A) Color flow image from a tortuous internal carotid artery, with flow going from right to left, shows the highest velocities beyond the bend (*point B*), represented in orange due to aliasing, skewed toward the outside of the bend. Spectral Doppler recordings showing that the peak velocity recorded on the outside of the bend (B) measure 70 cm/s compared to the peak velocity on the inside of the bend (C), which measures 55 cm/s.

If the vessel is circular, the cross-sectional area depends on the radius r of the tube ($A = \pi r^2$):

$$\frac{V_2}{V_1} = \frac{A_1}{A_2} = \frac{r_1^2}{r_2^2} \tag{5.8}$$

This relationship describes steady flow in a rigid circular vessel, but it does give us an indication as to how

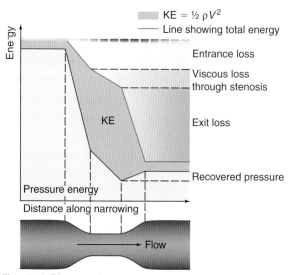

Fig. 5.16 Diagram showing how energy losses can occur across a narrowing. *KE,* Kinetic energy. (From Oates, 2008.)

pressure within the narrowing is therefore lower than the pressure in the portion of the vessel before the narrowing (this sometimes leads to confusion in understanding; if you squeeze on a hose to produce a jet of water, the pressure upstream of the narrowed hose may increase but the pressure in the jet of water is lower). As the fluid passes beyond the narrowing, the velocity slows again and the KE is converted back to pressure energy, which increases. Energy is lost as the fluid passes through the narrowing (Fig. 5.16), with the severity of the entrance and exit losses depending on the geometry and degree of the narrowing (Oates 2008). In normal arteries, very little energy is lost as the blood flows away from the heart toward the limbs and organs, and the mean pressure in the small distal vessels is only slightly lower than in the aorta. In minor stenoses, the conversion from pressure to KE and back may have very low loss and not adversely affect the circulation. However, in the presence of significant arterial disease, energy may be lost from the blood as it passes through tight narrowings or small collateral vessels around occlusions, leading to a drop in the pressure greater than that which would be expected in a normal artery. This can lead to reduced blood flow and tissue perfusion distally. Because the entrance and exit losses account for a large proportion of the pressure loss, it is likely that two adjacent stenoses will have a more significant effect than one long one (Oates 2008).

The conversion of pressure into a high-velocity jet has profound consequences for the circulation. If the pressure loss is not recovered distally, there will be a reduction in downstream pressure that will limit that available for the distal circulation. The velocity jet itself can lead to turbulence, disturbed flow, and areas of flow separation, possibly leading to thrombus. The changing pressure in the stenosis that varies throughout cycle can exert forces on plaque, leading to rupture. If stenosis is severe enough, then it can lead to:

- Flow reduction—for example, in claudication,
- Pressure reduction—for example, in renovascular hypertension,
- Embolism—for example, in carotid disease.

There are other consequences of the conversion of energy through the stenosis. The pressure loss is greatest when velocities are highest and so is greatest during systole. This results in a reduction in the pressure pulse which, if associated with a reduction in peripheral resistance to compensate, leads to damped flow downstream. Another consequence of the change from pressure to KE is that there is a limit to how fast arterial blood can travel; it is unusual to see velocities of greater than 6 m/s in the human circulation.

Because of the relationship between peak velocity and the reduction of pressure in a stenosis, there has been interest in using the measured peak velocity as an indication of pressure *loss* through a stenosis. This has been most successful in evaluation of renal artery stenosis (see Ch. 12), though there is also reported success for iliac artery disease. Even though specific values remain elusive, velocities remain useful in vascular ultrasound practice, and the ratio of the peak velocity is indicative of the anatomical severity of a stenosis, but it is the peak within the stenosis that gives more indication of its hemodynamic impact.

When a stenosis becomes very severe, for example, if it is long with a very small lumen, there is no longer conversion of energy from pressure to KE, and the stenosis itself becomes more and more resistant. In these cases, flow through very severely narrowed arteries declines drastically; velocities will depend on the pressure gradient through the narrowing and its vascular resistance.

The change in flow and velocity for carotid artery stenoses has been modeled to aid understanding of velocity values. Fig. 5.17 shows how the flow and velocity within an idealized stenosis vary with the degree of diameter

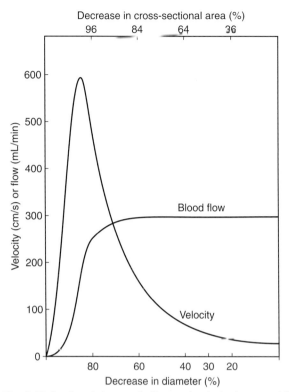

Fig. 5.17 Predicted changes in flow and velocity in a carotid artery as the degree of stenosis alters, predicted by a simple theoretical model of a smooth, symmetrical stenosis that includes the contralateral carotid. (From Spencer & Reid, 1979.)

reduction caused by the stenosis, based on the predictions from a simplified theoretical model of a carotid stenosis, which includes the contralateral carotid collateral flow, both supplying the cerebral arteries. On the right-hand side of the graph, where the diameter reduction is less than 70%–80%, the flow remains relatively unchanged as the diameter of the vessel is reduced. This is because the proportion of the resistance to flow due to the stenosis is small compared with the overall resistance of the vascular bed that the vessel is supplying. However, as the diameter reduces further, the resistance offered by the stenosis becomes a significant proportion of the total resistance, and the stenosis begins to limit the flow. This is known as a hemodynamically significant stenosis. At this point, the flow decreases quickly as the diameter is reduced.

The graph also predicts the behavior of the velocity as the vessel diameter is reduced and shows that the velocity increases with diameter reduction. Noticeable changes in velocity begin to occur at lower degrees of

stenosis than would produce a flow reduction; velocity changes are a more sensitive method of detecting moderate lumen reductions than measurement of flow. Measurements of velocity made using Doppler ultrasound are also more accurate than measurement of flow, as will be discussed later (see Ch. 6). Therefore, it is usually the change in velocity of blood within a diseased artery that is used to quantify the degree of narrowing. Eventually, in the internal carotid artery there comes a point at which the resistance to flow produced by the narrowing is so great, and the collateral side so dominant that the flow drops to such an extent that the velocity begins to decrease, as shown on the left side of the graph. Therefore, it is possible for there to be apparently normal or low velocities seen in a very tightly narrowed internal carotid artery; however, the presence of disease should be obvious on the color flow image.

As blood flow is pulsatile and arteries are nonrigid vessels, it is difficult to predict the theoretical velocity increase that would be seen for a particular diameter reduction. Instead, velocity criteria used to quantify the degree of narrowing are produced by comparing Doppler velocity measurements with arteriogram results, as arteriography has been considered to be the "gold standard" for the diagnosis of arterial disease.

Flow separation leading to flow reversal can also be seen in diseased arteries. As we have seen, pressure falls within a stenosis as the blood velocity increases. If the vessel lumen rapidly returns to its normal diameter distal to the stenosis, the mean velocity falls and the blood pressure rises. This "adverse pressure gradient" produces a force in the opposite direction to overall flow. As the flow near the vessel wall has a lower velocity, and therefore lower inertia, it will reverse, while the higher-velocity flow in the center of the vessel is reduced but not reversed. A schematic diagram of this effect is shown in Fig. 5.18. The color image in Fig. 5.19 demonstrates the increase in velocity as the blood flows through a stenosis, with flow reversal occurring along the distal wall beyond the stenosis as the vessel lumen returns to its normal diameter.

Transition From Laminar to Turbulent Flow

Turbulent flow occurs when laminar flow breaks down and the particles in the fluid move randomly in all directions with variable speeds. A schematic diagram of laminar flow and turbulent flow is shown in Fig. 5.20. Turbulent flow is more likely to occur at high velocities

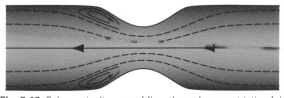

Fig. 5.18 Schematic diagram of flow through a constriction followed by a rapid expansion downstream, showing the regions of flow reversal. The velocity increases as the blood flows through a stenosis (from right to left) followed by an area of flow reversal beyond the narrowing. (After Caro et al. 1978, with permission.)

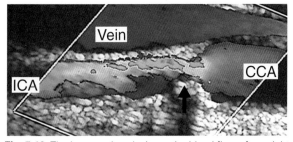

Fig. 5.19 The increase in velocity as the blood flows from right to left through a stenosis (*arrow*) produces the color change from red to turquoise (due to aliasing). Beyond the stenosis, flow reversal occurs along the posterior wall, represented by the deep blue, as the vessel lumen returns to its normal diameter. *ICA*, Internal carotid artery; *CCA*, common carotid artery.

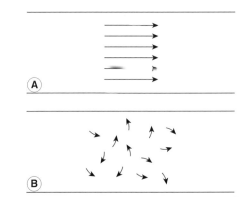

Fig. 5.20 Schematic diagram of (A) laminar flow and (B) turbulent flow.

TABLE 5.1 **Typical Values of the Reynolds Number in Various Arteries in the Body**	
Artery	**Reynolds Number**
Ascending aorta	1500
Abdominal aorta	640
Common carotid	217[a]
Superficial femoral	200
Posterior tibial	35[a]

[a]Estimated values.
With permission from Evans & McDicken, 1999.

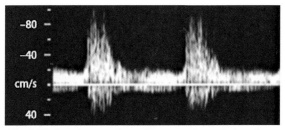

Fig. 5.21 Doppler waveform demonstrating turbulent flow.

(*V*), and the critical velocity at which flow becomes turbulent depends on the viscosity (μ) and the density (ρ) of the fluid and the diameter of the vessel (*d*). Reynolds described this relationship, which defines a value called the Reynolds number (*Re*):

$$R_e = \frac{dV\rho}{\mu} \qquad (5.9)$$

Once the Reynolds number has exceeded the critical value of approximately 2000, turbulent flow will occur. Table 5.1 gives typical values of the Reynolds number in various arteries in the body and shows that in normal vessels the velocity of blood is such that turbulent flow does not occur, with the exception of the proximal aortic flow during heavy exercise, for which cardiac output is increased. The presence of an increase in the blood velocity, due to arterial disease, can cause turbulent flow. Fig. 5.21 is a Doppler waveform demonstrating turbulent flow. In the presence of turbulence, not all the blood is traveling in the same direction, resulting in the angle of the beam to flow (angle of insonation) being smaller

for some parts of the blood flow. This results in turbulent spikes seen on the Doppler spectrum. It is possible for turbulent flow to occur only during the systolic phase of the cardiac cycle, when the systolic flow exceeds the critical velocity and the diastolic flow does not.

The presence of turbulent flow causes energy to be lost, leading to an increased pressure drop across the stenosis. It is thought that bruits in the tissue near a stenosis may be due to perivascular tissue vibration caused by turbulence, and this may also lead to post-stenotic dilatation of the vessel. Vortices or irregular movement of a large portion of the fluid are more correctly referred to as disturbed flow rather than turbulent flow.

VENOUS FLOW

The venous system acts as a low-resistance pathway for blood to be returned to the heart. Veins are collapsible, thin-walled vessels capable of distending to a larger cross-sectional area than their corresponding arteries, thus acting as a blood volume storage system that is important in the regulation of cardiac output. In addition, they also have a thermoregulation role in which blood is diverted to the superficial veins to reduce body temperature. The venous system can be divided into the central system (within the thorax and abdomen), the deep peripheral system, and the superficial peripheral veins.

An important structural feature of the vein is the presence of very thin, but strong, bicuspid valves that prevent retrograde flow away from the heart. The vena cava and common iliac veins are valveless. Valves are found in the external iliac, common femoral veins, internal jugular vein, and subclavian vein in a proportion of the population. Generally, the more distal the vein, the greater the number of valves.

Venous flow back to the heart is influenced by respiration, the cardiac cycle, and changes in posture.

Changes in Flow Due to the Cardiac Cycle

The central veins include the thoracic and abdominal veins, which drain to the right side of the heart via the inferior and superior venae cavae. The flow pattern and pressure in the central venous system are affected by changes in the volume of the right atrium that occur during the cardiac cycle. Reverse flow occurs in the thoracic veins when the right atrium contracts, as there is no valve in the vena cava. This flow reversal can also be seen in the proximal veins of the arm and neck (Fig. 5.22) due to their proximity to the chest. During ventricular contraction, the atrium expands, increasing venous flow into the right atrium, and then flow gradually falls during diastole, only increasing briefly as the tricuspid valve opens. Flow patterns in the lower-limb veins and peripheral arm veins are not significantly affected by the cardiac cycle due to vein compliance (which allows damping of the pressure changes), the

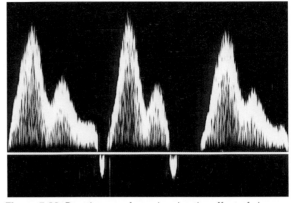

Figure 5.22 Doppler waveform showing the effect of changes in the pressure in the right atrium on blood flow in the jugular vein.

presence of valves, and changes in intra-abdominal pressure during respiration.

Effects of Respiration on Venous Flow

Respiration has an important effect on venous pressure and flow because of changes in the volume of the thorax brought about by movement of the diaphragm and ribs. Inspiration during calm breathing expands the thorax, leading to an increase in the volume of the veins in the chest, which in turn causes a reduction in the pressure in the intrathoracic veins. This creates a pressure gradient between the veins in the upper limb and head and those in the thorax, producing an increase in flow into the chest. Flow is decreased during expiration as the volume of the thorax decreases, leading to an increase in central pressure.

The reverse situation is seen in the abdomen as the diaphragm descends during inspiration, increasing intra-abdominal pressure. This leads to a decrease in the pressure gradient between the peripheral veins and the abdominal veins, thus reducing flow. During expiration the diaphragm rises, producing a reduction in intra-abdominal pressure, and the pressure gradient between the abdominal veins and peripheral veins increases, causing increased blood flow back to the heart. The effects of respiration are observed as phasic changes in flow in proximal deep peripheral veins (Fig. 5.23). Breathing maneuvers are often used to augment flow when investigating venous disorders (see Ch. 13).

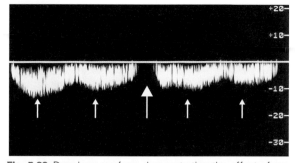

Fig. 5.23 Doppler waveform demonstrating the effect of respiration on the blood flow in the common femoral vein. The *large arrow* indicates the cessation of flow during inspiration and the *small arrows* show small changes in flow due to the cardiac cycle, which may not always be seen in the common femoral vein.

Changes in Venous Blood Pressure Due to Posture and the Calf Muscle Pump

Changes in posture alter hydrostatic pressure and can produce large pressure changes in the venous system (Fig. 5.1). If an individual is lying supine, for example, there is a relatively small pressure difference between the venous pressures at the ankle and right atrium. However, when an individual is standing, there is a column of blood between the right atrium and the veins at the ankle. If the hydrostatic pressure is assumed to be zero in the right atrium, the hydrostatic pressure at the ankle will be equal to the distance between the two, which is dependent on the person's height, but is usually between 80 and 100 mmHg. Therefore, in a standing position, there is a significant pressure gradient to overcome in order for blood to be returned to the heart; this is achieved by the calf muscle pump mechanism assisted by the presence of the venous valves.

The muscle compartments in the calf contain the deep veins and venous sinuses, which act as blood reservoirs. Regular small contractions occur in the deep muscles of the calf, causing compression of the veins, thereby propelling blood flow out of the leg, with the venous valves preventing the blood refluxing back down. This also generates a pressure gradient between the superficial and deep veins in the calf, and blood drains through the perforating veins and major junctions from the superficial to the deep venous system. The valves in the perforators prevent blood flowing from the deep to the superficial veins. During more active exercise, such as walking or running, the calf

muscle pump mechanism is able to produce a significant pressure reduction in the deep and superficial venous systems to approximately 30 mmHg. The pressure change that occurs during exercise is called the ambulatory venous pressure. At rest, because the hydrostatic pressure is the same on both the arterial and venous sides, the pressure drop across the capillary bed is the same whether the person is standing or lying down. However, after exercise the pressure on the venous side of the capillary bed will drop, but the pressure on the arterial side will remain the same, creating a pressure drop across the capillary bed and aiding the return of blood to the heart. Once the muscle contraction stops, the venous pressure in the lower leg will begin to rise due to filling of the venous system from the arterial system via the capillaries.

It is possible to measure the ambulatory venous pressure by inserting a small cannula into a dorsal foot vein, which is then connected to a pressure transducer and recorder. The pressure in the vein is first recorded with the patient standing. The patient is asked to perform 10 tiptoe maneuvers and then to stand still. The pressure recording demonstrates the pressure reduction during the exercise, and the venous refilling time can also be calculated. With normal veins, the refilling of the venous system occurs gradually by capillary inflow and takes 18 seconds or more to return to preexercise pressures (Fig. 5.24A). If there is significant failure of the venous valves in either the superficial or the deep venous system, reflux will occur, leading to a shorter refilling time and a higher postexercise pressure (Fig. 5.24B). Reflux in the deep or superficial venous systems, or in both, can lead to chronic venous hypertension in the lower leg and may result in the development of venous ulcers. Failure of the calf muscle pump due to poor flexion of the ankle and poor contraction of the calf muscle can lead to a reduction in the volume of blood ejected from the calf. This results in an inability to lower venous pressure adequately and can cause chronic venous hypertension. Patients at greatest risk due to poor calf muscle pump mechanism include those with limited ankle flexion due to chronic injury, osteoarthritis, or rheumatoid arthritis.

Abnormal Venous Flow

Venous disease can dramatically alter the flow patterns seen in the veins. Valve incompetence allows retrograde flow in the veins, which can easily be demonstrated

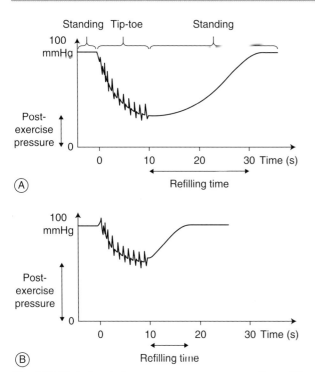

(A)

(B)

Fig. 5.24 Typical ambulatory venous pressure recordings. (A) Normal venous refilling. (B) Incompetent veins leading to a shorter refilling time.

with color flow imaging and spectral Doppler. Venous outflow obstruction results in the loss of the spontaneous phasic flow generated by respiration seen in normal veins. Congestive heart failure may lead to increased pulsatility of the flow in the femoral and iliac veins. Ultrasound now plays an important role in the diagnosis of venous disease, which is discussed further in Chapters 13 and 14.

Factors That Influence the Doppler Spectrum

INTRODUCTION

The shape of the Doppler spectrum can provide much useful information about the presence of disease and enables the sonographer to make measurements to quantify the degree of vessel narrowing. However, the shape of the spectrum will also depend on other factors, such as the velocity profile of the blood flow being interrogated and how evenly the ultrasound beam insonates the vessel. Factors that relate to the equipment rather than the blood flow can also affect the shape of the waveform. It is important to understand how these factors influence the waveform shape in order to be able to interpret the Doppler waveform. The sonographer

should also be aware of potential errors involved in any measurements made.

FACTORS THAT INFLUENCE THE DOPPLER SPECTRUM

Blood Flow Profile

The Doppler spectrum displays the frequency content of the signal along the vertical axis, which is converted to velocity using angle correction (see Figs. 3.14 and Fig 3.15). The relative brightness of the display relates to the proportion of back-scattered power at each velocity, and the time is displayed along the horizontal axis. The velocity profiles seen within arteries can be quite complex and

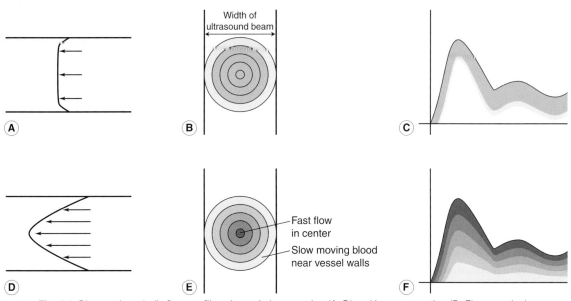

Fig. 6.1 Blunt and parabolic flow profiles shown in long section (A, D) and in cross-section (B, E) respectively. If a wide ultrasound beam is used to insonate the vessel, all the velocities present will be detected. Idealized Doppler spectra (C, F) show the difference in velocity/frequency distribution from these profiles.

will vary over time, as discussed in Chapter 5. The frequency content displayed in the Doppler spectrum will depend on the velocities of the cells present within the blood. If we assume that the vessel is uniformly insonated by the Doppler beam, all the different velocities of blood present within the vessel will be detected and displayed on the spectrum. If blood is traveling with a blunt flow profile, most of the blood cells will be moving with the same velocity, and the spectrum will show only a small range of frequencies (Fig. 6.1A–C). If, however, the blood is traveling with a parabolic flow profile, then the blood in the center of the vessel will be traveling faster than that near the vessel walls, and therefore the Doppler spectrum will display a wide range of frequencies (Fig. 6.1D–F).

The spread of frequencies present within the spectrum at a given point in time is known as the degree of spectral broadening. Fig. 6.1 shows the way in which the degree of spectral broadening depends on the velocity profile of the flow being interrogated, with greater spectral broadening seen in Fig. 6.1F than in Fig. 6.1C. The presence of turbulent flow (e.g., as a result of a stenosis) will increase spectral broadening, as the blood cells will be traveling with different velocities in random directions (see Fig. 5.21). Therefore, increased spectral broadening may indicate the presence of disease. However, the degree of spectral broadening can also

be influenced by Doppler instrumentation, and this is known as intrinsic spectral broadening (ISB, discussed later in this chapter).

Nonuniform Insonation of the Vessel

The examples of idealized spectra given in Fig. 6.1 assume that the beam evenly insonates the whole cross-section of the blood vessel in order to detect the correct proportions of all the blood velocities present. This is, however, an unrealistic situation, as the Doppler beam can be quite narrow, even in the elevation plane (of the order of 1–2 mm wide), and therefore may insonate only part of the artery or vein. If the beam passes through the center of the vessel (Fig. 6.2A), only part of the flow near the vessel walls (i.e., near the anterior and posterior walls) will be detected. The blood flow along the lateral walls will not be detected, as it is not insonated by the Doppler beam. Therefore, in the presence of parabolic flow, the low-velocity flow near the walls will only be partially detected, and the Doppler spectrum will no longer truly represent the low-velocity flow present within the vessel.

Sample Volume Size

The size and position of the sample volume, which can be controlled by the operator, will also affect the proportion of the vessel insonated. A small sample volume

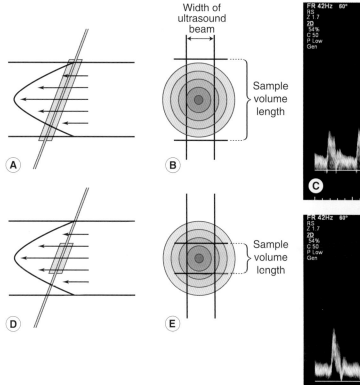

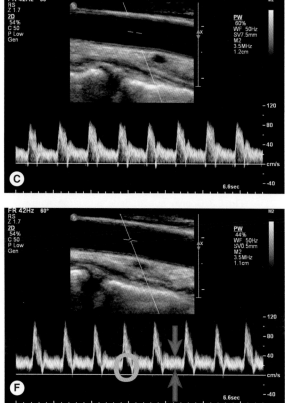

Fig. 6.2 Incomplete insonation of the vessel will occur when a narrow beam is used. The area within the vessel where flow is detected is shown when a large sample volume length (A and B) and a small sample volume length are used (D, E) along with typical Doppler spectra that may be obtained (C and F). Note the absence of low-velocity flow in (F) compared with (C) creating a window under the spectrum *(circle)*. The degree of spectral broadening is also reduced in (E) *(arrows)*.

placed in the center of a large vessel may not detect any of the flow near the vessel wall (Fig. 6.2D–F). However, a larger sample volume, which could cover the whole depth of the vessel (Fig. 6.2A–C), would detect the flow near the anterior and posterior walls but not the lateral walls. The size of the sample volume (i.e., the sensitive region of the beam) will therefore affect the range of Doppler frequencies detected and should be taken into account when interpreting the degree of spectral broadening. The Doppler spectrum obtained with the large sample volume in Fig. 6.2C displays low-velocity flow near the baseline, detected from near the vessel walls, and demonstrates spectral broadening. The spectrum obtained with a small sample volume, placed in the center of the vessel, shows none of the low flow but has a clear window beneath the detected velocities. A narrow Doppler beam with a small sample volume placed in

the center of the vessel may detect only the fast-moving blood and therefore, in normal circumstances, would not demonstrate much spectral broadening. However, in the presence of disease, increased spectral broadening may be seen due to the presence of turbulent flow.

Pulse Repetition Frequency, High-Pass Filter, and Gain

The high frequencies present in the Doppler signal will be incorrectly displayed on the Doppler spectrum if aliasing has occurred as a result of a low pulse repetition frequency (PRF) (see Fig. 3.12A). This results in misleading waveform shapes and errors in velocity measurement. The effect of aliasing is easily visualized, as the Doppler waveform appears to "wrap around" from the top of the spectrum to the bottom. Aliasing can be corrected by increasing the PRF.

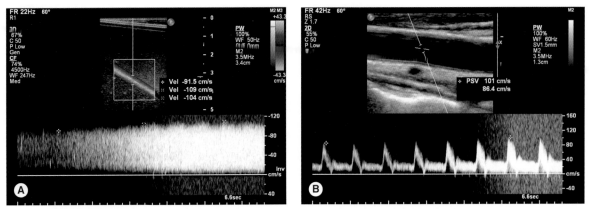

Fig. 6.3 Doppler spectrum detected from a flow phantom (A) with constant flow, and a normal carotid artery (B) obtained as the Doppler gain is increased from left to right. On the left, the gain is too low and the signal is barely detected. On the right, the gain is set too high, leading to saturation of the signal and increased spectral broadening that may lead to an overestimate of the peak velocity. The measured peak velocity can also be seen to change as the gain is increased (from 86 cm/s left side B to 101 cm/s right side B).

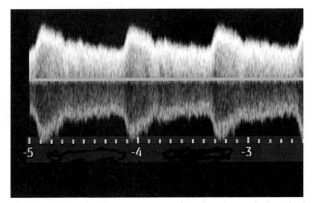

Fig. 6.4 Doppler spectrum demonstrating the appearance of a mirror image below the baseline, due to cross-talk between the forward and reverse channels, that may occur when the scanner's Doppler gain control is set too high.

The shape of the Doppler spectrum can also be altered if the high-pass filter is set too high, removing important information from the spectrum, such as the presence of low-velocity diastolic flow. The gain used to amplify the Doppler signal may also alter the appearance of the spectrum. If the gain is set too low, flow may not be detected. Increasing the gain can increase the appearance of spectral broadening, as shown in Fig. 6.3, and may also lead to errors in velocity measurements. An inappropriately high gain can also lead to overloading of the instrument, causing poor direction discrimination, and this may result in a mirror image of the spectrum appearing in the reverse direction on the display (see Fig. 6.4). The gain should be set so that the signal is detected, but saturation, i.e., complete whitening of the signal, as seen on the right-hand side of the signal in Fig. 6.3A and B, does not occur.

Intrinsic Spectral Broadening

ISB is broadening of the Doppler spectrum that is an artifact, related to the scanner rather than the blood flow interrogated. Linear and curvilinear array transducers use several elements to form the beam (see Ch. 2). Fig. 6.5 shows how the ultrasound beam from a linear array transducer can produce a range of angles of insonation, with the Doppler signals being detected at many angles. As the Doppler shift frequency detected is proportional to the cosine of the angle of insonation, θ,

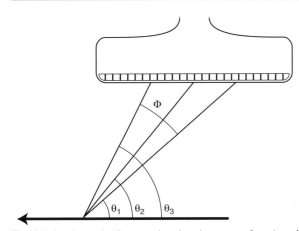

Fig. 6.5 A schematic diagram showing the range of angles of insonation produced by a linear array transducer when making blood velocity measurements. θ_1 and θ_3 represent the smallest and largest angles of insonation generated by the array, respectively, and θ_2 represents the angle produced by the midpoint of the active elements. Φ is the angle produced by the aperture of the active elements generating the Doppler beam. The *arrow* represents the direction of the blood flow. (Reprinted from Thrush & Evans, 1995, with permission from Elsevier.)

this will lead to a range of frequencies being detected even in the presence of a single target. A test object constructed of a string driven at a constant speed by a motor can be used to investigate this effect (Fig. 6.6A). The spectrum obtained from the moving string shows that a large range of Doppler shift frequencies have been detected despite the fact that the target is a single object moving at a constant velocity (Fig. 6.6B). This is due to the range of angles of insonation produced from different elements within the active portion of the probe and is the effect known as ISB. The degree of ISB depends on the range of angles over which back-scattered ultrasound is received by the transducer (Φ in Fig. 6.5)—i.e., it depends on the aperture of the transducer—and on the angle of insonation of the beam (θ). As the impact of spectral broadening is dependent on the cosineθ, the smaller the angle of insonation used to detect the blood flow, the smaller is the degree of ISB.

VELOCITY MEASUREMENTS

Converting Doppler Shift Frequencies to Velocity Measurements

The combination of imaging and spectral Doppler ultrasound allows an estimate of the angle of insonation (θ)

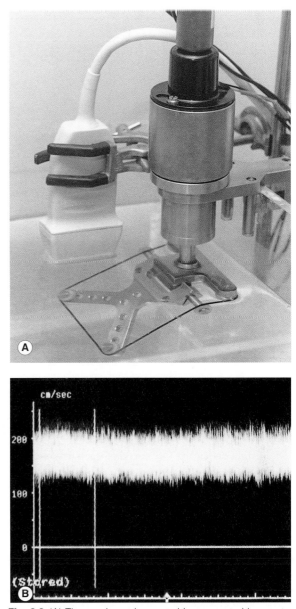

Fig. 6.6 (A) The moving-string test object mounted in a water tank at 45° to the ultrasound transducer. (B) A typical spectrum obtained from the moving string, showing the spread of frequencies detected. (Reprinted from Thrush & Evans, 1995, with permission from Elsevier.)

between the Doppler ultrasound beam and the blood flow. The angle of insonation is measured by lining up the angle correction cursor with the estimated direction of flow.

The Doppler equation (Eq. 3.1) can be used to estimate the velocity of the blood (V) from the measured

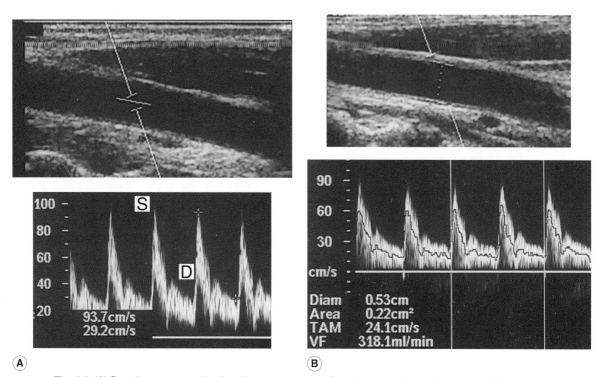

Fig. 6.7 (A) Doppler spectrum showing the measurement of maximum peak systolic velocity, *S*, and maximum end-diastolic velocity, *D*. (B) The mean velocity can be calculated from the Doppler spectrum, displayed by the *black line*. A large sample volume will allow the blood velocity at the anterior and posterior walls, as well as in the center of the vessel, to be estimated but may not detect the flow along the lateral wall. The time-averaged mean velocity (TAM), which is equivalent to time-averaged velocity (TAV), can be found by averaging the mean velocity over one or more complete cardiac cycles. Volume flow can be calculated by multiplying the TAM measurement by the cross-sectional area of the vessel (displayed *bottom left*).

Doppler shift frequency (f_d), as the transmitted frequency of the Doppler beam (f_t) is known and the speed of sound in tissue (c) is assumed to be constant (1540 m/s). As the velocity of the blood usually varies across the vessel, a range of velocities will be recorded at any given point in time. The velocity of blood also varies with time, due to the pumping action of the heart. This means that the velocity of the blood is not actually a single value. A choice has to be made as to which value to use to represent the velocity of the blood. The value most commonly used in vascular ultrasound is maximum peak systolic velocity (PSV). This is the maximum velocity recorded within the spectrum at the point in time that represents peak systolic flow, as shown on the sonogram in Fig. 6.7A. This velocity represents the fastest-moving blood in the vessel. The maximum velocity in the spectrum can similarly be measured at end diastole. These measurements do not take into account the slower-moving blood near the vessel walls.

An alternative is to measure mean velocity at any point in time. This can be calculated by the scanner by finding the average of all the velocities recorded at an instant in time, as shown as a black line superimposed on the Doppler spectrum in Fig. 6.7B. As with maximum velocity, the mean velocity will change during the cardiac cycle. If the mean velocity for each line of the sonogram is averaged over a complete cardiac cycle, this will give the value known as the time-averaged velocity (TAV). This can be used to estimate volume flow (discussed later in this chapter).

Many diagnostic criteria are based on velocity ratios rather than on absolute velocity measurements. For example, stenoses may be categorized by the velocity ratio of the maximum PSV within the stenosis, V_{sten},

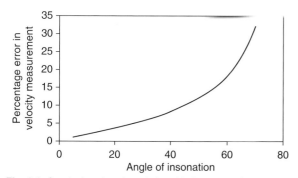

Fig. 6.8 Graph showing the relationship between the percentage error in the velocity measurements as the angle of insonation increases, for a 5° error in the placement of the angle correction cursor. (After Evans & McDicken, 2000. © John Wiley & Sons Limited, with permission.)

divided by the maximum PSV in the normal proximal vessel, V_{prox}:

$$\text{Velocity ratio} = \frac{V_{sten}}{V_{prox}} \quad \textbf{(6.1)}$$

Errors in Maximum-Velocity Measurements Relating to the Angle of Insonation

An estimate of the angle of insonation is required to convert the detected Doppler shift frequency into a velocity measurement. Any inaccuracy in placing the angle correction cursor parallel to the direction of flow will lead to an error in the estimated angle of insonation. This in turn will lead to an error in the velocity measurement. The velocity calculation depends on the $\cos\theta$ term, so the error created will be greater for larger angles of insonation. Fig. 6.8 shows the relationship between the percentage error in the velocity measurement as the angle of insonation increases where there is a 5° error in the placement of the angle correction cursor. For example, Fig. 6.8 shows that this 5° error in cursor placement causes an error in velocity measurement of 23% when the angle of insonation is 65°. In order to minimize this error, angles of insonation of greater than 60° should not be used. However, estimating the angle of insonation is not always straightforward, especially in the presence of disease. Some of the limitations are listed later.

Errors Relating to the Direction of Flow Relative to the Vessel Walls

The direction of the blood flow may not be parallel to the vessel wall, especially in the presence of a stenosis, vortices, or helical flow. Therefore, in these cases, aligning the angle correction cursor parallel to the walls may lead to large errors. If there is a clear image of the flow channel through a narrowing, for example, displayed on a color flow image, it may be possible to line up the angle cursor with the flow channel. However, the maximum velocity may be just beyond the stenosis, and the direction of flow may be less obvious at that point. The color image may be used to identify the site of maximum velocity, although this can be misleading, as the color image displays mean velocity of the blood in relation to the direction of the beam, and thus is dependent on the angle of insonation. What appears to be the maximum velocity on the image may instead be the site at which the angle between the Doppler beam and the direction of the blood flow is the smallest. It is important to consider this when estimating the site of maximum velocity and the direction of flow from the color image. The blood velocity may need to be measured at a few points through and beyond a stenosis to ensure the highest velocity has been obtained.

Errors Relating to the Out-of-Imaging Plane Angle of Insonation

It is important to remember that the interception of the ultrasound beam with the blood flow occurs in a three-dimensional space and not just in the two-dimensional plane shown on the image. An underestimate of the true velocity will be obtained if the out-of-imaging plane angle of insonation is not close to 0°. The transducer should be aligned with a reasonable length of the vessel, as seen on the image, to ensure a minimal error.

Creation of a Range of Insonation Angles by the Doppler Ultrasound Beam Aperture

The large aperture used by linear and curvilinear array transducers not only results in ISB but also leads to another problem. For velocity to be calculated from the Doppler shift frequency, the $\cos\theta$ term is required, but clearly only a single value for the angle can be used. Substituting the two extreme angles shown in Fig. 6.5 (θ_1 and θ_3) into the Doppler equation would give different values for the velocity. A decision has to be made as to which angle is most suitable for use in converting the detected Doppler frequency into velocity. Typically, ultrasound scanners use the angle between the center of the active elements and the direction of flow (i.e., angle θ_2).

This would be an appropriate angle to select for estimation of the mean velocity, but it leads to an overestimation of the calculated maximum velocity. In fact, in order to obtain a correct value for the peak velocity from the frequency spectrum, the smallest angle of insonation present (i.e., θ_1) should be used; however, this is not under the sonographer's control.

The larger the angle of insonation, the greater the potential source of error in velocity measurement, due to ISB. It is therefore important not to use a Doppler angle greater than 60°, with smaller angles of insonation giving smaller errors. The error produced due to spectral broadening can vary with changes in the active aperture, for example, when changing the position of the Doppler beam in relation to the transducer face, i.e., center, left, or right. It is worth avoiding making velocity measurements from a beam originating near the end of the transducer to reduce these errors, since fewer elements are used to form the beam at these locations. Fig. 6.9 shows the same blood flow velocity measured with (A) a beam originating from the far edge of the transducer and (B) a beam from a central location. Fig. 6.9A gives a significantly lower velocity measurement than Fig. 6.9B. The spectrum is also noisier in Fig. 6.9A compared to Fig. 6.9B).

Diagnosis of vascular disease often depends on velocity ratio measurements, and these are not affected by the errors produced by ISB as long as both measurements used to calculate the ratio are made with a similar angle of insonation.

Optimizing the Angle of Insonation

Ideally, the angle of insonation for estimating velocity measurement should be near zero to minimize errors; however, as peripheral vessels often lie parallel to the skin, this is not possible. No single choice of angle of insonation is completely reliable, especially when comparisons between velocity measurements are being made; however, the smaller the angle of the beam to flow, the smaller the possible error. Possible protocols used are discussed later.

Velocity Ratio Measurements

Ideally the angle of insonation used to make the velocity measurements proximal to and at the stenosis should be similar. This will result in the two velocities having similar systematic errors that will cancel out when calculating the ratio. However, the smaller the angles of insonation used for both measurements, the smaller the errors will be.

Absolute Velocity Measurements

Absolute velocity measurements are used to quantify disease in many situations, for example, peripheral arteries and carotid arteries. There are two schools of thought about selecting the angle of insonation when making absolute velocity measurements:

1. Always set the angle of insonation to 60°. This ensures that any error in alignment of the angle correction cursor only leads to a moderate error in the velocity estimate (Fig. 6.8) and that the errors caused by ISB

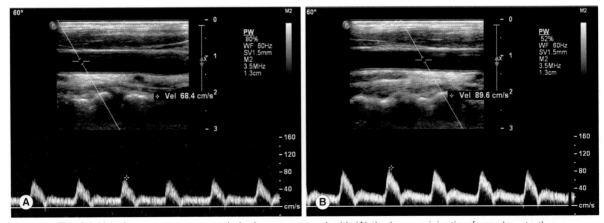

Fig. 6.9 Velocity measurements made in the same vessel with (A) the beam originating from close to the edge of the transducer and (B) from the center of the transducer with (A) giving a lower value of 68.4 cm/s compared to (B) 89.6cm/s. (Reprinted from Hoskins et al., with permission)

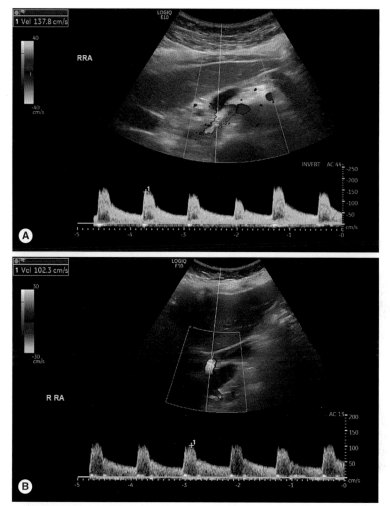

Fig. 6.11 Right renal artery (RRA) velocity in the same patient measured with an anterior approach (A) and flank approach (B). In the anterior approach the angle correction is 44°. Measured PSV is 138 cm/s. In the flank approach the angle correction is 13° and the measured velocity is 102 cm/s. Velocity measurements made from an anterior approach are often higher than from the flank, possibly due to intrinsic spectral broadening and from angle changes as the proximal renal artery curves in the image. From the flank, curvature has less impact because of the comparatively little change in the cosine of angles between 0° and 30°. *PSV*, Peak systolic velocity.

where vessels are usually stiffer. This cyclical variation in diameter will lead to errors in volume flow estimation, but it may be reduced by taking several diameter measurements and finding a mean value.

Noncircularity of the Vessel Lumen

The calculation of cross-sectional area from the diameter measurement assumes that the vessel lumen is circular, which may not be the case, especially in the presence of disease.

Errors in Measuring TAV

Incomplete insonation of the vessel will lead to an underestimation of the proportion of slower-moving blood at the vessel wall, which in turn will lead to errors in the mean velocity measurements. For example, if a Doppler recording is obtained from a vessel with parabolic flow using a narrow beam (as shown in Fig. 6.2A and B), the high-velocity flow in the center of the vessel will be adequately sampled, but a large proportion of the slower-moving blood at the vessel wall will not be detected. When the mean velocity is calculated from the spectra, this will be an overestimate of the true mean velocity due to the undersampling of the flow at the lateral edges of the vessel. This is true even if the sample volume is set to cover the near and far walls of the vessel as the out-of-imaging plane flow will not be sampled. Incomplete insonation of the vessel can lead to errors of up to 30% in the TAV (Evans & McDicken 2000).

If the wall thump filter is set too high, the low-frequency signals from the slower-moving flow will be removed, and this would lead to an overestimate in the mean velocity. Aliasing would lead to underestimation of the mean velocity due to the incorrect estimation of the high frequencies present within the signal. The presence of high-amplitude noise will bias the estimate of the mean velocity, as the Doppler system is unable to differentiate between the noise and the Doppler signals.

WAVEFORM ANALYSIS

As well as the blood velocity and flow changing with the presence of significant disease, the shape of the waveform will also be altered (as discussed in Ch. 5). The waveform may indicate whether the disease is proximal or distal to the site at which the Doppler signal is obtained. Over the years, several researchers have attempted to quantify these changes in waveform shape by defining various indices, and many modern scanners incorporate facilities to calculate such quantities, some of which are listed below.

Pulsatility Index

The pulsatility index (PI) can be used to quantify the degree of pulse wave damping at different measurement sites. It is defined as the maximum height of the waveform, S, minus the minimum diastolic, D (which may be negative), divided by the mean height, M, as shown in Fig. 6.12:

$$PI = \frac{S-D}{M} \quad \textbf{(6.4)}$$

Damped flow beyond significant disease will have a lower PI value than a normal pulsatile waveform.

Pourcelot's Resistive Index

The resistive index (RI) is defined as follows (Fig. 6.12A):

$$RI = \frac{S-E}{S} \quad \textbf{(6.5)}$$

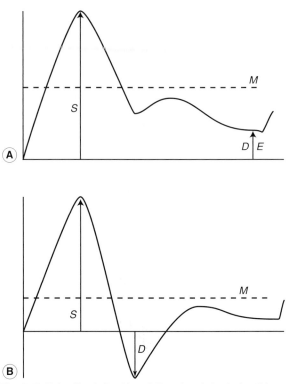

Fig. 6.12 Pulsatility index (A and B) and resistive index (A) can be calculated from the peak systolic *(S)*, minimum diastolic *(D)*, end-diastolic *(E)*, and mean velocity (or frequency) *(M)* shown here on two different waveforms.

where E is end-diastolic velocity. The value of RI can be calculated by the scanner and displayed on the screen. An example of the role of RI, in renal ultrasound, is shown in Chapter 12.

Systolic Rise Time/Acceleration Time

Systolic rise time, also known as acceleration time, is the time between the start of systole and peak systole.

Spectral Broadening

There have been several definitions of spectral broadening (SB) described over the years in an attempt to quantify the spread of frequencies present within a spectrum. One such definition is as follows:

$$SB = \frac{f_{max}-f_{min}}{f_{max}} \quad \textbf{(6.6)}$$

Increased spectral broadening indicates the presence of arterial disease but can, to some extent, also be introduced by the scanner itself, as in ISB (described earlier).

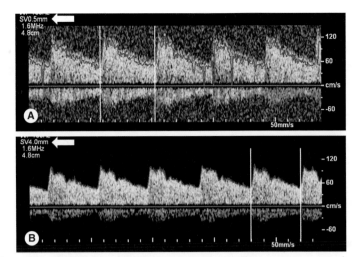

Fig. 6.13 Problems of automatic tracing of the sonogram part I. The sonograms are of a middle cerebral artery in transcranial Doppler ultrasound (TCD). (A) With a small sample volume, 0.5 mm *(arrow)*, there is noise in the sonogram and the maximum velocity trace *(blue line)* doesn't follow the maximum velocity reliably. (B) By increasing the sample volume size to 4 mm *(arrow)*, the spectral display is clearer and the automatic trace records a consistent flow waveform.

Spectral broadening may be visually inspected on a sonogram as show in Fig. 6.2F (arrows).

Measurements of Flow Waveform Velocities and Indices

Most scanners allow automated tracing of the Doppler spectral display. The accuracy of the trace depends on the consistency of the sonogram—whether the sample volume remains within the vessel—and the clarity of the sonogram. If the sonogram is weak or noisy, then the trace may be inconsistent and the indices measured inaccurate (Fig. 6.13). In very weak sonograms automated tracing may be impossible. Measurements made are also affected by settings, for example, the threshold or sensitivity (Fig. 6.14) that dictates what strength of the sonogram frequencies is included in the trace of maximum velocities. For measurements of mean velocity, for measuring volume flow, the presence of vessels with flow in the opposite direction can also lead to errors. Measurements of indices can be checked by manual tracing of the spectral display outline, but this is not possible for mean velocity.

Pulse Wave Velocity

The pressure pulse travels along the vessel at a different speed from the flowing blood; this is known as the pulse wave velocity (PWV). The speed at which the pulse is transmitted along the vessel depends on the elasticity of the vessel wall. For example, the pulse will travel much faster down the stiff-walled artery of a diabetic patient than down the normal artery of a younger person. PWV can be measured using two Doppler transducers to detect the transit time of the pulse along a known length of vessel. The transit time is given by the delay in the beginning of the pulse detected distally compared with that detected by the proximally positioned transducer (Fig. 6.15). PWV is given by the distance along the vessel between the two transducers divided by the transit time. Measurement of PWV has been used by researchers to study vessel wall elasticity changes (e.g., with age or diabetes).

Subjective Interpretation

Subjective interpretation of the Doppler spectrum can give many clues as to the level and extent of any disease. For example, changes in the pulsatility of the waveform shape can help to identify disease. The systolic rise time of the waveform is influenced by changes in the cardiac impulse and circulation proximal to the measurement site, whereas the decay of the velocity tends to relate to the distal circulation. Even if these various indices are not quantified, understanding the concept behind them can help when interpreting waveform shapes.

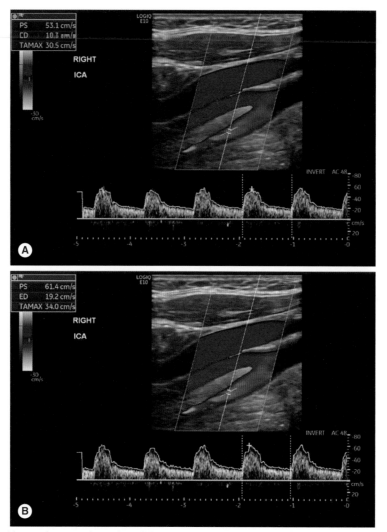

Fig. 6.14 Problems of automatic tracing of the sonogram part II. Automatic velocity measurements made in an internal carotid artery *(ICA)*. The spectral display is identical but threshold/sensitivity of the sonogram maximum velocity trace is set at different values. In image (B) it traces out weaker Doppler signals than in (A). The velocity measurements measured in image (B), PSV = 61 cm/s, are higher than in (A), PSV = 53 cm/s. *PSV*, Peak systolic velocity.

SPECTRAL DOPPLER ARTIFACTS

Like B-mode and CFI, spectral Doppler waveforms can suffer from artifacts whereby a signal may not be able to be detected due to bone or calcified plaque preventing penetration of the beam. It is also possible for a Doppler signal to arise from a location where a vessel is not present, when the pulse does not travel in a straight line, for example, due to a strongly reflective boundary that is not perpendicular to the beam. In Fig. 4.23 it would be possible to detect a spectral Doppler signal from within an artifactual vessel seen on the CFI, as the spectral Doppler pulse will follow the same path as the CFI pulse.

Aliasing (see Fig. 3.12) can be considered as an artifact, as high velocities are displayed incorrectly, preventing direct PSV measurements. Crosstalk on a spectral Doppler display (Fig. 6.4) can give a misleading mirror appearance of the waveform above and below the baseline and this can usually be overcome by reducing the gain. Spectral Doppler can detect movement that has

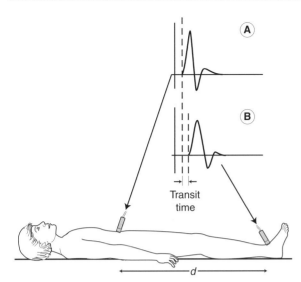

Fig. 6.15 The pulse wave velocity can be calculated using two transducers at a distance *d* apart along the vessel and measuring the transit time of the pulse. Although Doppler is used to measure the start of systole, the measurement made between two sites is the velocity of the pressure wave, not of flow itself.

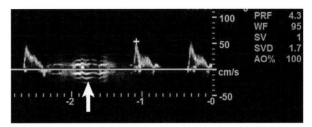

Fig. 6.16 Shows a movement artifact *(arrow)* detected during scanning a carotid artery when the patient was talking.

not arisen from the blood flow. Fig. 6.16 shows a movement artifact detected during scanning a carotid artery when the patient was talking. An understanding of the causes of artifacts will help the sonographer to recognize them when interpreting waveforms.

7

Approach to Scanning, Operational Policies, and Safety

INTRODUCTION

The preceding chapters have covered the basic scientific principles behind medical ultrasound, the Doppler effect, hemodynamics, and how ultrasound is used to form B-mode and color flow images. A sound understanding of these principals and how the scanner controls are adjusted to optimize the image are essential. However, it is also equally important that the sonographer understands their responsibilities within the operation and delivery of a service, regardless of the size or setting. This comes under the heading of clinical governance where organizations and the individuals within it are accountable for the quality and safety of their services by creating an environment that will provide the best outcome for patients. There are several key principles including education and training, risk management, safety including infection control and prevention, clinical audit, and the safe and effective use of information technology including data protection. The aim of this chapter is to introduce the sonographer to both the practical aspects of beginning a scan and some of the principles related to safe practice and clinical governance.

THE PATIENT

The well-being and interests of a patient are integral to every examination undertaken. It is an ironic fact that sonographer can be highly skilled in the use a state-of-the-art duplex scanner but fail to make an accurate diagnosis due to an inadequate approach to the examination and the patient. This may be primarily the fault of the sonographer or due to systemic failures such as poor departmental organization, inadequate training, or operating protocols.

When a patient enters the examination room, an introduction and explanation of the test will put them at ease, especially if they are nervous or in some discomfort. Local protocols that are rigid and do not allow any flexibility can lead to problems. For example, a protocol requiring patients to be completely flat with the head fully extended during carotid scans may lead to severe discomfort for patients with breathing difficulties, dizziness, angina, or spondylosis of the neck. It is possible they will not be able to tolerate the examination at all. An alternative would be to perform the scan with the patient sitting up on a low chair. It is still possible to obtain good images from this scanning position. Most problems can be solved with a little careful thought and the occasional inventive approach.

Patient Checklist

When first meeting a patient, it is good practice to make a simple introduction such as "my name is." It is then essential to check the patient's identity using unique identifiers such as date of birth and address to ensure that you will be examining the correct patient. Relying on the patient's name alone for identity is inadequate, as there could be two patients with the same name in the waiting area or a patient may have misheard another patient's name being called. The following steps are recommended as a useful checklist before, during, and at the end of the examination:

- Check available notes, referral documentation, and other relevant imaging studies
- Confirm the patient is expecting an examination and who has referred them for the test
- Discuss clinical history and context with the patient as appropriate
- Ensure the examination is appropriate and justified
- Provide an explanation of the test and an approximation of how long it will take
- Give the patient an opportunity to ask questions
- Confirm the patient consents for the test
- Consider chaperone requirements before beginning the test
- Ensure the patient is positioned comfortably on the examination table before starting the examination
- Monitor the patient during the test to ensure they are comfortable
- Provide tissue or cleaning wipes at the end of test to remove any residual ultrasound gel
- It is good practice to let the patient re-dress before explaining the outcome, and what happens next
- Dependent on local guidelines, inform the patient of the results or who will be doing this and in what time frame. Alternatively explain how they can obtain the results
- Answer any questions as appropriate within local guidelines
- Some patients may have additional needs that may be required to be taken into account, such as dementia, learning needs, or autism. This may affect the means by which you communicate with the patient and the support arrangements that may be required. For example, it may be beneficial to allow partners

and carers to sit with the patient during the examination. Most centers will have guidance on best practice relating to this issue.

STARTING THE SCAN

ADVICE

In most circumstances, start the scan with a cross-sectional survey of the region of interest before a longitudinal scan, as this helps to relate structures to each other and makes the anatomy easier to identify. For instance, the position of carotid bifurcation is easier to locate in cross-section by sweeping the transducer up the neck.

IMAGE ORIENTATION

Cross-Section
The general convention is to orient the image as if you are looking at the patient. For instance, the right saphenofemoral junction will appear on the right-hand side of the screen and the left saphenofemoral junction on the left side of the screen.

Longitudinal or Sagittal
The general convention is to have the direction of the patient's head on the left side of the screen and the foot direction toward the right side of the screen.

The scan should be carried out in a dimly lit room to optimize visualization of the screen and image. The transducer selected should usually be of the highest frequency that allows adequate penetration to the area to be examined. Ultrasound systems have exam-specific presets that broadly optimize the scanner settings for a specific application, for instance carotid imaging. Manufacturers' presets can be modified and stored to suit individuals' preferences. For new scanners it is essential to work with an applications specialist to optimize settings and understand the function of all the controls and options. Annotation lists can also be modified to suit department protocols and to aid work-flow.

It is important to adopt a logical approach when scanning. Using a systematic technique cuts down on examination time and ensures that pathology is less likely to be missed. Many departments have scanning protocols that include specific images that should be captured and stored during the examination. The scan is best started by examining the region of interest with B-mode imaging alone, to identify relevant structures. Avoid switching on the color flow or spectral Doppler straight away, unless they are essential for identifying vessels, as the imaging frame rate will be reduced, B-mode quality may be impaired, and the display may be confusing if anatomy has not been clearly identified. In a situation when you have made multiple adjustments to the controls but the image is not optimized or you are not sure, or forgotten which controls you have adjusted, it is often best to re-select the initial preset and then try to optimize the image from there.

SCANNER CONTROLS

The role of scanner controls has been described in Chapters 2 to 6. A summary list of the controls for B-mode, color flow, and spectral Doppler is provided in Appendix C. Many of these will be set for particular applications in the presets; sonographers may rarely alter dynamic range or color map during their scanning, although it is sometimes useful to be aware of what affects changes might make. However, there are a few controls that are used frequently during a scan, and these are reviewed here as a reminder of how to use ultrasound effectively.

B-Mode Controls

Optimize the overall image **gain** and, where required, the **time gain compensation** sliders, so that the returning echoes are of relatively uniform intensity throughout the image. In general, the gain should be set so that the lumen of any large nondiseased vessel appears clear or black but any further increase in gain would introduce noise or speckle. Adjust the **depth** so that the area of interest can be clearly defined without several centimeters of depth displayed below this point unless it is clinically necessary (Fig. 7.1). If the region of interest in the B-mode image is small, or very deep, consider using the **zoom** or **sector width** control to magnify the area. This will improve the frame rate and allow closer inspection of the anatomy. If the scanner has **transmit focus**, set the focal zones at the depth of interest on the scan image. B-mode frame rates of modern scanners are generally high even when multiple focus zones have been selected. Many vascular sonographers prefer B-mode images with high contrast using a lower dynamic range.

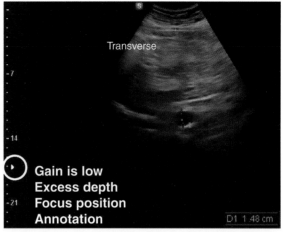

Fig. 7.1 Transverse B-mode image of the abdominal aorta. This image has several learning points. The overall B-mode gain could be increased. There is excess depth in the image, and this could be decreased to provide better resolution of the aorta. The focus position is set too low and should be positioned at the level of the aorta. The annotation tells us this is a transverse image but does not specify that is it is demonstrating the aorta. A body marker could also be useful.

Although presets are optimized for specific applications, variation in anatomy and ultrasound characteristic of the target leads to differences in image quality. It is worthwhile experimenting with different pre- and post-processing controls in order to understand the function of these controls and their effect on image appearance. Try this when imaging a carotid plaque and note the difference in the appearance of the image (Fig. 7.2).

Color Doppler Controls

Color flow imaging has been discussed in detail in Chapters 4 and 5. The main controls adjusted during most examinations are **color scale (or pulse repetition frequency), color box steering angle in linear arrays, color box size, transmit frequency, and color invert.** Appendix C summarizes these functions.

When using linear array transducers, it is possible to **steer** the color box to the left or right by 20° to 30° depending on the system. It is therefore possible to optimize the color box angle to the flow direction in order to demonstrate the flow (Fig. 7.3). This is frequently used in longitudinal scans. It is usually not used on transverse scans of arteries, and veins angulation is achieved by tilting the transducer (see Fig. 4.7). Inexperienced sonographers often find optimizing the color box steer

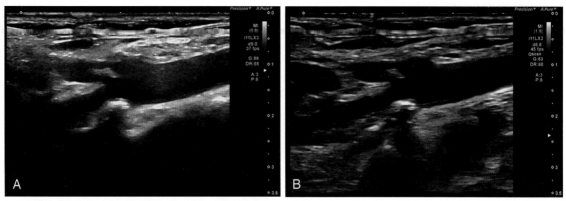

Fig. 7.2 Internal carotid artery plaque imaged with default carotid (A) and arterial (B) preset settings. The plaque is seen more clearly in image (B). Contrast and penetration are improved with a lower frequency and deeper focal setting. Presets can be altered and also saved to suit sonographer's preference, but they should have the confidence to adjust controls to improve image quality, as in this example. (Image courtesy of Ben Freedman.)

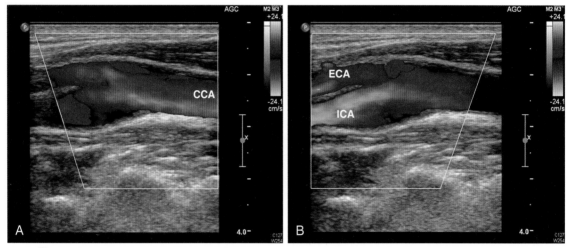

Fig. 7.3 Beam steering to optimize color flow imaging. In image (A), the color box is steered to the right. This gives a good angle between the beams and flow in the common carotid artery *(CCA)* as the artery becomes more superficial from right to left in the image. To image the external *(ECA)* and internal *(ICA)* carotid artery as shown in (B), the beam is steered in the other direction as the arteries now become deeper from right to left. Note that the color scale has inverted so that flow toward the beam in the CCA shown in (A) is displayed as red but in image (B), the color scale is switched to display flow away from the beam as red in the ICA and ECA. This normally happens automatically as the beam steering transitions between right and left.

challenging when learning color Doppler techniques. It is not always necessary to steer the color box from the square/rectangular position when a vessel courses at an angle through a square box, i.e., the vessel is not parallel to the transducer face. Increased steering angles lead to a longer path from transducer to target, and the beams may suffer from more distortion from refraction at more oblique angles (Fig. 7.4).

For curvilinear array transducers, it is necessary to optimize the angle of insonation. This can often be achieved by some rolling of the transducer and positioning of the color box to the edge of the image sector (see Fig. 9.8).

For trainee sonographers, a difficult aspect to master is determining the direction of blood flow from the appearance of the color flow image. Remember, the color

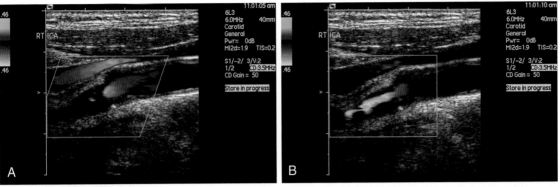

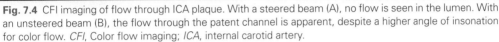

Fig. 7.4 CFI imaging of flow through ICA plaque. With a steered beam (A), no flow is seen in the lumen. With an unsteered beam (B), the flow through the patent channel is apparent, despite a higher angle of insonation for color flow. *CFI,* Color flow imaging; *ICA,* internal carotid artery.

displayed in the upper half of the color bar represents flow toward the transducer with respect to the beam, and color displayed in the lower half is flow away from the transducer with respect to the beam. The color assignment can be **inverted/reversed** to suit the application and the sonographer, but they should have confidence in the direction of flow by reconciling the direction of the vessel and the color within it with the color bar indication.

The **scale** or **PRF** is often altered during an examination. This is displayed as the maximum mean flow velocity (that can be displayed without aliasing) in centimeters per second in the direction of the beam on the top and bottom of the color bar, although some systems also show the PRF in hertz at the side of the screen.

For most arterial applications the aim is to show the peak systolic phase of the cardiac cycle toward the top of the color range so that an increase in velocity, particularly in a stenosis, is displayed as aliasing. A typical scale will be 25 to 30 cm/s for many arterial investigations, but for high velocity flows this may result in aliasing in undiseased arteries. The influence of change in flow direction in the image also leads to change in color hue and even aliasing in undiseased arteries (see Fig. 4.11), and the sonographer may increase the scale to avoid overinterpretation of stenoses. By optimizing the PRF or scale for the flow velocities present in a vessel, it is possible to investigate longer segments of an artery using color flow imaging, reducing the amount of time spent taking spectral Doppler measurements. In situations in which there is significant pathology, the flow velocities may be much lower than normal distal to a stenosis or occlusion, the PRF or scale should be lowered to demonstrate the low-velocity flow.

For venous flows, the color scale is set to optimize sensitivity to low flows and velocities; here sensitivity to flow is usually more important than local velocity changes within the venous lumen.

Color sensitivity is also affected by **transmit frequency** (see Fig. 4.18) and the **area of color investigation (color box)** (see Fig. 4.17). As well as increasing frame rate, reducing the size of the color box often leads to better line density and ensemble lengths, the number of pulses sent down each line, which will lead to improved spatial resolution and sensitivity. Sonographer modification to these individual parameters is possible in some systems, as are other minor controls, such as persistence and write priority, which can alter sensitivity to low-velocity flow.

Spectral Doppler Controls

The major controls altered during the examination are **steering, gain, scale, invert, sample volume size, and beam/flow angle correction**.

Beam steering in linear array follows similar rules for color flow imaging, although the spectral Doppler beam should be able to be steered independently.

The spectral Doppler **scale** should be set to avoid aliasing and show the flow waveform to best advantage in the spectral display. It is possible to make measurements with a flow waveform displayed below the baseline, but most of us prefer to use the **invert** control. The high-pass filter should be set to remove wall thump but not useful Doppler signals (this is normally optimized for a specific preset). The selection of the size of the **sample volume** is an important consideration. If detailed investigation of flow within a stenosis is to be performed, a small sample volume may be required, although using a slightly larger sample volume can lead to a clearer Doppler sonogram in some systems (see Fig. 6.13). The sample volume should be placed in the center of the vessel or at the point of maximum velocity indicated by the color image. However, if the presence of flow within a vein is to be detected, a large sample volume may be more appropriate. The issue of spectral Doppler angle correction remains a contentious subject, and this is reviewed in Chapter 6. The position of the **angle correction** cursor should be carefully lined up with the vessel wall or the direction of blood flow, as indicated on color flow imaging, to minimize angle-related errors. There are four possible reasons why a Doppler signal may be displayed both above and below the baseline, and the sonographer should be able to identify these:

1. Aliasing (see Fig. 3.12)
2. Mirroring due to the gain being set too high (see Fig. 6.4)
3. Flow reversal during the cardiac cycle (see Fig. 5.5)
4. The sample volume is wide and covers an artery and adjacent vein (see Fig. 3.5).

Many systems will automatically calculate and display the maximum velocity of the waveform in real time and when the image is frozen. Use caution when quoting these measurements, as sometime the scanner will make an error and measure noise or simply fail to measure maximum or minimum systolic velocity (see Ch. 6). In this case, a manual measurement should always be made.

B-mode, color flow, and spectral Doppler can all be used simultaneously on most scanners; the control is usually referred to as **triplex** or **simultaneous imaging**. If all three modes are used concurrently, the performance of each is limited by the time needed for the different pulses. Image quality is generally better if B-mode and color flow are used to guide placement of the spectral Doppler cursor and the update key is then used to switch between the imaging and spectral Doppler modes.

IMAGE CAPTURE, STORAGE, AND REPORTING

Acquisition and storage of images and reporting will vary depending on national protocols or local guidelines, and the information technology infrastructure available within departments. In general, most protocols require sonographers to save appropriate annotated images that are a representation of the ultrasound examination including abnormal pathology. This has a number of advantages:

- It demonstrates that protocols for the examination were followed
- The images provide evidence that the examination was carried out to a competent standard
- The images will support a written report or drawn diagrams
- They can be useful for teaching and training
- They can be reviewed for a second opinion (note, however, they only represent part of the examination)
- They can be used as part of audit and quality assurance processes and as a benchmarking tool
- They can be a reference for comparison with subsequent scans.

When recording images, it is important that demographic information and machine information are included so the patient, machine, sonographer, and department can be identified. Most departments have electronic patient management systems and picture archive and communication systems (PACS) that make the process of image storage and retrieval easy and secure. There may be legal requirements on how long images should be stored (either print or electronic) before they can be destroyed or deleted.

The report is ideally written by the sonographer performing the examination, although in some health care settings the initial report and images may be reviewed, and a final report issued by a qualified medical doctor. It is important that the report is written immediately after the examination, as it is possible to forget important points if it is written at the end of the scanning session consisting of many patients. The report should be concise, avoiding ambiguous language or double negatives. It is advisable to avoid abbreviations such as L for left as they can be misread or misinterpreted in the report. It is essential that the report includes the name of the person writing the report and the examination date and the time. The time is important for in-patient scans, as it can demonstrate the timeline in the patient's investigations and treatment, especially if there are complications, complaints, or adverse events. National ultrasound societies and professional bodies have published guidance on standards for reporting ultrasound investigations, and further reading and resourced are provided at the end of the chapter.

INFECTION CONTROL AND PREVENTION

Infection control and prevention are one of the key pillars in the delivery of safe health care. Hospital-acquired infection can be a significant cause of mortality and morbidity. All ultrasound departments should have policies related to infection control and prevention. The outbreak of the SARS CoV-2 pandemic (COVID-19) in early 2020 has had a profound impact on the practice of infection control and prevention in clinical practice, including imaging services.

Within the ultrasound department, the main sources of infection and cross-infection are from ultrasound probes and the scanner system due to lack of cleaning and decontamination, poor hand hygiene, inadequate cleaning of the local environment, or random mixing of patients with infectious diseases with noninfected patients on the same list. Equipment and transducers should be cleaned and disinfected at the start of a session, between patients, and at the end of a session. The manufacturers' guidelines should be followed in conjunction with local infection control and prevention policies. Ultrasound transmission gel should be removed from the transducer at the end of an examination using a soft tissue or wipe. Many transducers have notches or indents to aid orientation during scanning. These areas can accumulate gel and can be difficult to clean, or overlooked. Transducer faces can be delicate, and the use of abrasive tissues should be avoided. Once cleared of gel, an appropriate disinfectant can be used. The machine should then be disinfected using wipes or approved cleaning solutions. In some cases, it is possible to use disposable keyboard and control covers in high-risk environments. If the scan is to be performed near an open wound, a sterile probe cover and sterile gel should be used. As an extra precaution, a sterile transparent plastic dressing may be used to cover the wound, ensuring no air bubbles are trapped under the dressing that would prevent imaging.

High-touch and contact areas such as the examination table and patient chairs should also be cleaned between patients. The use of personal protective equipment (PPE) will depend on local protocols, but practitioners should be experienced in the use of this equipment, including gloves, scrubs, aprons, face masks, goggles, or

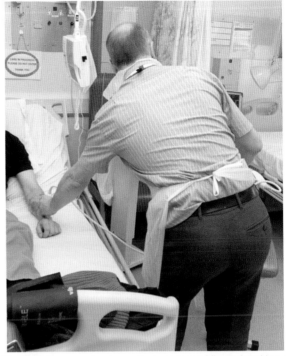

Fig. 7.5 An example of very bad posture while undertaking a ward-based portable ultrasound scan. Prolonged bending or twisting is likely to result in work-related musculoskeletal disorders.

eye shields. Hand hygiene is essential and can include alcohol-based hand gel if hands are not soiled or washing with soap and water for at least 20 seconds.

REPETITIVE STRAIN INJURY AND OCCUPATIONAL HAZARDS

It is recognized that sonographers are at high risk of developing occupational injuries including work-related musculoskeletal disorders (WRMSD) due to poor posture or technique during ultrasound examinations (Fig. 7.5). These can include prolonged periods of twisting, bending, neck extension and rotation, holding an uncomfortable static position for a long period of time, repetitive motions, and application of probe pressure. In extreme cases this can lead to chronic symptoms and injury, forcing individuals to leave the profession. It is the responsibility of both the employer and the sonographer to minimize the risk of WRMSD. To achieve this, it is essential that vascular ultrasound units are equipped with variable-height examination tables that have adjustable upper and lower sections. Ideally, it should be possible to tilt the table, especially for venous examinations. The operator's chair should have a variable-height adjustment, adjustable back rest, and swivel capability. The ultrasound scanner should have an ergonomic design with height-adjustable and swivel console and screen. Portable systems are less flexible, especially if they are placed on dressing trolleys, and this should be avoided. Sonographers should vary the workload and types of scans performed during the day and take regular breaks, including micro breaks where they can rest for a few minutes. The ability to scan with the nondominant hand also reduces strain on one side of the body. The probe should not be gripped too hard, and use of excessive probe pressure should be avoided. The scanning environment is also important. There should be the ability to adjust the ambient lighting in the room, the room temperature, and ventilation. Visual display equipment and workstations in the department should also be ergonomic and staff assessed for any additional measures or provision of equipment that will reduce the risk of WRMSD. If the sonographer develops problems, these should be treated at an early stage, as long-term chronic problems may be difficult to resolve.

SCOPE OF PRACTICE AND AUDIT

Ultrasound services must ensure that their practice and staff working within the service meet the standards defined by their health care institution, national bodies, regulatory or statutory authorities, or accrediting organizations. This also includes training, professional registration or accreditation, and ongoing personal development for staff providing the service. The department should have accessible protocols in place for all aspects of service delivery including scanning, reporting, infection control, health safety, and quality assurance. These should be updated and reviewed on a regular basis. Scope of practice should also be clearly defined to ensure that individuals are only practicing in the areas that they have appropriate knowledge, skills, and experience for. Policies related to duty of candor, to be open and honest with patients and other individuals when something goes wrong that causes harm or potential for harm, should also be in place.

Services must undertake clinic audit, where ultrasound images and reports can be reviewed and compared to other imaging modalities. Attendance at multidisciplinary team meetings is recommended as an effective way of aiding and supporting the audit process and should be a standard for all providers. Additional resources and reference material are provided in further reading.

SAFETY OF DIAGNOSTIC ULTRASOUND

During the scan, the patient is exposed to ultrasound energy, and it is important that the sonographer be aware of the possible risks and how to minimize them. Regulations and user guidelines have been produced to ensure that operators are able to conduct scans at safe outputs without adverse effects.

There are three main effects of ultrasound passing through on tissue:
- Heating. Ultrasound is absorbed in tissue, which causes heating dependent on the acoustic properties of the beam, the absorption characteristics of tissue, its heat capacity, and heat clearance.
- Cavitation. Small gas cavities respond to changes in the acoustic pressure of the pulse. At low amplitudes the bubbles change diameter, expanding at low pressure and contracting at high pressures. At higher pressures the bubble can become unstable, collapsing and causing local shock waves and high temperatures. This is described as internal cavitation.
- Streaming. Ultrasound produces a weak radiation force that can sometimes be observed in fluid collections as it pushes fluid. It is not a safety risk.

The effects on tissue will be the highest where there is maximum intensity, defined as the energy crossing a unit area (usually cm^2). This varies at different locations in the beam; the intensity can be described as the spatial peak I_{sp}, the maximum in the image, or spatial average I_{sa}. It also varies with time; the instantaneous peak I_{tp} is the peak intensity in the pulse whereas the temporal average I_{ta} will be the average intensity over time, more relevant to heating. In combination, for example, the spatial peak temporal average intensity, I_{spta}, is the peak within the beam averaged over time. Another value of intensity that is used is the spatial peak pulse average intensity, I_{sppa}, which is the spatial peak intensity averaged over the duration of the pulse. These have been used by the US Food and Drug Administration (FDA) to define the upper limit of exposure produced by ultrasound systems for diagnostic use (Table 7.1). Manufacturers supply data on the maximum I_{spta} and I_{sppa} in the operator's manual.

Over the years there has been an increase in the output power and intensities generated by ultrasound scanners.

TABLE 7.1 Guidance on the Upper Limits of Exposure for Manufacturers Seeking Marketing Clearance of Ultrasound Systems That Have an On-screen Display of Output Display (TI and MI).				
Application	**Derated I_{spta} (mW/cm^2)**	**Derated I_{sppa} (W/cm^2)**	**MI**	**TI**
All applications except ophthalmology	720	190	1.9	(6.0)[a]
Ophthalmology	50	NS	0.23	1.0

I_{spta}, Spatial peak temporal average intensity; I_{sppa}, spatial peak intensity averaged over the duration of the pulse; *MI*, mechanical index; *TI*, thermal index; *NS*, not specified.
Issued by the United States Food and Drug Administration FDA 2019.
[a]The upper limit of 6.0 is advisory. At least one of the quantities MI and I_{sppa} must be less than the specified limit.

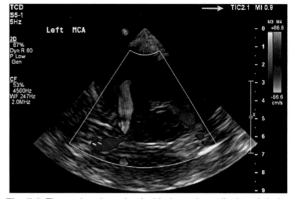

Fig. 7.6 Thermal and mechanical index values displayed during a transcranial Doppler scan. The TIC is selected because bone is immediately beneath the probe face. *TIC*, Cranial thermal index.

The use of color flow imaging with longer pulses of higher amplitude, pulsed wave Doppler with concentration of energy in the sample volume, and harmonic imaging where the nonlinear propagation increases with higher pressures all contributed to higher outputs.

These developments were amongst the factors that led to the development of output display standards (ODS), designed to give the sonographers a guide as to the output at any time and an indication of risk.

Output Display Standards—Mechanical and Thermal Indices

The output power produced by a system will vary with the modality used and the control settings. To make the user aware of the potential risks of any given scanner setup, two indices have been developed. These are the thermal index (TI) and the mechanical index (MI). These indices are displayed on the screen (Fig. 7.6) of modern scanners in real time and will demonstrate any changes in the potential risk as the scanner modalities or controls are altered.

The TI has been developed to indicate the potential risk of producing thermal effects during the scan. It is the ratio of acoustic power emitted at the time to the power required to heat the tissue by 1°C (degrees centigrade). A TI of 1 would therefore indicate the potential to heat the tissue in the beam by 1°C. An ultrasound exposure that does not produce a temperature rise of greater than

1.5°C above normal body temperature of 37°C is not thought to pose any risk of producing thermal damage. The power required to heat the tissue will depend greatly on what tissue is lying in the path of the ultrasound beam and is especially affected by the presence of bone, as bone is a strongly absorbing medium. For this reason, three models for the TI have been developed:

1. Soft tissue (TIS)
2. Tissue with bone present at the focus (TIB)
3. The cranial thermal index (TIC), used in transcranial Doppler.

The appropriate TI should be displayed depending on the scanner examination setup selected. The development of these indices suffers from some limitations, as it is not straightforward to estimate the heat lost from the various regions of the body that are scanned.

MI indicates the likelihood of the onset of inertial cavitation. It is related to the peak negative pressure of the ultrasound pulses being used at the time. For an MI of 0.7, the physical conditions probably cannot exist for bubble growth and collapse to occur (Duck & Shaw 2003). However, if this threshold is exceeded, it does not mean that bioeffects due to cavitation will occur. The higher the value of MI above this threshold, the greater the potential risk. There is currently no evidence that diagnostic ultrasound causes cavitation in soft tissue, except in the presence of gas, such as in the lung and intestines, and in the presence of contrast agents.

Another potential thermal hazard of which the sonographer should be aware is heating of the transducer itself, which may occur if the transducer has been damaged. Malfunction of the scanner may potentially lead to a higher than expected power output.

User's Responsibility

Diagnostic ultrasound has been used for many years with no reported evidence of harmful effects. However, it is prudent to keep patient exposure to the minimum required to obtain an optimal diagnostic result. This can be done by keeping the time of the examination of a particular area to a minimum, especially when using color and spectral Doppler ultrasound, as these modes are more likely to cause heating. Controls such as the gain should be optimized before increasing the output power. Changes in the TI and MI with changes in scanner setup should be monitored. It is important to keep up to date with current guidelines on the safe use of diagnostic ultrasound. National and International Organizations, AIUM, BMUS, EFSUMB, and WFUMB, provide safety statements and recommendations to guide good practice and include free access to literature for further reading (Ter Haar 2012). Vascular ultrasound applications are generally in the lower risk of diagnostic applications, but particular care should be taken if imaging through the eye where lower limits apply (see Table 7.1).

MAINTAINING EQUIPMENT

Equipment must be fit for purpose. This is particularly true for ultrasound scanners, the tool for vascular sonographers. The lifecycle of medical equipment, from investing in and choosing a scanner to its disposal and replacement, is the subject of entire books. The selection of equipment for high-standard imaging across a range of applications is complex, and evaluation will consider its image quality in all modes: how easy it is to use, its size and agility, what probes are available and how they perform, and even how much noise it makes. It will also depend on how much it costs to buy and maintain.

Departments must have some level of support and quality assurance for their scanners. Support may come from an in-house engineering team or from the manufacturers or other external companies. The level of support required will depend on operational requirements and costs.

Maintaining the scanner performance is the responsibility of all operators. Ultrasound scanners perform

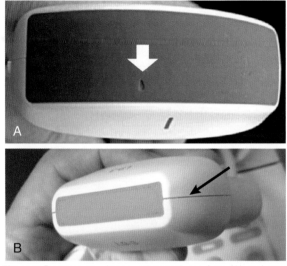

Fig. 7.7 Damage to ultrasound transducer face (A) and case (B). Damage to the lens of the probe will result in deterioration of the beam focusing. Damage to the case produces increased pockets for infection risk and the possibility of ingress of fluids into the transducer.

self-checks on the circuity and software, and the resulting error logs can be accessed by technical teams. Faults and poor performance are most likely to arise from damage to transducers, their leads and connectors, and from physical damage to the control panel. The operator will be the first to notice when a control is stiff or does not function. They should be the first to note that the transducer has damage (Figs. 7.7 and 7.8) or has nonfunctioning elements (Fig. 7.9) or faults in the lens (Fig. 7.10). Simple housekeeping can prolong the life of a scanner, keeping cables tidy in their housing (Fig. 7.11), cleaning the keyboard from gel, and clearing the filters so that the scanner circuits do not overheat. A checklist of daily and less frequent actions is suggested (Table 7.2). Ultrasound phantoms also known as test objects, usually consisting of fine wires embedded in a tissue mimicking gel with the wires imaged in transverse section, can also be used to assess image quality, as seen in Fig. 7.12. More sophisticated QA using ultrasound phantoms requires training and can be difficult to do consistently; development of phantoms has lagged behind those of scanners, but they can be useful to evaluate changes in performance; an extreme example is shown in Fig. 7.12.

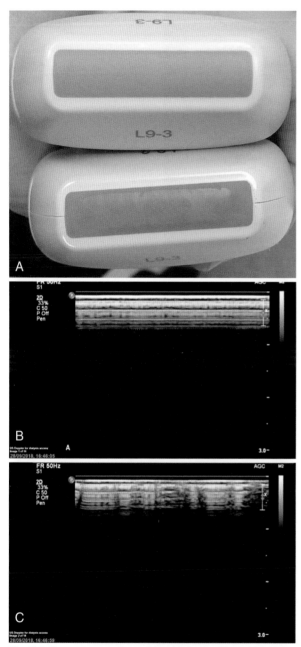

Fig. 7.8 Severe wear of an ultrasound transducer. The lower transducer (A) has severe abrasion damage, presumably from prolonged wiping of the face. The images (B) and (C) are of the reverberation pattern when transmitting into air. The pattern from the damaged transducer (C) shows deterioration with differences in sensitivity along the array.

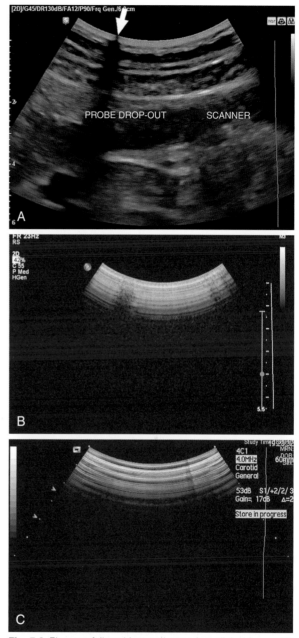

Fig. 7.9 Element failure (drop-out) seen in a clinical image (A) and when the transducer is transmitting into air (B and C). Single element drop-out (C) may have comparatively little effect on image quality, but large areas of damage (B) will lead to regions of poor spatial and contrast resolution in the image and poor Doppler sensitivity.

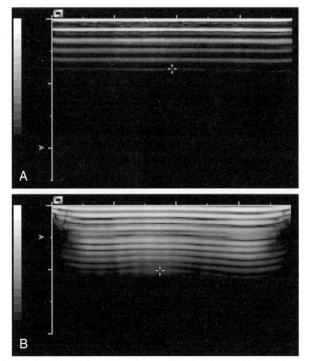

Fig. 7.10 Reverberation in air patterns from transducers. The depth to the last seen reverberation (A) can be used as a guide to transducer performance if carefully measured using standardized parameters. The variation in the pattern across the image in (B) shows evidence of damage to the layers of the transducer surface.

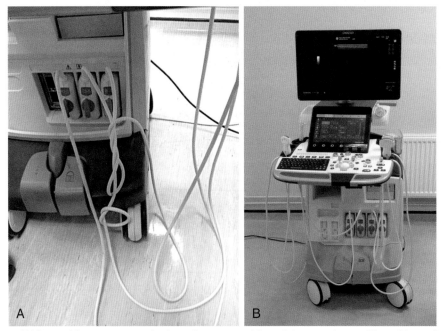

Fig. 7.11 (A) Poor cable management leads to damage to cable and the transducers. The cables trail on the floor; moving the scanner may cause these to be trapped in the wheels. The entwined cables and knots restrict the length of cable available and risk pulling other transducers off their storage. (B) Cables and transducers securely stowed. However, note that main cables trailing on the floor can be a trip hazard.

TABLE 7.2	Practical User Maintenance and Tests for Ultrasound Scanners
Clean ultrasound gel and any body fluids from console, cable, and transducers after every patient. Disinfect probe, cable, and controls with appropriate cleaning agent or wipes after every patient	Multi-daily
Ensure transducers are stored securely when not in use	Multi-daily
Ensure cables are properly stowed and not at risk of being run over by the scanner	Multi-daily
Clean monitors of dust/gel, etc.	Daily
Check correct operation of main scanner controls	Daily
Inspect transducers used for damage	Daily
Inspect reverberation images (in air) for shadows and streaks cause by dropout for all transducers	Daily
Air reverberation pattern (sensitivity)	Monthly
Element drop-out tests	If fault seen/monthly
Electrical safety testing	Yearly

Adapted from Dudley et al., BMUS Guidelines Ultrasound 2014. 22; 8–14

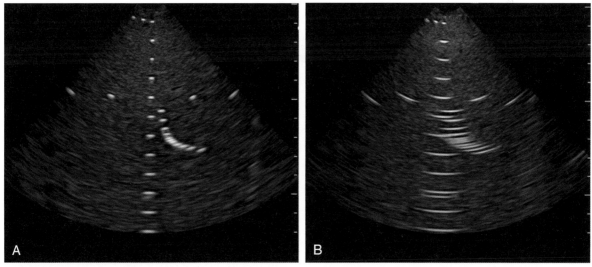

Fig. 7.12 Comparison of two transducers on an ultrasound phantom. The transducer in image (B) was suspected of poor performance, but images of patients were hard to quantify compared with another identical transducer (A). Scanning a phantom revealed severe deterioration of lateral resolution.

8

Ultrasound Assessment of the Extracranial Cerebral Circulation

INTRODUCTION

Ultrasound can be used to evaluate the extracranial cerebral circulation in order to investigate patients with suspected stroke or transient ischemic attack (TIA) or patients who have already suffered a stroke. Stroke is one of the leading causes of death in the world. Approximately 85% of strokes are ischemic (i.e., thrombotic or embolic or both) as opposed to hemorrhagic. MRI (magnetic resonance imaging) or CT (computerized tomography) are used to identify if a stroke is ischemic or hemorrhagic, as treatment differs greatly between the two. Up to 80% of ischemic strokes occur in the carotid territory, the area of the brain supplied by the carotid arteries; however, not all these strokes are due to carotid artery disease. Trials have shown that patients with significant carotid artery disease and relevant symptoms benefit from surgery in order to prevent a stroke. The majority of carotid artery disease develops at the carotid bifurcation, and in the presence of a significant stenosis, carotid endarterectomy (CEA) can be performed. In this procedure, the diseased inner arterial wall (plaque) is removed, thus eliminating a potential source of emboli or a flow-limiting stenosis. Carotid ultrasound examinations can be used to screen symptomatic patients for carotid artery disease before further investigation, such as computed tomography angiography (CTA). Alternatively, some centers use ultrasound examination to select patients directly for surgery without the use of further imaging. If the ultrasound scan is inconclusive and further imaging is required, CTA is normally used. Some centers perform CEA for significant asymptomatic carotid disease prior to or combined with coronary artery bypass graft (CABG) surgery, with the aim of reducing the stroke rate associated with CABG surgery. In these centers the cardiologist or cardiac surgeons will require access to a carotid scanning service to detect the presence of any significant disease.

ANATOMY

The brain is supplied by four vessels—the right and left internal carotid and vertebral arteries—and receives 15% of the cardiac output. The term *extracranial cerebral arteries* refers to all the arteries that carry blood from the heart up to the base of the skull. The left and right sides of the extracranial circulation are not symmetrical (see Fig. 8.1). On the left side, the common carotid artery (CCA) and subclavian artery arise directly from the aortic arch, whereas on the right side the brachiocephalic artery, also known as the innominate artery, arises from the aorta and divides into the subclavian artery and CCA. The CCA, which has no branches, divides into the internal and external carotid arteries (ICA and ECA), but the level of the carotid bifurcation in the neck is highly variable. In approximately 90% of cases, the ICA lies posterolateral or lateral to the ECA and, unlike the ECA, has no branches below the skull. The proximal branches of the ECA are the superior thyroid, lingual, facial, and maxillary arteries. The carotid artery widens at the level of the bifurcation to form the carotid bulb. In some cases, the carotid bulb may only involve the proximal ICA, and not the distal CCA, and the degree of widening of the carotid bulb is quite variable. Within the skull, the distal segment of the ICA follows a U-shaped curved path, known as the carotid siphon. The most important branch of the ICA is the ophthalmic artery, which supplies the eye. The terminal branches of the

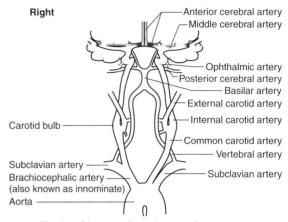

Fig. 8.1 Diagram of cerebrovascular anatomy.

ophthalmic artery, the supratrochlear, and supraorbital arteries unite with the terminal branches of the ECA. The ICA finally divides into the middle cerebral artery (MCA) and the anterior cerebral artery (ACA).

The posterior circulation of the brain is mainly supplied by the left and right vertebral arteries, via the basilar artery. The vertebral artery is the first branch of the subclavian artery, arising from the highest point of the subclavian arch. At the sixth cervical vertebra, the vertebral artery runs posteriorly to travel upward through the transverse foramen of the cervical vertebrae. It is common for one vertebral artery to be larger than the other, with the left more often being larger than the right. The two vertebral arteries join, at the base of the skull, to form the basilar artery, which then divides to form the posterior cerebral arteries. Fig. 8.2A shows how the circle of Willis, situated at the base of the brain, joins the cerebral branches of the ICAs and basilar artery via the anterior and posterior communicating arteries. There is further discussion of the anatomy and assessment of the intracerebral arteries in Chapter 17. Blood flow to the brain is regulated by changes in cerebrovascular resistance, with carbon dioxide playing a major role in vasodilation.

Collateral Pathways and Anatomical Variants

In the presence of severe vascular disease, the cerebral circulation has many possible collateral (alternative) pathways, both extracranially and intracranially. Not all of these can be assessed using ultrasound. The pathways that can be visualized using ultrasound are the following:

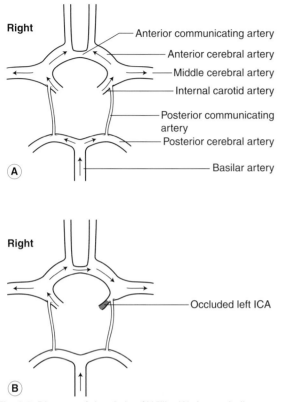

Right

- Anterior communicating artery
- Anterior cerebral artery
- Middle cerebral artery
- Internal carotid artery
- Posterior communicating artery
- Posterior cerebral artery
- Basilar artery

(A)

Right

- Occluded left ICA

(B)

Fig. 8.2 Diagram of the circle of Willis. (A) *Arrows* indicate normal flow direction. (B) *Arrows* indicate cross-over flow from the right internal carotid artery *(ICA)* to the left middle cerebral artery in the presence of a left ICA occlusion.

- The ophthalmic artery. The ECAs do not normally supply blood to the brain, but in the presence of severe ICA disease, branches of the ECA can act as important collateral pathways. One such pathway is via the terminal branches of the ECA, communicating with the terminal branches of the ophthalmic artery. This collateral pathway can be observed using continuous-wave (CW) Doppler to detect reversal of flow in the supraorbital artery, a terminal branch of the ophthalmic artery, toward the brain. This can lead to waveform shape changes in the ECA with the spectral Doppler demonstrating lower resistance flow waveforms than typical for the ECA.
- The circle of Willis. In the normal circulation, there may be little blood flow through the communicating arteries in the circle of Willis, but in the presence of severe vascular disease they perform an important

role in flow distribution. For example, in the presence of a left ICA occlusion, it is possible for the right ICA to supply blood flow to the left MCA via the right ACA, the anterior communicating artery, and the left ACA, with flow reversal occurring in the left ACA (see Fig. 8.2B). This could lead to higher than expected flow velocities in the common and ICAs contralateral (opposite side) to an occlusion.

- The vertebral arteries may also supply flow to the MCA via the posterior communicating arteries of the circle of Willis. If the circle is well developed, it is possible for a single extracranial artery to provide adequate cerebral blood flow. However, in about 75% of the population, parts of the circle may be hypoplastic (very small) or absent, making the circle incomplete and therefore preventing the development of good collateral flow (von Reutern & von Büdingen 1993), but this may only become apparent in the presence of severe disease. Adequate collateral pathways have a better chance of developing in the presence of slowly developing disease.
- In the presence of a CCA occlusion, it is possible for reversal of flow in the proximal ECA supplied by one of its proximal branches to supply a patent ipsilateral (same side) ICA, discussed later (see Fig 8.23). Severe narrowing or occlusion of the proximal subclavian or brachiocephalic artery can result in a collateral pathway that "steals" blood from the brain to supply the arm. In this case, blood will be seen to flow retrogradely down the ipsilateral vertebral artery to supply the distal subclavian artery beyond the diseased segment (Fig. 8.3). This is known as subclavian steal syndrome. Assessment of vertebral arteries is discussed later in the chapter (Figs. 8.13 and 8.42).

There are few variations in the extracranial circulation. In rare cases, the left CCA and subclavian artery may share a common origin or a single trunk. Other anomalies are the left vertebral artery arising directly from the aortic arch and, even more unusually, the right vertebral origin arising from the aortic arch.

SYMPTOMS OF CAROTID AND VERTEBRAL ARTERY DISEASE

Patients with carotid artery stenosis may suffer from TIA, stroke, or amaurosis fugax (a form of transient monocular visual disturbance/blindness). A TIA has

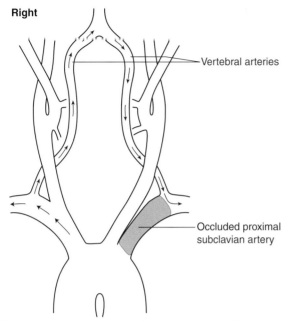

Right

Vertebral arteries

Occluded proximal subclavian artery

Fig. 8.3 *Arrows* indicate the direction of collateral flow in sub-clavian steal syndrome, via reverse flow in the vertebral artery to supply the arm, in the presence of a severe stenosis or occlusion of the proximal subclavian artery.

been defined as a transient episode of neurological dys-function caused by focal brain, spinal cord, or retinal ischemia, without acute infarction (Easton et al. 2009). Symptoms of TIA may only last a few minutes and the patient will make a full recovery within 24 hours, whereas patients suffering from a stroke will have symp-toms lasting more than 24 hours and may not make a full recovery. Patients suffering from a TIA are at high risk of suffering an early stroke. Therefore, the occur-rence of a TIA requires urgent investigation and treat-ments to reduce the risk of stroke. Symptoms of carotid territory TIA include single or multiple episodes of loss of power or sensation in an arm or leg (monoparesis), in both (hemiparesis), or in one side of the face; slurring or loss of speech (dysphasia); or visuospatial neglect.

As the right side of the brain controls the left-hand side of the body and the converse, the symptoms will relate to the contralateral carotid artery. Speech is usu-ally controlled by the dominant side of the brain (i.e., a right-handed patient's speech will typically be controlled by the left side of the brain). Patients suffering from epi-sodes of amaurosis fugax often complain of "a curtain drawing across one eye" lasting for a few minutes, which is usually due to reduced blood flow within the retinal

circulation, possibly due to emboli. In this situation, the symptoms in the eye will relate to the ipsilateral carotid artery. Typical carotid territory and vertebrobasilar symptoms are shown in Box 8.1. Vague symptoms, such as dizziness and blackout, are not usually associated with carotid artery disease. Subclavian steal syndrome does not usually cause significant symptoms. Only about 15% of patients suffer symptoms of TIA before a stroke. The causes of TIA include large-vessel cervical or intracra-nial atherosclerosis with stenosis (16%), cardioembolic (29%), lacuna (16%), uncertain cause (36%), and other 3% (BMJ best practice online resource). It is therefore appropriate that these alternative causes are investigated as the different causes require different medical or sur-gical treatment. For example, as part of the TIA patient pathway, an ECG can be used to assess the possibility of a cardioembolic cause. Only 1% to 2% of all strokes are hemodynamic strokes (i.e., due to flow-limiting steno-ses) (Naylor et al. 1998).

There are various classifications for stroke. An exam-ple is the Bamford stroke classification (Bamford 2000). It defines four subcategories of cerebral infarction on the basis of presenting symptoms and signs (Table 8.1). It is useful for the sonographer to be familiar with the acro-nyms as these are often used on imaging request forms.

Patients with symptoms of TIA or minor stroke are at a cumulative recurrent risk of a stroke due to large-vessel disease of 4% at 7 days following symptoms, 12.6% at 1 month, and 19.2% at 3 months (Naylor 2008). Ultrasound can be used to help select those patients who

TABLE 8.1	**Bamford Stroke Classification**		
Total anterior circulation stroke (TACS)	**Partial anterior circulation stroke (PACS)**	**Lacunar syndrome (LACS)**	**Posterior circulation syndrome (POCS)**
Criteria	*Criteria*	*Criteria*	*Criteria*
All three of the following:	**Two** of the following:	**One** of the following:	**One** of the following:
• Unilateral weakness (and/or sensory deficit) of the face, arm, and leg • Homonymous hemianopia • Higher cerebral dysfunction (dysphagia, visuospatial disorder)	• Unilateral weakness (and/or sensory deficit) of the face, arm, and leg • Homonymous hemianopia • Higher cerebral dysfunction (dysphagia, visuospatial disorder)	• Pure sensory stroke • Pure motor stroke • Sensorimotor stroke • Ataxic hemiparesis	• Cranial nerve palsy and a contralateral motor/sensory deficit • Bilateral motor/sensory deficit • Conjugate eye movement disorder (e.g., gaze palsy) • Cerebellar dysfunction (e.g., ataxia, nystagmus, vertigo) • Isolated homonymous hemianopia or cortical blindness

would benefit from CEA to reduce the risk of stroke (method discussed later in the chapter). It has been shown that the benefit of CEA is greatest when the surgery is performed within 2 weeks of the patient's symptoms and that the benefit is reduced by almost a third if surgery is performed more than 4 weeks following the last symptom (Rothwell et al. 2004). In symptomatic patients with a 70% to 99% stenosis, the absolute risk reduction of CEA is 23% if surgery is performed within 2 weeks compared to 7.4% if performed at more than 12 weeks after symptoms.

Guidelines produced by the National Institute for Health and Care Excellence (NICE) Stroke and TIA in over 16s: diagnosis and initial treatment: (NG 128 [published: 1 May 2019]) recommend immediate referral of people who have had a suspected TIA for specialist assessment and investigation, to be seen within 24 hours of the onset of symptoms, and that everyone with TIA who after specialist assessment is considered as a candidate for CEA should have urgent carotid imaging. Symptomatic patients with a 50% to 99% (The North American Symptomatic Carotid Endarterectomy Trial [NASCET]) stenosis should be referred urgently to vascular surgery for consideration for CEA alongside best medical treatment. This, therefore, requires patients suffering TIA or minor stroke to have rapid access to carotid duplex scanning to enable early diagnosis and treatment.

Symptoms similar to TIA can also be caused by other neurological problems, such as epilepsy, intracranial tumor, multiple sclerosis, or migraine (sometimes known as TIA mimics). Referral to a neurologist can be made to confirm appropriate symptoms and investigations.

Asymptomatic carotid disease can be discovered clinically by the presence of a carotid bruit, heard as a murmur when listening to the neck with a stethoscope. However, the presence of a carotid bruit may not be due to an ICA stenosis but could instead relate to an ECA or aortic stenosis or to no stenosis at all. A large proportion of patients with a >70% stenosis will not have a carotid bruit, and therefore its presence or absence is not accurate enough to predict the presence of disease.

Trauma to the neck, such as whiplash, can lead to dissection of the carotid artery wall, possibly causing the vessel to occlude, resulting in symptoms of stroke. This condition may be suspected in patients suffering a stroke following a neck injury, especially younger patients. Dissection may involve the brachiocephalic artery, CCA, or ICA. Dissection of the CCA can also occur as an extension of aortic arch dissection. The possible extent of dissection and difficulty of imaging the proximal and very distal arteries with ultrasound means that alternative imaging is usually required to confirm the diagnosis. Ultrasound examination may also be requested in the presence of a pulsatile swelling in the neck to identify the presence of a carotid aneurysm or carotid body tumor (CBT), both of which are quite rare. A more common cause for prominent pulsatile swelling particularly at the base of the right side of the neck is vessel tortuosity at the right CCA origin. This occurs most frequently in older patients and can relate to changes in body shape and posture. In rare situations the carotid bifurcation is dilated and lying very superficially under the skin surface.

SCANNING

Objectives and Preparation

> **PURPOSE OF SCAN**
>
> The purpose of the carotid scan is to identify the extent of any atheroma or, on rare occasion, thrombus within the common carotid artery and extracranial internal and external carotid artery and to determine the degree of narrowing of the vessels. The examination can also provide evidence of possible arch disease indicated by the appearance of carotid waveforms. The examination should also demonstrate the presence and direction of flow in the vertebral arteries.

No specific preparation is required, but the patient must be capable of lying or sitting still during the examination. The optimal position for scanning the carotid arteries is with the sonographer sitting behind the patient's head. This allows easy access to the neck and enables the sonographer to rest their arm on the examination table while performing the scan and avoids the sonographer twisting their back. Alternatively, the sonographer can sit by the side of the patient. The patient should lie supine on the examination table with the head resting on a thin pillow. The neck should be extended and the head turned in the opposite direction to the side being examined. If the patient has difficulty in breathing or has back problems, it may be necessary to sit the patient in a more upright position. If the patient is in a wheelchair (e.g., following a disabling stroke), it may be easier to do the scan with the patient remaining in the wheelchair with their head resting on a pillow for support, preventing unnecessary movement of the patient. However, being in an upright position may affect the velocity values recorded, and more care may be required in grading any significance disease (Pemble 2008).

The examination can be performed with a medium- to high-frequency flat linear array transducer, depending on the size of the patient's neck. The higher the frequency, the better the resolution of the vessel wall structure; however, in some cases the carotid bifurcation lies deep in the neck, requiring a lower-frequency transducer for visualization. Blood flow velocities detected in the majority of normal and diseased carotid arteries are reasonably high, so the scanner should be configured to visualize high-velocity pulsatile flow. A nominal color scale of 20 to 30 cm/s (or pulse repetition frequency [PRF] of 3000 Hz) is typical. Most ultrasound systems have examination presets available that are suitable for most carotid examinations, but it may be necessary to alter these to enable the detection of low-velocity flow when differentiating carotid artery occlusion from a subtotal occlusion. A small spectral Doppler sample volume is usually used to interrogate the carotid arteries, as it allows for more selective investigation of areas of velocity increase or flow disturbance.

Technique

The carotid arteries are best visualized through the sternocleidomastoid muscle, which provides a good ultrasonic window, and this is done using a lateral rather than an anterior approach. The procedure is as follows:

1 Using B-mode imaging only, the CCA should be visualized in transverse section (Fig. 8.4A), starting in the lower neck as this is the easiest area to identify the artery. On the right side, as the probe is moved to the base of the neck it is usually possible to visualize the distal brachiocephalic artery and the origin of the CCA and subclavian artery. On the left side, the origin of the CCA cannot normally be visualized, as it lies too deep in the chest. The CCA should be scanned along its length, in transverse section, up to the bifurcation, and along the ICA and ECA (Fig. 8.4B) as high up the neck as can be seen. This allows the sonographer to ascertain the level and orientation of the carotid bifurcation and also gives the first indications of the presence and location of any arterial disease. The jugular vein lies over the CCA (Fig. 8.4A) and is usually easily compressed. However, it is important not to apply too much transducer pressure when scanning the carotid arteries as there is a possibility of dislodging an embolus from the vessel wall. If B-mode is suboptimal, it can be helpful to use color flow imaging to locate the bifurcation and orientation of the vessels.

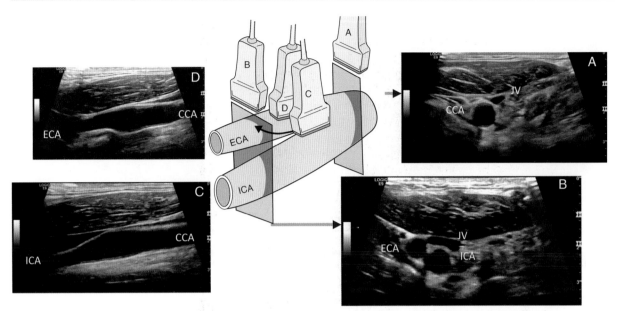

Fig. 8.4 Schematic diagram of the carotid bifurcation showing possible longitudinal and transverse imaging planes alongside images. (A) Transverse image of the CCA; (D) transverse image of the ICA and ECA, distal to the carotid bifurcation; (C) the ICA in longitudinal section; and (D) the ECA in longitudinal section. *CCA,* Common carotid artery; *ECA,* external carotid artery; *ICA,* internal carotid artery; *JV,* jugular vein.

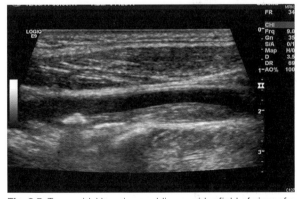

Fig. 8.5 Trapezoidal imaging enabling a wider field of view of a diseased common carotid artery.

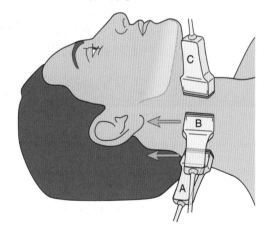

Fig. 8.6 Longitudinal transducer positions that can be used to visualize the carotid arteries. (A) Posterior. (B) Lateral. (C) Anterior. (The jaw line is clearly demonstrated.) The *arrows* show it is normally possible to image above the jaw *(arrows)* using the posterior and lateral positions.

2   The CCA is now visualized in longitudinal section using B-mode imaging, starting at the base of the neck. It is useful to use an extended field of view by selecting trapezoidal imaging (also known as virtual convex, see Ch. 2), as this will cover a wider region of tissue (Fig. 8.5). A longitudinal image of the CCA can be easily obtained by imaging the CCA in transverse section and then, keeping the CCA in the center of the image, rotating the probe so the CCA first appears as an ellipse and finally can be seen in longitudinal section. Prior knowledge of the orientation of the ICA

and ECA gained from transverse imaging is helpful for locating the correct longitudinal imaging plane to view the ICA and ECA (Fig. 8.4C and D). It is necessary to use a range of longitudinal scan planes to visualize the carotid arteries, especially at the bifurcation (see Fig. 8.6). Typically, the ICA lies posterolateral or

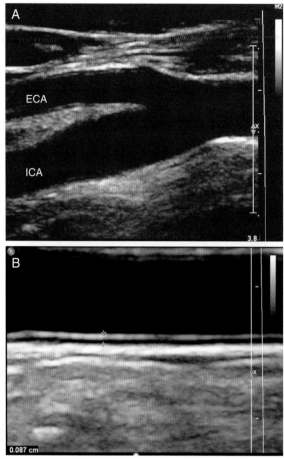

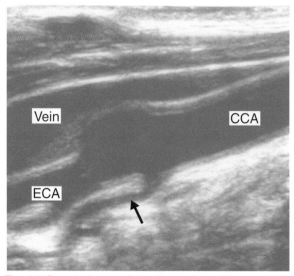

Fig. 8.8 B-mode image of the external carotid artery *(ECA)* showing the superior thyroid branch *(arrow)*. *CCA*, Common carotid artery.

Fig. 8.7 (A) Longitudinal B-mode image of the carotid bifurcation with the internal and external carotid arteries (*ICA* and *ECA*) seen in the same plane. (B) Zoomed image showing the intima-media layer *(crosses)* of the posterior common carotid artery wall.

lateral to the ECA and is usually the larger of the two vessels; however, the orientation of the vessels is quite variable. In a small percentage of cases, the bifurcation will appear as a tuning fork arrangement (Fig. 8.7A) easily viewed in one plane, but in the majority of cases the ECA and ICA will have to be imaged individually. This is achieved by keeping the lower portion of the probe face over the CCA and slowly rotating the upper portion through a small angle to image first the ICA and then the ECA, or vice versa. Only small probe movements are required when imaging the ICA and ECA, as the vessels usually lie close together.

3 Having located the three vessels and observed any evidence of disease in the B-mode image, color flow imaging can be used to investigate the flow from the proximal CCA up into the ICA and ECA. Identification of ECA branches (either on B-mode or color imaging) serves as a further indication as to which vessel is the ECA, as the ICA has no branches below the jaw (Fig. 8.8). The jugular vein can sometimes pass between the ICA and ECA at the bifurcation, which can complicate the identification of the ICA and ECA, or the jugular vein may be mistaken for one of the arteries. Color flow imaging can provide evidence of disease, such as velocity changes due to stenosis, areas of filling defects due to the presence of atheroma, and the absence of flow due to occlusion. Diagnosis should not be made based on the color flow imaging alone, but it greatly aids the sonographer in selecting areas that require close investigation with the spectral Doppler.

4 The spectral Doppler is now used to observe the inflow to the carotid arteries by placing the sample volume in the proximal CCA at the base of the neck. The shape of the waveform may suggest the presence of proximal or distal disease, such as an ICA occlusion. In the absence of significant distal or proximal disease, the left and right CCA waveforms should appear symmetrical.

5 The examination so far has provided many clues as to which of the two vessels beyond the bifurcation is

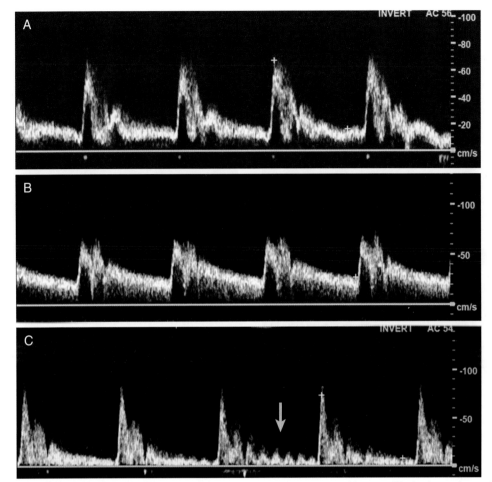

Fig. 8.9 Typical normal Doppler spectra obtained from the common carotid artery (A), the internal carotid artery (B), and the external carotid artery (ECA) (C). The effect of tapping the temporal artery which can be seen on ECA diastolic flow is marked with the *arrow*. However, this test should be interpreted with caution.

the ICA, such as the relative size and position of the two vessels and the presence of ECA branches. Spectral Doppler can now be used to confirm the identification of the ICA and ECA, as the ICA waveform shape is less pulsatile and has higher diastolic flow than the ECA (see Fig. 8.9). It is imperative that the ICA and ECA should be correctly identified, as it is the presence of disease in the carotid bifurcation and ICA, not the ECA, that is the possible cause of carotid artery symptoms. If significant disease is present in the ICA, the upper limit of the disease in relation to the level of the jaw should be assessed. If no endpoint to the disease in the ICA can be seen, alternative imaging, such as CTA, will be required to identify this, if CEA is being considered.

6 Using spectral Doppler flow is assessed in the proximal, mid, and distal CCA. Peak systolic velocity (PSV) and end-diastolic velocity (EDV) measurements should be made in the disease-free section of the distal CCA (approximately 1 cm proximal to the bifurcation), and in the ICA at the site of the maximum velocity increase within any stenoses, to allow the degree of narrowing to be graded. If no stenosis is seen, the ICA waveform should be obtained in the proximal ICA, a short distance from the bifurcation, beyond the carotid bulb as any localized flow disturbance from the bulb should have dissipated. Atypical waveform shapes should also be noted.

7 If no flow is detected in the ICA (Fig. 8.10) or CCA (Fig. 8.11) using the default carotid pre-set scanner settings, it is necessary to rule out the presence of low

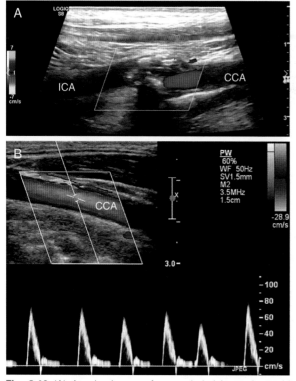

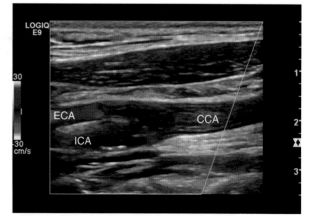

Fig. 8.11 Image of an occluded common carotid artery *(CCA)* and internal carotid artery *(ICA)*. The external carotid artery *(ECA)* is filling via retrograde flow in an ECA branch, not seen in this image.

Fig. 8.10 (A) A color image of an occluded internal carotid artery *(ICA)* showing flow in the common carotid artery *(CCA)* with an absence of flow in the ICA. (B) Doppler spectrum obtained from a CCA proximal to an ICA occlusion showing high-resistance flow with reduced diastolic flow.

velocity due to a critical stenosis or subtotal occlusion or under perfusion (Fig. 8.12) before reporting the vessel to be occluded. This is achieved by optimizing the scanner controls to detect low-velocity flow (i.e., by lowering the PRF/scale and high-pass filter setting, increasing the gain and ensuring a good angle of insonation). A typical color scale of 8 to 10 cm/s (PRF < 1000 Hz) is a good starting point. If no flow is still detected, the power Doppler mode (see Ch. 4) can be used to confirm occlusion, as this is sensitive to low velocity. Other flow modalities such as B-flow (see Ch. 4) can also be useful. If low-velocity flow is detected, the cause should be identified. For example, low-velocity, higher-resistance flow, often demonstrated as reduction or absence of end-diastolic flow but with rapid systolic rise time, may be detected in the CCA because of an ICA occlusion (Fig. 8.10B). Low-velocity damped flow may be detected in the ICA due to a severe

stenosis of the ICA origin. An occlusion in a distal vessel such as the MCA can also lead to low-velocity, high-resistance flow being detected in the proximal ICA (see Fig. 8.25).

8 To conclude the first side of the examination, the vertebral artery should be located using B-mode or color flow imaging. The patient's head should be turned slightly to one side but more centrally than when imaging the carotid arteries. First image the mid-CCA in longitudinal section and then slowly angle the transducer into a more anteroposterior plane. The vertebral processes, seen as bright echoes, should slowly be seen to stand out. Only short sections of the vertebral artery and vein can be seen at this level as they run through the transverse foramen of the vertebrae. The walls of the vertebral artery and vein can often be seen on the B-mode image, but color flow imaging can also help visualize the vessels (see Fig. 8.13). Spectral Doppler is then used to confirm the flow direction and to assess the flow waveform shape seen in the vertebral artery.

9 Having completed the first side of the examination, the patient is asked to turn the head in the opposite direction, and the other side is examined in the same way. It is important to remember that the carotid and vertebral arteries on both sides are linked via several possible collateral pathways, and that the presence of severe disease in one extracranial vessel may affect flow in another extracranial vessel if it is supplying a collateral pathway.

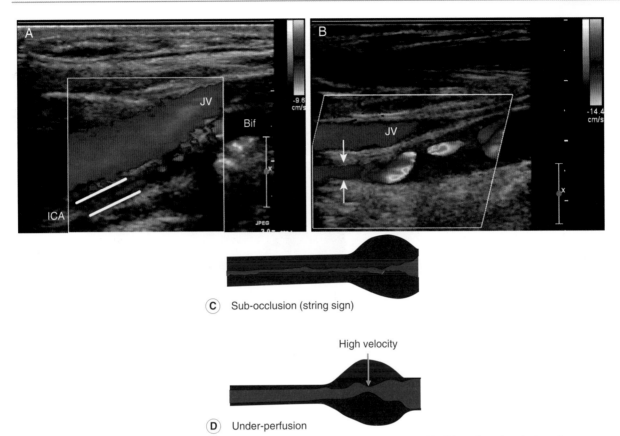

Fig. 8.12 Color image showing a narrow channel of low-velocity flow detected in (A) a subtotal occlusion of the internal carotid artery *(ICA)* and (B) an underperfused internal carotid artery. The *solid white lines* in (A) and *arrows* in (B) show the position of the ICA wall. A low pulse repetition frequency/scale is required to detect the low-velocity flow. Diagram showing the difference between (C) a subocclusion and (D) underperfusion. *Bif*, Carotid bifurcation; *JV*, jugular vein.

RECOMMENDATION

The peak systolic velocity (PSV) and end-diastolic velocity (EDV) should be measured in the common carotid artery 1–2 cm below the bifurcation and at the site of maximum velocity within any internal carotid artery (ICA) stenosis. If no narrowing is seen in the ICA, the PSV and EDV should be measured in the ICA just beyond the carotid bulb. These velocity measurements and ratios obtained from the measurements can be used to grade the degree of narrowing within the bifurcation.

B-MODE IMAGING

Normal Appearance

The normal vessel walls will often appear as a double-layer structure when imaged in longitudinal section (Fig. 8.7), especially if a high-frequency transducer is used. This represents the intima-media layer and adventitia (see Ch. 5) and is most clearly seen on the posterior wall in the CCA, when the vessel lies at right angles to the ultrasound beam. The normal thickness of the intima-media layer is of the order of 0.5 to 0.9 mm, when measured on ultrasound and is dependent on age. A normal vessel lumen should appear hypoechoic; however, it is possible for the sonographer to remove echoes, such as those due to reverberation artifacts, from within the lumen by adjusting the scanner controls, for example, reducing the time gain compensation or using harmonic imaging (see Ch. 2), so careful optimization of the imaging controls is important. The B-mode imaging focal zone should be placed in the region of the vessel to ensure optimal imaging of the vessel walls. Occasionally, it is difficult to obtain adequate B-mode images of the

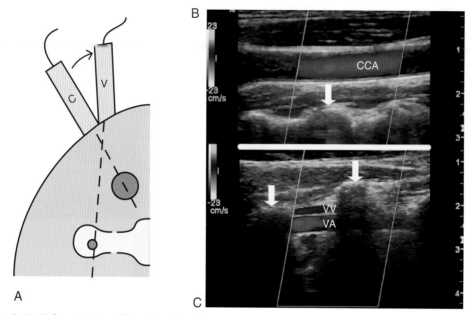

Fig. 8.13 (A) Showing the different imaging planes required to visualize (B) the common carotid artery *(CCA)* (imaging plane c in A) and (C) vertebral artery *(VA)* and vein *(VV)* (imaging plane v in A). The vertebral processes of the spine are marked by the *arrows*.

bifurcation. In this case, color flow imaging may help locate the vessels and enable spectral Doppler measurements to be made.

> **CAUTION**
>
> Reverberation artifacts can give the appearance of structures within the lumen. Reverberation artifacts can be generated from large boundaries within the imaging plane, such as muscle or vein wall, overlying the carotid artery. Changing the angle at which the carotid artery is viewed, either by heel-toeing the transducer or using a different scan plane, can minimize these artifacts or enable differentiation of artifacts from true structures, as the reverberation artifact will change location on the image if the scanning angle is changed (see Fig. 2.37).

Abnormal Appearance

The ultrasound appearance of the early stages of carotid artery disease is a thickening of the intima-media layer. As the disease progresses, more substantial areas of atheroma can be visualized, and this is most likely to occur at the carotid bifurcation. However, in a small proportion of patients, significant disease may be seen in the CCA (Fig. 8.5) and may also involve the CCA origin. It is important to remember the way ultrasound interacts with tissue and the effects of scanner setup, such as gain control, compression curve, harmonic imaging, compound imaging, and adaptive image processing (see Ch. 2), before drawing conclusions about the appearance of plaque surface or composition. Fig. 8.14 shows how the appearance of an image of a plaque can change depending on the equipment setup. A high-frequency transducer should ideally be used when investigating plaque composition, as a high transmit frequency gives better axial resolution. However, if the vessel lies deep in the neck, a lower transmit frequency or lower-frequency probe may be necessary to give adequate penetration to obtain an image.

Many studies have been carried out comparing the ultrasound appearance of atheromatous plaque with histological investigation of specimens removed during CEA (Fig. 8.15) in an attempt to use ultrasound to predict which plaques are more likely to be the source of emboli. Several of these studies show an association between the symptoms and the presence of intraplaque hemorrhage (i.e., bleeding into the plaque). If the surface of a plaque containing intraplaque hemorrhage or lipid pools ruptures, the contents of the plaque are discharged into the vessel lumen, causing distal embolization and possibly leading to symptoms such as TIA or

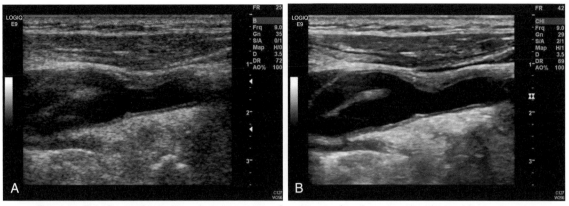

Fig. 8.14 This figure shows how the appearance of an image of a plaque can be changed by equipment setup. (A) Fundamental ultrasound only. (B) Harmonic imaging with compound imaging and adaptive imaging.

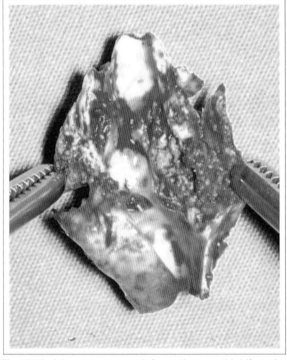

Fig. 8.15 Atheroma removed from the carotid bifurcation during carotid endarterectomy.

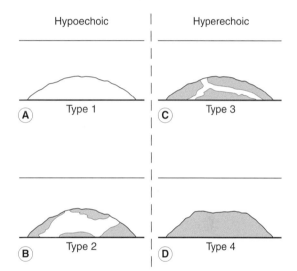

Fig. 8.16 Plaque categorization based on ultrasound imaging described by Bock & Lusby. (Bock and Lusby in Labs et al. [eds], *Diagnostic Vascular Ultrasound* [Hodder Arnold, 1992]. Reprinted by permission of Edward Arnold (Publishers) Ltd.)

stroke. On B-mode ultrasound, hypoechoic areas (seen as near black) have been shown to relate to either lipid or intraplaque hemorrhage with hyperechoic plaques (seen as white) considered to be more benign (Bock & Lusby 1992). Fig. 8.16 shows the plaque categorization based on ultrasound images described by Bock and Lusby.

A multicenter European study (European Carotid Plaque Study Group 1995) showed that the echogenicity on the B-mode image was inversely related to the content of soft tissue (including hemorrhage or lipid) and directly related to the presence of calcification. The plaques were also described as being homogeneous or heterogeneous. Irregularity of the plaque surface was not found to relate well to the presence of ulceration.

These and many other studies over recent years suggest that the most useful quality of the B-mode appearance of a plaque is the proportion of hypoechoic areas or

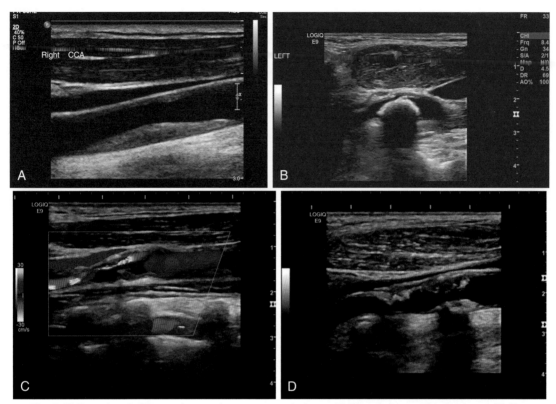

Fig. 8.17 Examples of different ultrasound appearances of plaque. (A) Smooth homogeneous plaque. (B) Predominantly hyperechoic calcified plaque with shadowing seen behind the plaque. (C) Heterogeneous plaque with hypoechoic areas suggesting possible areas of lipid pool or intraplaque hemorrhage. (D) Irregular heterogeneous plaque with areas of calcification demonstrated by shadowing behind the plaque. *CCA,* Common carotid artery.

areas of low echogenicity within the plaque. Clearly the appearance of a plaque is dependent on the scanner controls being set to give an optimal image. Several research centers have used computer-assisted image analysis methods in an attempt to quantify features in images of plaques objectively (Gronholdt et al. 2001; Fosse et al. 2006).

Fig. 8.17 demonstrates the ultrasound appearance of a range of hypoechoic and hyperechoic plaques, with both heterogeneous and homogeneous appearances. Fig. 8.18 shows an example of a stenosis with an unusual web appearance with minimal plaque seen, which may be due to an internal flap or tear. In Fig. 8.19 images of plaques with crater-like defects can be seen that have the appearance of an ulcer on (a) a B-mode image with (b) associated CTA image. Fig. 8.19C gives an example of how power Doppler imaging can help identify flow within the crater.

The Guidelines of the European Society for Vascular Surgery (Naylor ESVS 2018) have not included plaque morphology as a feature to use when selecting symptomatic patients who would benefit from surgery. These guidelines have, however, suggested plaque echolucency may confer an increased risk, along with other features, in asymptomatic patient with 60% to 99% stenosis. With further research, plaque morphology may play a greater role in patient selection for CEA, but currently the degree of narrowing and symptoms are the main features that impact clinical decision making.

COMMENT

Large areas of atheroma will often be seen in the origin of an occluded internal carotid artery and, if the occlusion is long-standing, the occluded internal carotid artery may appear much smaller as its lumen contracts over time (see Fig. 8.20). The ICA can sometimes be seen to move to and fro, laterally in time with arterial pulsation as the flow abruptly encounters the occlusion.

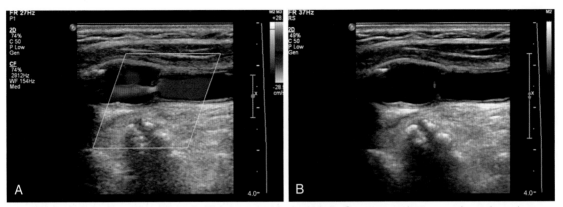

Fig. 8.18 Color flow (A) and B-mode (B) images at the carotid bulb. On rare occasions, stenosis can have the appearance of a thin web with minimal plaque seen. It is not always clear if this is a true plaque, intimal tear or flap.

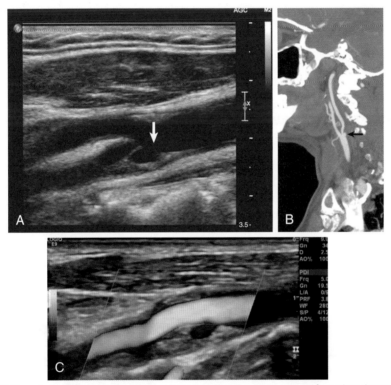

Fig. 8.19 (A) B-mode image of plaque with a crater that has the appearance of an ulcer *(arrow)* confirmed on (B) computed tomography angiogram image *(arrow)*. (C) Power Doppler image of another plaque with the appearance of a crater showing flow within the crater.

COLOR IMAGING

Normal Appearance

Flow in normal carotid arteries is pulsatile, with forward flow present throughout the cardiac cycle. With the appropriate PRF/scale selected, color should continually fill the vessel lumen up to the walls and the PSV should be represented by a color near to the top of the color scale. For some patients, it may be necessary to optimize the PRF/scale from the pre-set value. For younger patients

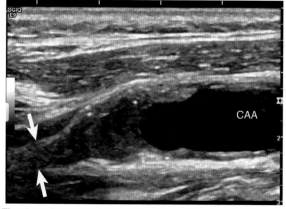

Fig. 8.20 A long-standing internal carotid artery (ICA) occlusion. *Arrows* show ICA walls. *CCA,* Common carotid artery.

this often involves an increase in PRF and for older patients, a decrease. The flow usually appears more pulsatile in the ECA than in the ICA and CCA. At the bifurcation, changes in the vessel geometry often lead to areas of flow reversal within the bifurcation, on the opposite side of the vessel to the ECA origin, giving the normal appearance seen in Chapter 5 (see Figs. 5.10 and 5.11).

Abnormal Appearance

The lack of color filling to the vessel wall may indicate the presence of atheroma. However, it is important to ensure that filling defects are not due to a poor Doppler angle, inappropriately high PRF/scale or high-pass filter setting, or the presence of an image artifact preventing the color from being displayed. Fig. 8.21A shows a color flow image of a proximal ICA, which has an area with no color filling giving the appearance of a hypoechoic (echo

lucent) plaque. However, the apparent absence of flow here is due to a poor angle of insonation of 90° resulting in no flow detection (see Fig 4.10). Even if the scale/PRF is lowered as seen in Fig. 8.21B, to enable detection of low flow, the flow is still not detected due to the poor angle of insonation. However, when the angle of insonation is optimized (Fig. 8.21C), flow can now be detected in this area, ruling out the presence of a large hypoechoic plaque. The area of flow reversal seen in this minimally diseased CCA origin (Fig. 8.21C) is due to local hemodynamics seen in the carotid bulb and is a common finding (see Figs. 5.10 and 5.11) in normal or minimally diseased ICAs. It is therefore essential when an area of poor color filling is seen, to ensure the angle of insonation and PRF/scale are appropriately optimized. Once the image has to be optimized, if a filling defect is still present at the vessel wall, where atheroma is not apparent on the B-mode image, this would indicate an area of hypoechoic atheroma.

The angle of insonation is also very important when imaging in transverse section, and the sonographer should ensure that the flow is being imaged at an angle of less than 90° by tilting the probe toward or away from the flow to enable good color filling (see Fig. 4.7).

Increased velocity within a stenosis usually causes a change in the color displayed on the image, often associated with aliasing (Fig. 8.22B yellow arrow) and sometimes with flow recirculation (Fig. 8.22B orange arrow). The color flow image can help to locate the area of greatest narrowing within a diseased segment of a vessel, which should then be investigated with the spectral Doppler (Fig. 8.22B). Velocity measurements in the CCA (Fig. 8.22A) and ICA (Fig. 8.22B) can be made to

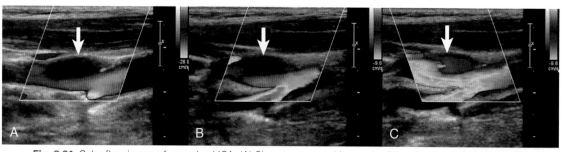

Fig. 8.21 Color flow image of a proximal ICA. (A) Shows an area with no color filling *(arrow)* giving the appearance of a hypoechoic (echo lucent) plaque that is actually due to a poor angle of insonation of 90° resulting in no flow detection. (B) PRF/scale is lowered, to enable detection of low flow, the flow is still not detected due to the poor angle of insonation. (C) The angle of insonation is optimized, flow can now be detected in this area, ruling out the presence of a large hypoechoic plaque. *ICA*; Internal carotid artery; *PRF*, pulse repetition frequency.

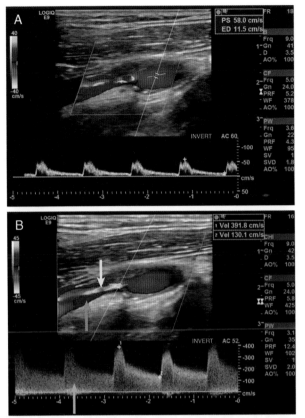

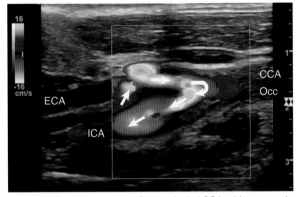

Fig. 8.23 Color flow image of an occluded CCA with antegrade flow seen in the ICA, filling via retrograde flow in the proximal ECA and an ECA branch. *Arrows* indicate the direction of flow. *CCAOcc,* Common carotid artery occlusion; *ECA,* external carotid artery; *ICA,* internal carotid artery.

Fig. 8.22 Color flow images and velocity waveforms from (A) the distal common carotid artery and (B) within the stenosis in the proximal internal carotid artery in the presence of an ICA stenosis. Velocity measurements show a PSV of 58 cm/s in the CCA and a PSV in the ICA of 392 cm/s, ICA PSV/CCA PSV ratio of 6.7, and ICA PSV/CCA EDV ratio of 34 suggesting a narrowing of ≥90%. (B) Also shows increased spectral broadening due to the stenosis with the loss of the "window" under the spectrum. (Aliasing: *yellow arrow,* flow recirculation: *orange arrow,* spectral broadening/loss of "window": *green arrow*).

assist with quantifying the degree of narrowing and this will be discussed later in the chapter. High-velocity jets may be seen within and just beyond a stenosis, and the path of the flow may no longer be parallel to the vessel wall. In this case, the color image allows more accurate angle correction for velocity measurements. An area of flow reversal may be seen distal to a stenosis where the vessel lumen opens up again beyond the narrowing (see Ch. 5 and Fig. 8.22B orange arrow). Turbulent flow may also be seen beyond a stenosis (Ch. 5). The complete absence of color filling within a vessel could indicate that the vessel is occluded, but this should be confirmed by optimizing the color controls for detection of low-velocity

flow (reducing the scale to ≤10 cm/s and adjusting the wall filter) to rule out the presence of a very tight stenosis somewhere along the vessel. The apparent lack of color filling within the CCA or ICA during diastole may indicate high-resistance flow due to an occlusion or tight stenosis distal to that point. Spectral Doppler should be used to confirm the absence of diastolic flow, and both color and spectral Doppler should be used to investigate the distal vessels carefully. It is also important to understand the difference between the concepts of subocclusion, often called string sign (Fig. 8.12A) and underperfusion (Fig. 8.12B), as surgery is often not possible for subocclusion but maybe possible in cases of underperfusion. With underperfusion, the ICA lumen has become small due to a low pressure resulting from a proximal critical stenosis. In a subocclusion there is a very narrow channel of flow in the center of the vessel, surrounded by diseased vessel wall with no endpoint to the diseased vessel wall seen below the jaw line. Doppler waveforms often show a high-resistance, very low flow or no net flow waveform. In underperfusion, the lumen appears larger than a subocclusion but collapsed down compared to a normal vessel, and there is color filling of the lumen to the walls with a damped flow waveform shape.

Color flow imaging also has the potential to detect collateral pathways that have developed in the presence of occlusion or severe stenosis. Fig. 8.23 shows an image of an occluded CCA with a patent ICA filling via retrograde flow in the proximal ECA that is filling via retrograde flow in an proximal ECA branch. The presence of this collateral pathway seen on the color flow image will help to confirm the presence of the CCA occlusion, indicated by the absence of flow detected in the CCA, and the patency of the ICA. Interpreting this image can be challenging due to the path of the flow changing within the image, resulting in changes in the angle of insonation at different locations within the vessel; however, careful consideration of this will enable interpretation. Arrows displayed in Fig. 8.23 show the path of the flow in the vessels with the area of blue on the right side of the image showing the flow changing direction, at the bifurcation, due to the CCA occlusion.

SPECTRAL DOPPLER WAVEFORMS

Normal appearance

Spectral Doppler recordings obtained from the ECA show a higher-resistance flow pattern with a pulsatile waveform shape and low diastolic flow (Fig. 8.9C) compared with the low-resistance waveform shape seen in the ICA (Fig. 8.9B). The normal CCA waveform (Fig. 8.9A) has a shape somewhere between that of the ICA and the ECA. The PSVs seen in the carotid arteries depend on the relative size of the vessel but are typically between 50 and 90 cm/s, although it may be higher in younger people. The flow profiles in the normal bifurcation seen in color flow imaging (see Fig. 5.10) will affect the spectral Doppler waveform shapes detected in the ICA origin, which may appear disturbed or demonstrate areas of reverse flow. Distal to the bifurcation and carotid bulb, the waveform shapes should no longer appear disturbed. However, where spikes are seen on the ICA waveform, due to flow disturbances generated in the carotid bulb (see Ch. 5), the maximum PSV should be measured without including these spikes as shown in Fig. 8.24. Fig. 8.24 shows appropriate measurement caliper location, and the arrow shows a spike due to flow disturbance in the bulb.

Abnormal Appearance

The presence of a narrowing within the carotid arteries will lead to an increase in the velocity of the blood across the stenosis. Once the vessel is narrowed by a ≥50% reduction in diameter, velocity measurements are used for quantifying the degree of stenosis. This can be measured using spectral Doppler. The increase in velocity is related to the degree of narrowing (see Ch. 5). These velocity changes can be used to grade the degree of narrowing. The Doppler waveforms obtained within

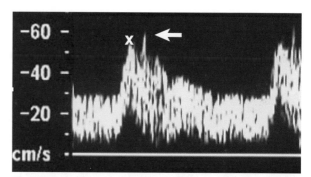

Fig. 8.24 An ICA waveform with a spike *(arrow)* seen due to flow disturbances generated in the carotid bulb. The maximum ICA PSV should be measured without including the spike (as shown by the *cross*). *ICA*, Internal carotid artery; *PSV*, peak systolic velocity.

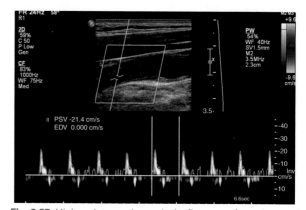

Fig. 8.25 High-resistance, low-velocity flow waveform detected in an internal carotid artery proximal to ipsilateral distal disease such as a middle cerebral artery occlusion. With these low velocities it can be difficult to obtain good color filling on the image even with low PRF/scale settings. *PRF*, Pulse repetition frequency

or just beyond a significant stenosis usually demonstrate an increase in spectral broadening (Fig. 8.22B) seen as a loss of a clear window under the peak systolic flow waveform.

Unusually low velocities can indicate the presence of disease proximal or distal to the site at which the Doppler recording is made. High-resistance waveforms, with an absence of flow during diastole, obtained from the CCA may indicate a severe ICA stenosis or occlusion (see Fig. 8.10B). Fig. 8.25 shows another example of a high-resistance waveform, obtained from an ICA proximal to distal disease, such as an ipsilateral MCA occlusion. A reversal of flow during the whole of diastole in the carotid arteries (Fig. 8.26) may relate to a heart

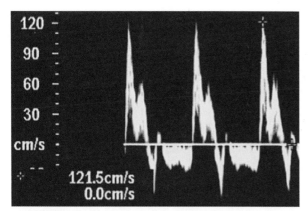

Fig. 8.26 Common carotid artery waveform showing reverse diastolic flow in the presence of aortic valve regurgitation.

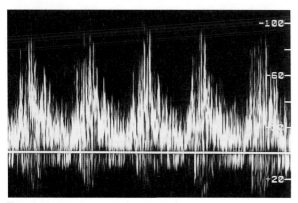

Fig. 8.27 Doppler recording demonstrating turbulent flow beyond a significant stenosis.

problem, such as aortic valve regurgitation (Malaterre et al. 2001). In this case this abnormal appearance will be seen in both the left and right carotid arteries and not be associated with only one side. The waveform detected distal to a very severe, flow-limiting stenosis will often demonstrate turbulent flow with an increased systolic rise time (Fig. 8.27). Fig. 8.28 shows a Doppler waveform from a CCA in the presence of an ipsilateral significant brachiocephalic artery stenosis, demonstrating damped flow with poststenotic turbulence, as indicated by spectral broadening. Proximal left common carotid and brachiocephalic disease can often be difficult to image; however, the presence of abnormal waveforms can indicate the need for alternative imaging to assess for proximal disease.

These various abnormal waveform shapes can give the sonographer useful clues as to the presence of significant disease proximal or distal to the site of the Doppler recording. The total absence of flow within a vessel, as demonstrated by color flow imaging, can be confirmed using spectral Doppler. However, it is sometimes possible to pick up low-velocity signals, due to wall thump, at a point just within the occluded vessel. The presence of small veins in the area of the bifurcation can also produce misleading Doppler signals, as venous flow in the neck can appear pulsatile.

COMMENT

It is possible for the carotid artery bifurcation to appear normal on B-mode and color imaging but for the spectral waveforms to appear abnormal due to disease proximal or distal to the bifurcation.

SELECTION OF TREATMENT FOR CAROTID ARTERY DISEASE

The results from two large multicenter trials, the NASCET Collaborators (NASCET 1991, 1998) and the European Carotid Surgery Trialists' Collaborative Group (ECST 1998) have had a large influence on the management of atherosclerotic carotid artery disease. These trials compared the benefits of carotid surgery, which carries some risk of mortality and morbidity, with the best medical treatment for patients with symptomatic carotid artery disease. The carotid artery disease was quantified using angiography (which has now routinely been replaced by CTA or MRA). However, the method used to report the degree of narrowing from an angiogram differed between the European and North American trials. In the ECST trial, the degree of stenosis was measured by comparing the residual lumen diameter with the estimated diameter of the carotid bulb, whereas the NASCET trial compared the residual lumen diameter with the diameter of the normal distal ICA, as shown in Fig. 8.29. Using these two different methods can lead to significant differences in grading the disease. For example, the narrowing in Fig. 8.29 would be reported as a 70% diameter reduction by the European method but as only a 50% reduction by the North American method. Fig. 8.29 also gives the approximate equivalent degree of stenosis, measured (from the same stenoses) using the different methods employed by the NASCET and ECST trials. Fig. 8.30A shows an ultrasound B-mode image of a plaque with a diameter measurement made using the NASCET method, by comparing the lumen diameter with the ICA diameter distal to the carotid bulb. Fig. 8.30B shows the

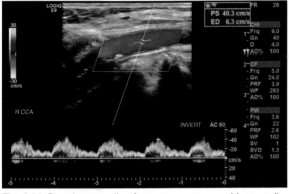

Fig. 8.28 Doppler recording from a common carotid artery distal to an ipsilateral significant brachiocephalic artery stenosis. This demonstrates a damped waveform shape with poststenotic turbulence due to the proximal disease.

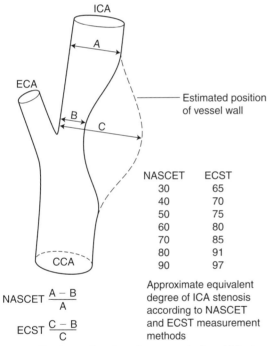

NASCET	ECST
30	65
40	70
50	75
60	80
70	85
80	91
90	97

$$\text{NASCET } \frac{A - B}{A}$$

$$\text{ECST } \frac{C - B}{C}$$

Approximate equivalent degree of ICA stenosis according to NASCET and ECST measurement methods

Fig. 8.29 The North American Symptomatic Carotid Endarterectomy Trial Collaborators *(NASCET)* and European Carotid Surgery Trialists' Collaborative Group *(ECST)* trials used different methods of reporting the degree of narrowing seen on carotid angiograms. *CCA*, Common carotid artery; *ICA*, internal carotid artery; *ECA*, external carotid artery. (Reprinted with permission from Elsevier. Donnan et al. Surgery for prevention of stroke. *The Lancet*, 1998, 351: 1372–1373.)

same plaque with the diameter measurement made with the ECST method, giving a significantly different result from the NASCET method used in Fig. 8.30A. When quoting diameter reduction measurement in the ICA, it

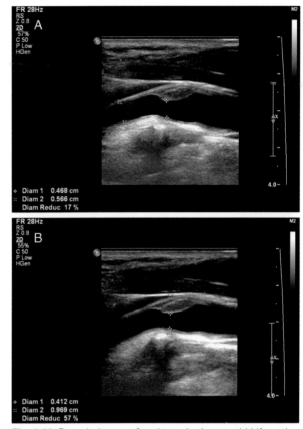

Fig. 8.30 B-mode image of a plaque in the carotid bifurcation showing a diameter reduction measurement made using (A) the North American Symptomatic Carotid Endarterectomy Trial Collaborators (NASCET) method and (B) European Carotid Surgery Trialists' Collaboration Group (ECST) method.

is essential to specify if the NASCET or ECST method of measurement has been used. The Joint recommendation for reporting carotid ultrasound investigations in the UK (Oates et al. 2009) is based on NASCET measurements. However, it is possible, in a patient with a large carotid bulb, for the bulb to contain a large plaque and hence a large plaque volume without it causing a significant stenosis, for example <50%, by the NASCET method. In this situation it is important to describe this in the scan report, and it can be useful to quote an ECST method estimation, clearly specifying that the ECST method has been used, as this may affect the choice of treatment, especially if the patient is symptomatic.

The difference in methods used to grade the degree of narrowing has made the comparison of the results from the two trials complicated. The ECST study showed that surgery reduced the risk of stroke in patients with

[ECST]80%–99% stenosis. However, the NASCET reported similar results for patients with [NASCET]70%–99%, which is equivalent to an [ECST]80%–99% stenosis. Rothwell et al. (2003) remeasured the ECST angiograms using the NASCET method and, analyzing the results of both trials together, concluded that CEA was of marginal benefit in symptomatic patients with a [NASCET]50%–69% and was highly beneficial in those with a [NASCET] ≥70% stenosis but without near occlusion. Rothwell et al. (2003) indicate that it would be necessary to operate on about six patients to prevent one stroke; however, surgical procedures and patient selection may have improved, thus reducing this number. The trials suggest that surgery did not provide any significant benefit in patients with the string sign, near occlusion.

An alternative treatment for significant carotid disease is carotid angioplasty and stenting (CAS). Stents are expandable mesh tubes that can be used to keep a diseased vessel patent. Although stent placement does not involve a general anesthetic, sometimes used in CEA, there is a potential risk of stroke during the procedure. CAS may be an appropriate treatment in a specific group of high-risk patients (Naylor et al. 2018).

The NASCET and ECST trials were reported over 20 years ago since when medical treatment has developed, the quality of surgical intervention has been improved and audited along with a fuller understanding of the benefit of rapid diagnosis, review, and intervention. Large stroke centers have been established, where outcomes are reviewed. The algorithm shown in Fig. 8.31 (Aboyans et al. 2017, Naylor et al. 2018) shows how the degree of stenosis and symptoms may be used to judge the risk/benefit to a patient for either CEA + BMT (best medical therapy) or BMT alone. For symptomatic within <6 months having a 70% to 99% (NASCET) stenosis, CEA and BMT is recommended. For symptomatic patients within <6 months having a 50% to 69% (NASCET) stenosis, CEA + BMT should be considered. The risk/benefit for surgery may vary depending on many factors, for example, on the life expectancy of the patient, patient's general health, the local perioperative stroke/death rates, and developments in BMT. CAS can be considered in patients at high risk with CEA.

A trial studying patients with significant (60%–99%) asymptomatic stenosis, the Asymptomatic Carotid Atherosclerosis Study (ACAS) (1995) showed limited benefit of surgery in this group. Redgrave & Rothwell (2007) reviewed the evidence for medical and surgical intervention in these patients and concluded that the absolute benefit from endarterectomy for asymptomatic carotid stenosis is small but can sometimes be justified in men. As the benefits for CEA are small, screening for asymptomatic disease is not recommended in the Guidelines of the European Society of Vascular Surgery (ESVS) (Naylor et al. 2018). Future developments in patient selection may enable the group of patients at high risk of stroke to be more closely targeted.

COMMENT

It is important that the sonographer is up to date with the criteria for selection of treatment for patients with carotid artery stenosis as the ultrasound scan results will form an important part of the diagnostic process.

GRADING THE DISEASE

Imaging

Angiographic grading of carotid artery disease, as with other arterial disease, is described in terms of diameter reduction. Therefore, as ultrasound criteria were developed by comparing with angiography as the gold standard, ultrasound grading of stenoses is also typically described in terms of diameter reduction. Table 8.2 gives the percentage area reduction associated with a given percentage diameter reduction, assuming a symmetrical lumen reduction; however, these values are not correct in the presence of eccentric disease. B-mode imaging is the most appropriate method to evaluate the degree of narrowing, if the degree of lumen diameter reduction is less than 50%. However, if disease is eccentric, it is possible to overestimate the degree of narrowing if the atheroma lies on the anterior or posterior wall when imaged longitudinally. It is equally possible to underestimate the degree of narrowing on a longitudinal image if the plaque is situated on the lateral walls. Fig. 8.32 shows the change in appearance of the plaque when imaged in different scan planes. Therefore, the diseased vessel should be visualized in transverse section first, in order to select the optimal longitudinal imaging plane, especially in the presence of eccentric plaques, although possible scan planes are limited (see Fig. 8.6). Fig. 8.33 is a schematic diagram showing a range of possible under- and overestimations of the disease when imaging eccentric disease in longitudinal section alone.

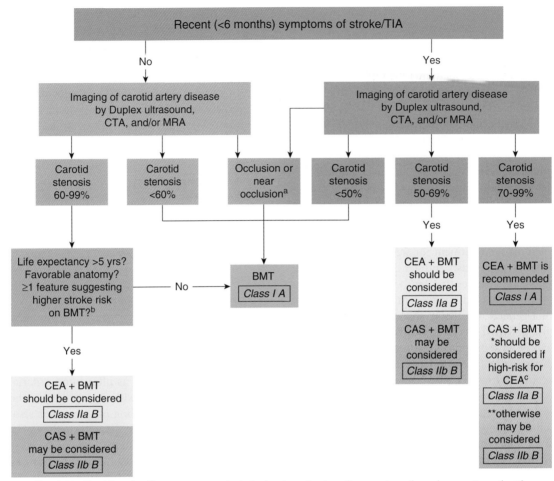

Fig. 8.31 Algorithm detailing management strategies in patients with symptomatic and asymptomatic atherosclerotic extracranial carotid artery stenosis. *Green boxes* denote level 1 recommendations, *yellow boxes* denote level 11a and 11b recommendations. *BMT*, Best medical therapy; *CAS*, carotid artery stenting; *CEA*, carotid endarterectomy; *CTA*, computer tomography angiography; *MRA*, magnetic resonance angiography; *TIA*, transient ischemic attack. (Aboyans et al. 2018) (Reproduced with permission.)

TABLE 8.2 **Relationship Between Diameter Reduction and Cross-Sectional Area Assuming a Concentric Stenosis**	
Diameter Reduction (%)	**Cross-Sectional Area Reduction (%)**
30	50
50	75
70	90

The percentage diameter reduction can be estimated from diameter measurements as follows:

$$\% \text{ diameter reduction} = (1-[\text{diameter of patent lumen}/\text{total diameter of vessel}]) \times 100$$

Scanners have the facility to enable both diameter and area reduction measurements to be made manually from the B-mode image, and it is essential not to confuse these two methods (see Table 8.2).

Color flow imaging and power Doppler can also help in identifying any lumen reduction (see Fig. 8.34). It is

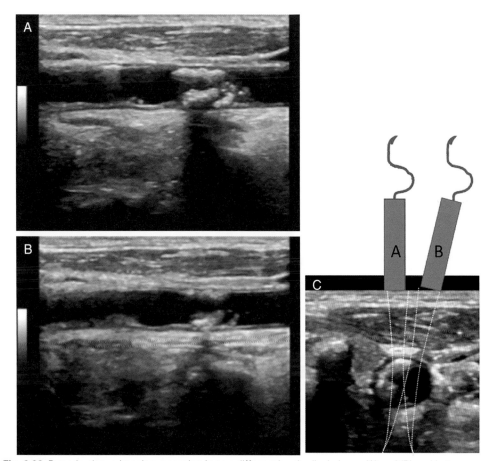

Fig. 8.32 B-mode plaque imaging, scanning in two different longitudinal planes (A) and (B) and in transverse (C). In the longitudinal images (A) and (B) the stenosis appears very severe (A) and less severe (B). The transverse view (C) shows the approximate position of the beam (*white lines A* and *yellow lines B*) of these longitudinal scans.

possible to obtain a color flow image in longitudinal and transverse section, and this may help in estimating the degree of narrowing, but there are potential pitfalls. Spurious flow voids can be created due to a poor angle of insonation or inappropriate PRF or filter settings, which may lead to an overestimate of the degree of narrowing. If the color gain is set too high, it is possible for the color to appear to "bleed" out of the vessel lumen or over the plaque, and this can lead to an underestimate of the degree of narrowing.

Spectral Doppler

As the quantity of atheroma in the vessel increases, it becomes more difficult to estimate the degree of narrowing from the B-mode image, especially in the presence of calcified or hypoechoic atheroma. However, velocity criteria are used to grade the degree of stenosis once the vessel becomes narrowed by a ≥50% reduction in diameter. Over the years, several criteria have been produced for grading carotid artery disease, many of which have been published, by comparing Doppler measurements with those of angiography, which has its own limitations, as the gold standard.

Velocity criteria for grading carotid stenoses are based on the PSV and EDV in the ICA, and the ratio of the PSV in the ICA to that in the CCA. Unlike the grading of stenosis in other parts of the arterial system, where there is often a proximal segment of normal vessel that can be used to calculate a velocity ratio, the geometry of the carotid bulb makes the situation less straightforward. The

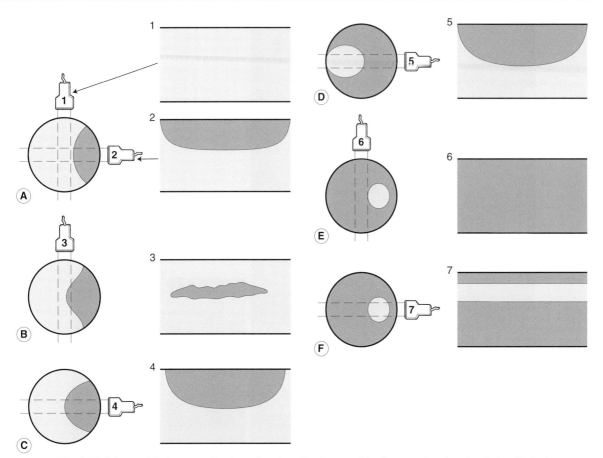

Fig. 8.33 It is possible to overestimate and underestimate eccentric disease when imaging in longitudinal section. The schematic diagrams show examples of disease imaged in transverse and longitudinal section from the numbered transducer positions. (A) An area of atheroma may not be seen in one longitudinal plane *(1)* and may appear more significant in another *(2)*. (B) Atheroma on the lateral walls may protrude into the center of the vessel and give the appearance of atheroma floating in the vessel. (C, D) These longitudinal images give a similar appearance despite very different degrees of narrowing. (E, F) The longitudinal image may give the appearance of the vessel being occluded (E) or stenosed (F) depending on the imaging plane used.

ratio of the PSV in the ICA to that in the CCA will partly depend on the relative dimensions of the CCA and ICA, and this is further complicated by the variable geometry of the carotid bulb. The presence of a large branch in the form of the ECA also complicates matters. Using a combination of absolute velocity measurements and velocity ratios potentially reduces the pitfalls of using absolute velocity criteria alone. For example, an increase in PSV can arise due to hypertension, age-related changes in vessel wall compliance, or increased flow to supply a collateral pathway. However, an increase in velocity would be seen in both the CCA and ICA, and the absence of a significant velocity increase along the vessel would reassure

the sonographer that there was no significant evidence of a stenosis. Conversely, an abnormal velocity ratio in the presence of low velocities, possibly due to low cardiac output, may help to identify a stenosis.

COMMENT

Some centers choose to overcome angle-dependent variations in velocity recordings by using a fixed insonation angle of 60°. In practice this may not always be possible. Aiming to take measurements with an angle between 45° and 60° is a practical solution.

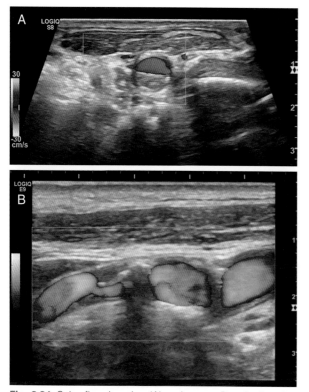

Fig. 8.34 Color flow imaging (A) and power Doppler imaging (B) can help identify the diameter reduction (A) in transverse section and (B) longitudinal section.

Table 8.3 shows a summary of reporting criteria given in the recommendations for carotid ultrasound investigations in the UK (Oates et al. 2009) and US (Grant et al. 2003). The table is color coded to show the source of the different velocity grading criteria. These criteria can be used in conjunction with the appearance of the stenosis on B-mode and color Doppler ultrasound. Oates et al. (2009) also provide advice on measurement technique and situations where caution is required in quantifying disease using these criteria. Table 8.3 includes the St Mary's ratio, the ICA PSV to CCA EDV ratio, published by Nicolaides et al. (1996), with the advice that this ratio should not be used in the absence of CCA diastolic flow or the presence of reversal of CCA diastolic flow, for example, due to aortic valve disease (see Fig. 8.26). The US recommendations for reporting carotid ultrasound investigations (Grant et al. 2003) include ICA EDV in the velocity criteria, although these have not been included in the UK recommendations (Oates et al. 2009). The criteria listed in Table 8.3

have both been correlated against angiography using the NASCET method of reporting angiographic findings. When reporting results from a carotid ultrasound scan, it is important to specify whether any ≥50% stenosis reported is based on NASCET or ECST measurements. To fit with the velocity criteria in Table 8.3, any diameter reduction measurements made on B-mode should be made using the NASCET method shown in Fig. 8.30A.

Each center should verify its criteria locally by comparing the ultrasound findings with alternative imaging such as CTA or magnetic resonance angiography (MRA). If a department has more than one scanner, it is necessary to check the criteria used on each machine, as different models of scanner may give different results. It is important for sonographers to understand how the results of their scans are used by the surgical or medical teams that have requested them and that these teams are aware of the method the sonographers use to define the degree of disease. It is also important that other departments involved in carotid artery imaging, for example, radiology providing MRA or CTA imaging, use similar measurements methods (e.g., NASCET) when comparing results with ultrasound imaging.

COMBINING B-MODE, COLOR IMAGING, AND SPECTRAL DOPPLER INFORMATION

The information obtained from all three modalities should be used to estimate the degree of narrowing, as all modalities have their strengths and weaknesses. Fig. 8.35 gives an example of how this can be done. Fig. 8.35A shows a transverse image of a diseased ICA, with evidence of atheroma, part of which appears calcified (shown by the arrow). This image suggests a diameter reduction of 50% to 70%. Fig. 8.35B shows a longitudinal image of the same vessel with an absence of flow seen in the proximal ICA. However, when the same vessel is imaged in a different longitudinal plane (Fig. 8.35C), the flow can now be seen within the vessel. Although the vessel lumen appears to be only slightly narrowed on this color image (Fig. 8.35C), the presence of a velocity increase, demonstrated by aliasing, should alert the sonographer to the possible presence of a more significant narrowing. Spectral Doppler velocity measurement (Fig. 8.35D) gives a PSV of 200 cm/s and an EDV of 75 cm/s in the ICA. Using the velocity criteria of Grant et al. (2003) (Table 8.3) these velocity measurements

TABLE 8.3 Summary of reporting criteria given in recommendations for carotid ultrasound investigations in the UK (Oates et al. 2009) and USA (Grant et al. 2003)

Percentage Stenosis Diameter reduction (NASCET)	Internal Carotid Peak Systolic Velocity cm/s	Peak Cystolic Velocity Ratio ICA$_{PSV}$/CCA$_{PSV}$	Internal Carotid Artery End Diastolic Velocity cm/s	St Mary's Ratio[‡] ICA$_{PSV}$/CCA$_{EDV}$
<50	<125[*]	<2[*]	<40	<8
50–59	>125-230	2–4[*]	40-100	8–10
60–69				11–13
70–79	>230[*]	>4[*]	>100	14–21
80–89				22–29
>90	>400[†]	>5[†]		>30
Near occlusion	High, low, or string flow	Variable	Variable	Variable
Occlusion	No flow detected	Not applicable	Not applicable	Not applicable

NASCET, North American Symptomatic Carotid Endarterectomy Trial Collaborators; *ICA*, internal carotid artery; *PSV*, peak systolic velocity; *CCA*, common carotid artery; *EDV*, end-diastolic velocity.
[*]Grant et al. (2003).
[†]Filis et al. (2002).
[‡]Nicolaides et al. (1996).

Color code:

	Criteria recommended by Grant et al (2003) and Oates et al (2009)
	Criteria recommended by Grant et al (2003)
	Criteria recommended by Oates et al (2009)

would indicate a narrowing of 50% to 69% (NASCET) diameter reduction. An ICA PSV to CCA PSV ratio should be measured to support this conclusion. Fig. 8.22 shows how absolute velocities can be combined with velocity ratios to quantify a stenosis.

By using the appearance of both B-mode and color images in transverse and a variety of longitudinal imaging planes, along with velocity measurements and velocity ratios, the sonographer is able to estimate the degree of narrowing. There will be situations where the different grading criteria may give conflicting results. For example, in the presence of a tight stenosis or occlusion, the velocities may be raised throughout in the contralateral CCA and ICA, if they are providing collateral flow. However, if the ICA PSV/CCA PSV ratio remains below 2, this would indicate that no significant stenosis is present on that side. This makes the ICA PSV/CCA PSV ratio especially useful in the presence of contralateral or bilateral disease or situations that may lead to increased velocities that do not relate to stenosis. There

will, however, be occasions in which imaging and velocity measurement are limited or give conflicting results that cannot be explained, preventing the sonographer from making a quantification of the severity of the disease, and this should be made clear in the scan report.

PREFORMING CEA ON THE BASIS OF DUPLEX ULTRASOUND ALONE

When ultrasound is to be used to select patients for surgery, without the use of any other alternative imaging, it is essential that at least two independent sonographers have undertaken a scan of the patient and that their findings are in agreement. The examination and report should cover the points listed in Box 8.2. It is also important that the final duplex scan is within 1 day of surgery in case there have been any changes in the diseases such as progression or occlusion. An area that is sometimes overlooked is the identification of a tongue of posterior wall plaque extending along the wall of the

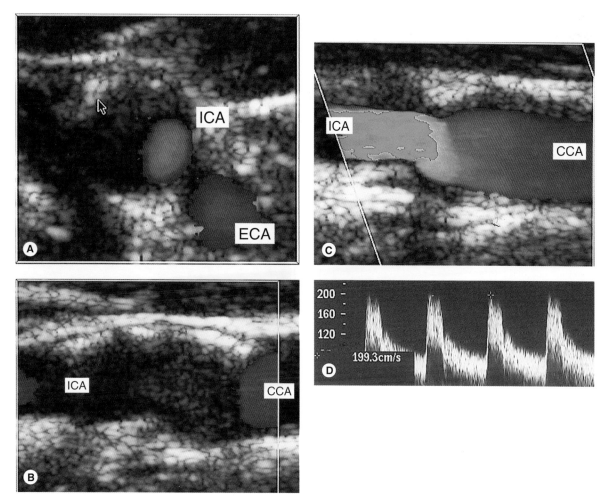

Fig. 8.35 A combination of B-mode, color flow imaging, and spectral Doppler can be used to assess carotid disease. (A) A transverse image of a diseased internal carotid artery *(ICA)*, with atheroma, part of which appears calcified *(arrow)*, with the appearance of a 50%–70% diameter reduction (external carotid artery, *ECA*). (B) A longitudinal image of the vessel with an absence of flow seen in the proximal ICA. (C) When the vessel is imaged in a different plane, flow can be seen within the vessel. Although the vessel lumen appears to be only slightly narrowed in this plane, a velocity increase, demonstrated by aliasing, is seen. (D) Spectral Doppler velocity measurement gives a peak systolic velocity of 200 cm/s in the ICA, indicating a 50%–69% (North American Symptomatic Carotid Endarterectomy Trial Collaborators: NASCET) diameter reduction.

ICA. It is useful for the surgeon to know if this is present as it may require more extensive dissection than anticipated.

PROBLEMS ENCOUNTERED IN IMAGING CAROTID ARTERY FLOW

Calcified Atheroma

Extensive calcified plaque within the carotid bifurcation leading to significant shadowing on the image can cause problems with grading the disease. Calcification may prevent any B-mode, color, or spectral Doppler information from being obtained from within the vessel. The initial appearance of the absence of flow detected by the color flow imaging may mislead the sonographer into thinking that the vessel is occluded. However, the presence of bright echoes on the anterior wall and an absence of echoes below this should suggest calcification (see Fig. 8.36). Images of the vessel distal to the calcification should be obtained and the presence of flow established.

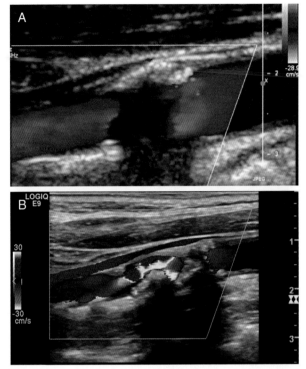

Fig. 8.36 Calcification of the anterior arterial wall can prevent B-mode imaging, color flow imaging, and spectral Doppler recordings within the calcified segment of vessel. (A) Color flow imaging does not suggest a significant change in velocity across the calcified segment. (B) Marked flow disturbance (increased velocity and flow recirculation) is seen beyond the area of calcification, suggesting a significant stenosis at the site of the calcification.

If the distal vessel can be seen clearly, with no evidence of further calcification, but no flow is detected even when the scanner is optimized to detect low-velocity flow, the vessel is probably occluded. If flow is detected distal to a calcified area, the spectral Doppler waveform may assist in grading the degree of stenosis present within the calcified area. It is also important to image the carotid artery from anterior medial and medial-posterior positions as there may be a clearer view.

The presence of extensive calcified atheroma may not necessarily relate to a significant narrowing. If the calcified atheroma only extends a short way along the vessel wall, the presence of a normal Doppler waveform beyond it would suggest that it was not causing a severe stenosis. If, however, the calcification extends for more than 1 cm, a normal waveform beyond it cannot be used to indicate the absence of any significant narrowing, as normal flow waveforms and velocities can be established within a short distance distal to a stenosis. If an abnormal waveform is detected beyond the calcification, the presence of a significant stenosis can be more confidently predicted. High PSV and EDV (Fig. 8.22B) produced by a jet extending beyond a stenosis, poststenotic flow turbulence (Fig. 8.27), or low-velocity, damped flow would all suggest the presence of a significant stenosis. If any doubt about the presence or absence of significant disease remains at the end of the examination, the sonographer should make this clear in the report, as alternative imaging would be required to clarify the degree of narrowing. In cases of less severe calcification, the sonographer may be able to overcome poor imaging by viewing the vessels in a different plane (see Fig. 8. 35).

Vessel Tortuosity

Imaging tortuous vessels can be a problem, as the vessel may not appear in a single plane. Its path may run

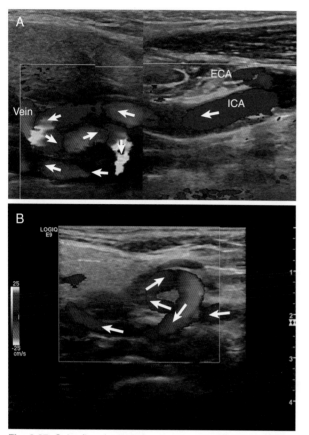

Fig. 8.37 Color flow image of a tortuous internal carotid artery *(ICA)* due to (A) a kink and (B) a loop. *Arrows* show direction of flow. *ECA,* External carotid artery.

parallel to the ultrasound beam, thus producing poor B-mode images of the vessel walls. Color Doppler imaging can be used to assist in following tortuous arteries, but the changing direction of the vessel may require regular changes in the steering angle of the color box to allow the flow to be visualized. Fig. 8.37 shows two examples of tortuous ICAs: (A) a kink and (B) a loop. It is important that these findings should be included in the ultrasound report, in the presence of significant carotid stenosis. Vessel tortuosity may have an impact on plans for surgery, especially if a shunt is required. The end of the shunt may not pass across the kink or loop and could become obstructed against the vessel wall.

Poor Doppler angles may limit the color flow imaging, and in this situation, power Doppler may help to image the vessel and assist in ruling out filling defects in the vessel due to the presence of atheroma.

Imaging Vessels at Depth

In patients with large necks and/or with high carotid bifurcations, clear images of the carotid bifurcation and ICA may be difficult or impossible to obtain. While the carotid bifurcation for most patients typically lies within 3 cm of the skin, deeper arteries pose challenges to standard linear arrays, since their transmit frequency and focusing in the elevation plane will be suboptimal at depth. This may lead to poor B-mode imaging and limitations with color sensitivity, especially in the ICA. It is useful to have a lower-frequency curved array transducer to hand for these patients. The image quality may not have the spatial resolution of high-frequency linear arrays, but the penetration and sensitivity to flow will usually be able to indicate if there is disease and whether there are velocity changes. Manufacturers now also have higher frequency curvilinear arrays optimized to 4 to 5 cm depth and are increasing the availability of matrix arrays that allow more flexible focusing in the elevation plane at a range of depths. Probes capable of imaging at greater depths are also useful to assess the proximal CCAs and brachiocephalic artery and the distal extracranial ICA where indicated.

POSTOPERATIVE CAROTID ARTERY APPEARANCE ON ULTRASOUND

Only a small percentage of patients develop severe recurrent stenosis or occlusion following surgery, and of these, only a few suffer from any symptoms. It has been shown that routine postoperative ultrasound surveillance does not significantly affect patient management, and patients are often rescanned only if symptoms recur. The scan procedure is the same as that already described, but the postoperative appearance differs slightly from the appearance of a normal carotid bifurcation. First, the vessel wall no longer has the double-layer appearance where the plaque has been removed. It is often possible to see a step in the posterior CCA wall at the beginning of the site of the endarterectomy (Fig. 8.38A). A vein or prosthetic patch may be used to close the site of the endarterectomy, as it is thought that this may reduce the risk of early postoperative thrombosis or late restenosis. If a patch has been used to widen the vessel, it will often produce a slightly dilated bifurcation compared to normal. A prosthetic patch produces a brighter echo than a vein patch or adjacent arterial wall, and it can therefore usually be easily seen on the image. It is also normally possible to observe sutures associated with the patch as bright pin-point echoes. Vein patches can be susceptible to rupture whereas prosthetic patches can be susceptible to infection, which can produce a rucked appearance to the patch (Fig. 8.38B). Ultrasound can be used to measure the dimensions of the endarterectomy site and investigate any recurrent disease.

POST CAROTID ARTERY ANGIOPLASTY AND STENTING APPEARANCE ON ULTRASOUND

Ultrasound can also be used to follow up patients who have had a carotid stenosis treated by angioplasty and stenting. Fig. 8.39A shows how with B-mode imaging the stent can be clearly seen within the carotid artery

with evidence of the plaque seen between the stent and the carotid artery wall. Color flow imaging and spectral Doppler (Fig. 8.39B) can be used to assess the residual lumen post stenting and to monitor any restenosis within the stent. One issue that has arisen with ultrasound assessment of stented carotid arteries is that the velocities detected in the stented vessels without significant narrowings are, on average, higher than the velocities seen in normal carotid arteries. Lal et al. (2008) found that velocity criteria developed for native arteries overestimate the degree of in-stent restenosis. It has been suggested that this may be due to the difference in the mechanical properties, specifically the wall compliance, of the stent compared to the native vessel. New velocity criteria, specifically for assessing stented carotid arteries, have been developed, and two of these

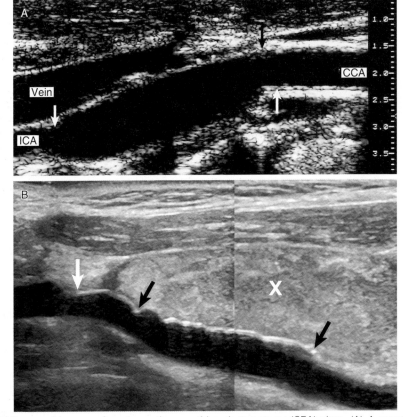

Fig. 8.38 Ultrasound images of postoperative carotid endarterectomy (CEA) sites. (A) A montage image of a CEA site. The *downward-pointing arrows* demonstrate the length of the endarterectomy site. The *upward-pointing arrow* demonstrates the intima-media layer proximal to the endarterectomy site. (B) A rucked CEA patch. The *black arrows* show sutures. The *white arrow* shows the distal extend of the patch, and the X is a large area of hematoma overlying the CEA site. *CCA,* Common carotid artery; *ICA,* internal carotid artery.

(Lal et al. 2008, Zhou et al. 2008) are shown in Table 8.4. Significant restenosis of the stent, especially in the presence of further symptoms, will probably require further treatment.

NONATHEROMATOUS CAROTID ARTERY DISEASES

Nonatheromatous extracranial carotid diseases include aneurysms, CBTs, dissection, and traumatic AV-fistula with the internal jugular vein (IJV), but all are relatively rare. Patients may have a pulsatile swelling in the neck that can be investigated with ultrasound to rule out an aneurysm. The carotid arteries should be scanned along their length, especially in the area of the suspected swelling, and the cross sectional diameter measured. Any unusual appearances relating to the arteries should be reported. In many cases, the "pulsatile swelling" is due to a superficial brachiocephalic bifurcation or carotid bifurcation, often associated with tortuous vessels, leading to the vessel being easily palpated. Ultrasound can be used to monitor aneurysms found by other imaging modalities.

Another possible cause of a pulsatile swelling is the presence of a CBT. The carotid body is a small chemoreceptor organ located within the vessel wall in the posteromedial aspect of the carotid bifurcation and is responsible for detecting blood gases and pH. CBTs, which are also termed chemodectomas, are rare neoplasms with a reported incidence of one in 30,000.

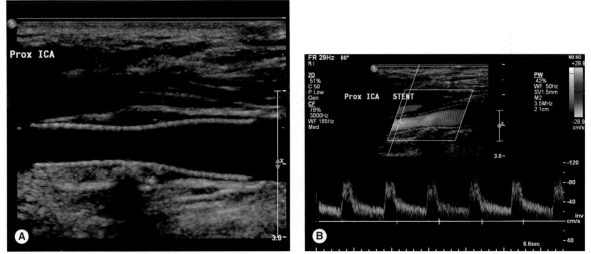

Fig. 8.39 (A) B-mode image showing a carotid artery that has been treated with angioplasty and stenting. (B) Color flow imaging and spectral Doppler can be used to assess the residual lumen post angioplasty and stenting. *ICA*, Internal carotid artery.

TABLE 8.4 **Two Criteria Developed for Assessing Stenosis in Stented Carotid Arteries (ICA PSV Measured From Within Stented Segment)**

Author	Percentage Stenosis Diameter Reduction	ICA PSV (cm/s)	ICA EDV (cm/s)	ICA PSV to CCA PSV Ratio
Lal et al. (2008)	0%–19%	<150[a]		<2.15[a]
	20%–49%	150–219		
	50%–79%	220–339		≥2.7
	80%–99%	≥340		≥4.15
Zhou et al. (2008)	>70%	>300	>90	>4

CCA, Common carotid artery; *EDV*, end-diastolic velocity; *ICA*, internal carotid artery; *PSV*, peak systolic velocity.
[a]PSV and EDV measurements for stented carotid arteries are performed within the stented segments.

However, they make up 65% of all head and neck paragangliomas (Robertson et al. 2019).

As a CBT grows, it causes the ICA and ECA to be splayed apart, and the tumor usually appears highly vascular on color flow imaging (see Fig. 8.40). However, further investigation is required to confirm any ultrasound findings.

Carotid artery wall dissection, which can be due to trauma such as whiplash, can create a false lumen within the carotid arteries (see Fig. 8.41). This may remain patent and be seen as a second flow lumen on color flow imaging. Alternatively, the false lumen may occlude, causing a reduction in the residual vessel lumen or possibly a complete occlusion of the vessel. An intimal flap may be seen on the image as a fine line within the lumen that may move due to the pulsatile blood flow; however, it can be difficult to image.

NORMAL AND ABNORMAL APPEARANCES OF VERTEBRAL ARTERY FLOW

The vertebral artery and vein can be seen between the vertebral processes. The vein lies above the artery, and flow in the artery is normally seen traveling toward the head (cephalad flow) (Figs. 8.13 and 8.42). It is not uncommon to see a larger vertebral artery or higher velocities on one side, usually the left, compared with the other. Occasionally, it may only be possible to visualize one of the vertebral arteries. The Doppler spectrum obtained from the vertebral artery demonstrates

a low-resistance waveform shape with high diastolic flow (Fig. 8.42A). It is not possible to scan the entire length of the vertebral artery because sections of it are obscured by the vertebral processes; however, if indicated, it is sometimes possible to image the vertebral artery origins in the base of the neck, although this can be quite difficult.

Reverse flow (i.e., flow away from the head) in one of the vertebral arteries would suggest subclavian steal syndrome (see Fig. 8.3). Doppler recordings obtained from the ipsilateral distal subclavian artery will appear damped (see Ch. 10), and sometimes it is possible to

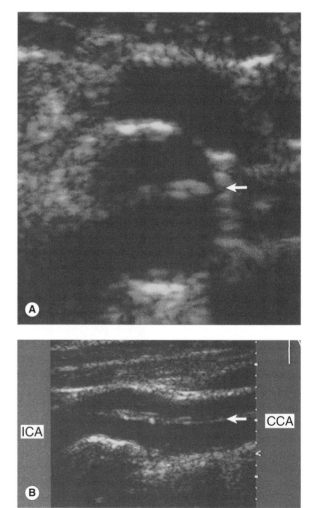

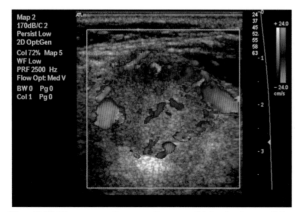

Fig. 8.40 Transverse image of a carotid body tumor lying between the internal carotid artery *(right)* and external carotid artery *(left)*.

Fig. 8.41 B-mode image of a carotid artery wall dissection *(arrows)* showing a false lumen imaged in transverse section (A) and in longitudinal section (B). *CCA*, Common carotid artery; *ICA*, internal carotid artery.

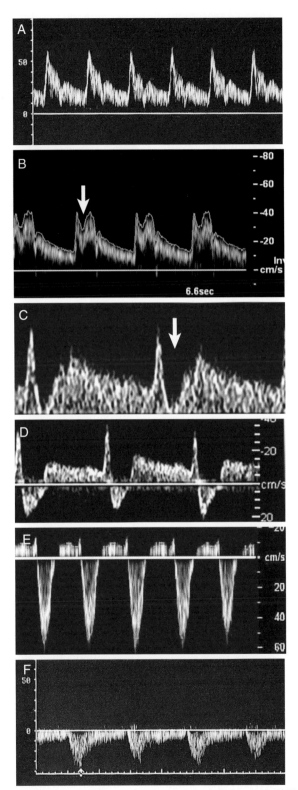

Fig. 8.42 Waveforms recorded in vertebral arteries showing varying degrees of subclavian steal. (A) Flow seen in a normal vertebral artery with cephalad flow throughout the cardiac cycle. (B and C) Peak systolic hesitation *(arrow)* suggesting insipient or latent steal indicating moderate brachiocephalic disease or proximal subclavian artery disease. (D and E) Partial flow reversal seen in the vertebral artery indicating partial subclavian steal and (F) total flow reversal indicating subclavian steal due to varying degrees of proximal significant disease or occlusion.

detect a stenotic jet in the proximal subclavian artery due to a stenosis. In some cases, the appearance of the vertebral artery flow can be confusing, showing flow away from the head during systole and toward the head during diastole. Examples of the effect of differing degrees of subclavian steal on the vertebral artery waveform are shown in Fig. 8.42. When the pressure drop across the diseased subclavian artery is not sufficient to cause flow reversal in the vertebral artery throughout the whole cardiac cycle, further assessment can be performed by asking the patient to exercise their arm, ipsilateral to the abnormal vertebral flow, by bending the forearm toward the shoulder once per second for 1 minute. Alternatively, a sphygmomanometer cuff can be used to induce hyperemia by inflating the cuff around the upper arm to a pressure above systolic pressure for 2 to 3 minutes and then deflating. The exercise or hyperemia will increase the blood flow to the arm and cause an increase in reverse flow in the vertebral artery.

REPORTING CAROTID ULTRASOUND SCANS

The ultrasound report should describe the presence, location, and appearance of any atheroma seen within the CCA and ICA. In the presence of extensive disease (Fig. 8.43), the lower and upper extent of the disease should be clearly stated in the report. Any significant velocity increases along the carotid arteries should be reported and interpreted to estimate the degree of narrowing present. Abnormal waveforms seen within the CCA, ICA, or ECA should also be described, along with a suggestion as to what they may indicate. The presence and direction of vertebral artery flow should be noted. The report should make it very clear if there was any limitation of the carotid examination, such as the following:
- Inconclusive identification of an occlusion or subocclusion
- Calcification obscuring the vessel for more than 1 cm
- No visible endpoint to ICA disease
- Whether the scan was otherwise suboptimal
- Whether waveforms obtained suggest possible significant vascular disease proximal or distal to the bifurcation which may require further investigation.

The report can consist of a written report alone or may include images of atheroma and waveforms seen. Alternatively, a diagrammatic representation of the disease

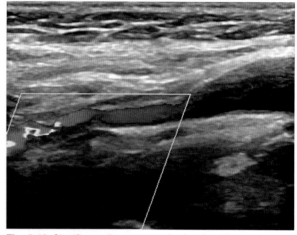

Fig. 8.43 Significant disease seen in the distal internal carotid artery, near the level of the jaw, needs to be highlighted in the scan report.

seen can be produced. Fig. 8.44 is an example of a diagrammatic method of producing a report. It is important that the department has a written protocol, including the criteria used to interpret the Doppler findings and the method of reporting to be used. With guidelines now recommending rapid access to carotid ultrasound imaging, it is of vital importance that reports are available to the referring medical team immediately after the scan. This diagnostic service is often done as part of a single visit TIA clinic, whereby the patient will see a stroke specialist or a neurologist, have any relevant diagnostic tests, and is then seen by the stroke specialist or neurologist again, on the same day, to decide on a treatment plan.

ULTRASOUND IN LARGE-VESSEL VASCULITIS

Takayasu's arteritis and giant cell arteritis (GCA) are both forms of large-vessel vasculitis where inflammation of arteries can lead to a reduction in flow. Although less common than atherosclerotic disease, ultrasound is useful in the diagnosis and for following up both types of arteritis. Practitioners should be aware of the presentation and appearance of arteritis, which differs in appearance and distribution when compared with atheromatous disease. It is included in the chapter for carotid arteries because these are among the arteries affected and, in these cases, symptoms can be severe.

Takayasu's arteritis affects the aorta and its branches, most commonly in young (<40 years) Asian women. Symptoms depend on the arteries affected but include

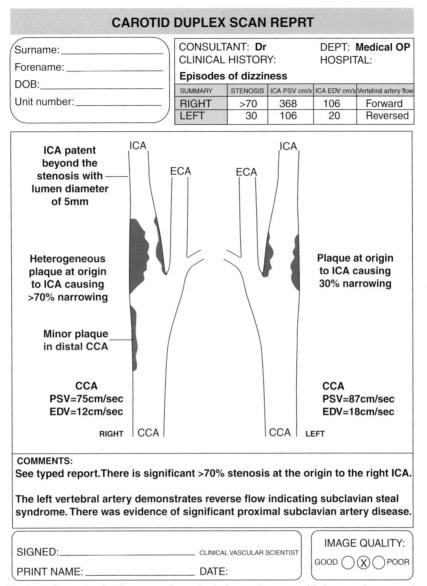

Fig. 8.44 Example of a diagrammatic method of reporting a carotid ultrasound scan result.

The figure contains the following:

CAROTID DUPLEX SCAN REPRT

Surname: _____
Forename: _____
DOB: _____
Unit number: _____

CONSULTANT: **Dr**   DEPT: **Medical OP**
CLINICAL HISTORY: HOSPITAL:
Episodes of dizziness

SUMMARY	STENOSIS	ICA PSV cm/s	ICA EDV cm/s	Vertebral artery flow
RIGHT	>70	368	106	Forward
LEFT	30	106	20	Reversed

ICA patent beyond the stenosis with lumen diameter of 5mm

Heterogeneous plaque at origin to ICA causing >70% narrowing

Minor plaque in distal CCA

CCA PSV=75cm/sec EDV=12cm/sec

Plaque at origin to ICA causing 30% narrowing

CCA PSV=87cm/sec EDV=18cm/sec

RIGHT CCA   CCA LEFT

COMMENTS:
See typed report. There is significant >70% stenosis at the origin to the right ICA.

The left vertebral artery demonstrates reverse flow indicating subclavian steal syndrome. There was evidence of significant proximal subclavian artery disease.

SIGNED: _____ CLINICAL VASCULAR SCIENTIST

PRINT NAME: _____ DATE: _____

IMAGE QUALITY:
GOOD ◯ (X) ◯ POOR

reduced or absent radial artery pulses if the proximal arm arteries are narrowed, hypertension if the renal arteries are stenosed, and neurological symptoms including dizziness, vertigo, syncope, and stroke if flow to the brain is impaired.

The appearance of arteritis is of an enlarged artery medial wall with uniform echogenicity and a circumferential distribution. In severe cases, the lumen is small and can restrict flow (Fig. 8.45). In transverse, the hypoechoic wall thickening forms a halo around the lumen. Depending on the severity and symptoms, ultrasound can be used to examine for arteritis of the carotid, subclavian, and axillary arteries by direct B-mode imaging with color flow imaging (CFI) and Doppler confirmation. For investigation of narrowing of abdominal branches, CFI and Doppler measurements can be used to assess the severity of stenosis and any hemodynamic consequences.

Ultrasound in GCA/Temporal Arteritis

Vascular sonographers increasingly find themselves asked to provide services for the investigation of GCA. GCA can affect many arteries including the aorta and its branches, and the axillary and carotid arteries. However, it is the temporal

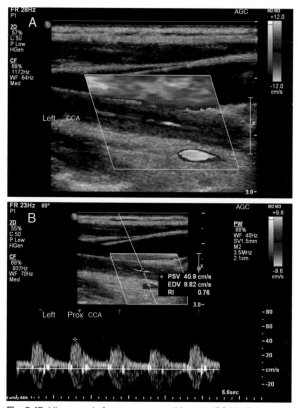

Fig. 8.45 Ultrasound of a common carotid artery *(CCA)* in Takayasu's arteritis. (A) The inflammation causes uniform narrowing of the artery with a severe reduction in lumen as demonstrated by the small residual lumen. In this example (B), the tight narrowing along the length of the CCA causes high resistance resulting in low velocities.

arteries where there are specific high-risk symptoms, where diagnosis is made using biopsy, and it is in temporal arteries that studies have shown ultrasound to be effective in diagnosis of GCA. For these reasons it is also commonly described as an investigation for temporal arteritis.

GCA causes inflammation of the arteries leading to a swelling and constriction of the lumen with loss of flow. In temporal arteries this can lead to headaches on one or both sides of the forehead, tenderness on the scalp and temples, pain during jaw movement—jaw claudication— and visual impairment such as double vision or loss of vision in an eye. Untreated, GCA can lead to blindness in one or both eyes, TIA, and stroke. Treatment with steroids is effective but depends on accurate and timely diagnosis.

High-frequency ultrasound was proposed as an effective alternative to temporal artery biopsy (TAB) in 1997 (Schmidt et al. 1997). TAB has a very high specificity, but its sensitivity is impaired by sampling errors, delays in performing the test, and the inconsistent distribution along the temporal artery. It is also an invasive procedure. The advantage of ultrasound investigation is that it can look along the entire length of the temporal artery and its main two branches and that it can be repeated safely.

The investigation is made on the superficial temporal artery (STA) and the frontal and parietal branches (Fig. 8.46). A high-frequency transducer is essential to image these superficial arteries, and the "hockey stick" type of probe allows easy manipulation along the vessels. Normal arteries exhibit a thin arterial wall, and the clarity of

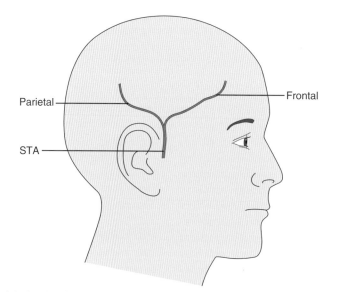

Fig. 8.46 Diagram of the location of superficial temporal artery *(STA)* and branches for investigation of giant cell arteritis.

the intima depends on the size of the artery and resolution of the transducer. The STA outer to outer diameter is typically 2 to 2.5 mm with slightly smaller diameters for the frontal and parietal branches. The appearance of arteritis is a general thickening of the artery wall, with the resulting edema causing a hypoechoic ring around the lumen, described as a "halo sign" when imaged in a transverse section. Images of normal appearance of the temporal artery and an example of the halo sign are shown in Fig. 8.47.

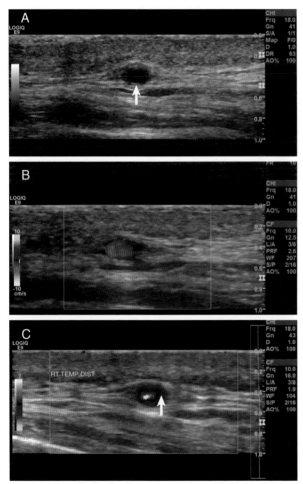

Fig. 8.47 (A) Transverse images of a frontal branch of the temporal artery. In B-mode the arterial wall is seen (arrowed) with normal appearance. (B) In a scan of the normal temporal artery, color flow fills the lumen. There is slight CFI overwriting of the artery walls, even though gain has been reduced. There is no indication of arterial inflammation. (C) Halo sign in a temporal artery exhibiting GCA. The dark area surrounding the lumen shows the presence of inflammation (arrow). CFI, Color flow imaging; GCA, giant cell arteritis.

Other arteries may show signs of inflammation; studies have shown that the sensitivity of the test is improved if the axillary arteries are also imaged and measured.

Scanning Technique

The STA, a branch of the ECA, is located anterior to the patient's ear at the level of the tragus. By scanning in transverse, the probe can be moved to locate the artery and position it at the center of the image. High imaging fundamental frequencies (>12 MHz) are used with an image depth of around 1 cm and the focus placed around 5 mm depth. Only very light pressure is required, as the artery is superficial and readily compressed. Color flow imaging parameters should be set so that flow fills the lumen but does not overwrite or bleed into the artery wall. The artery is scanned in transverse plane to its bifurcation into the frontal and parietal branches and any thickening of the wall identified and noted. The probe is then turned to image the artery along its axis and the color flow parameters are set (steering, gain, PRF/scale) so that an increase in velocity leads to aliasing. The artery is then imaged in long section along its length to examine for wall thickening and stenosis; if a stenosis is suspected, it should be confirmed by an increase in velocity; the threshold for a stenosis is a twofold increase in PSV. The process is repeated for the parietal and frontal branches. If a halo sign is suspected, then compression of the artery distinguishes the lumen from the surrounding arterial wall. Halo thickness is measured longitudinally from the edge of the artery wall to the lumen as displayed by color flow (see Fig. 8.48). The axillary arteries are imaged, wall thickness measured, and Doppler measurements of velocities recorded.

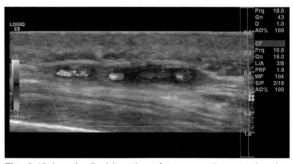

Fig. 8.48 Longitudinal imaging of a temporal artery showing thickening of the arterial wall with halo size 0.61 mm.

Thresholds for Indications of GCA

The sonographer should report the presence and patency of the STA and branches bilaterally, since absence of a segment may indicate an occlusion. The presence of a halo sign is the most important indicator of GCA; the intima-media wall thickness (IMT) of the hypoechoic halo is ≥0.3 mm in GCA. Compression of the artery in transverse is used to confirm the presence of the hypoechoic wall; the lumen itself is compressed but the wall remains visible. Brighter hyperechoic irregular arterial walls are indicative of atheromatous disease, which can vary in severity. Atheroma can be present independently of the halo sign indicative of GCA; both can lead to stenosis that causes a velocity increase and both can lead to occlusion. For the axillary artery, homogeneous wall swelling of at least 1.5 mm is definitive for arteritis (Schmidt et al. 2008). A more recent study has indicated that cutoffs for IMT, above which GCA is indicated, are 0.42 mm in the common STA, 0.34 mm in the frontal branch, 0.29 mm in the parietal branch, and 1 mm in the axillary artery (Schafer et al. 2017).

The effectiveness of ultrasound has been evaluated in the TABUL study (Luqmani et al. 2016) in which operators were trained to perform ultrasound to a common standard and where results were compared with TAB. These results and the findings of several other studies are summarized in a review that includes technical tips for good ultrasound practice (Monti et al. 2018).

9

Duplex Assessment of Lower-Limb Arterial Disease

INTRODUCTION

Lower-limb arterial disease (LLAD) is a common condition in the older population, and estimates suggest it affects at least 1 in every 10 people over the age of 60, although many may not experience any significant symptoms (Criqui & Aboyans 2015; Aboyans et al. 2017). Additionally, there is increasing prevalence of younger people with diabetes presenting with foot ulcers associated with diseased arteries of the calf and foot. This area is a diagnostic challenge for the vascular imaging department. The symptoms of LLAD can range in severity from mild muscle pain on exercise (claudication), relieved by rest, to severe ischemia resulting in potential amputation. The vascular laboratory has an established role dating back to the 1980s for the noninvasive diagnosis of peripheral arterial disease enabling vascular clinicians to formulate management and treatment plans. These can range from conservative management, thus avoiding unnecessary intervention, to complex procedures requiring radiological and surgical reconstruction of the circulation. Postprocedural imaging, to confirm the patency of angioplasty sites, stents, and bypass grafts, or to identify false aneurysms, is also an important function of the vascular laboratory. Fig. 9.1 summarizes the current role of ultrasound. Recent innovations have also seen the development of acute limb salvage and acute diabetic foot services, involving a multidisciplinary team approach, including members of the vascular laboratory to assess blood flow. The aim of these services is to provide urgent assessment within 24 hours of referral to enable rapid treatment, thereby preventing limb and foot loss.

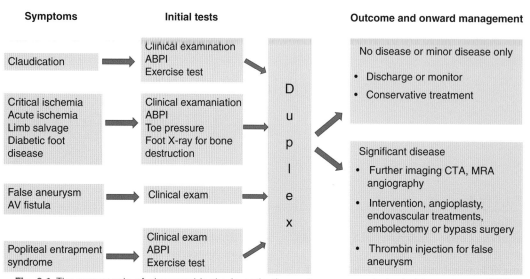

Fig. 9.1 The current role of ultrasound in the investigation and management of arterial symptoms. *ABPI*, Ankle–brachial pressure index; *CTA*, computed tomography angiography; *MRA*, magnetic resonance angiography.

This chapter provides an overview of LLAD and disorders and offers practical advice on investigation and diagnosis using duplex ultrasound. It also covers some nonimaging techniques.

ANATOMY OF THE LOWER-LIMB ARTERIAL SYSTEM

The anatomy of the lower-limb arterial system is demonstrated in Fig. 9.2. The abdominal aorta has been included in this section, as it can be a source of lower-limb symptoms.

The aorta lies slightly to the left of the midline in the abdomen, and its bifurcation is located at the level of the fourth lumbar vertebra in the region of the umbilicus. The aorta divides into the left and right common iliac arteries (CIA) at the aortic bifurcation. The CIA is variable in length (3.5–12 cm) and in some cases it is very short, with the iliac bifurcation occurring close to the aorta. The CIA divides into the external and internal iliac arteries at the iliac bifurcation, which lies deep in the pelvis. The internal iliac artery supplies blood to the pelvis and pelvic viscera. The external iliac artery varies in length (6–12 cm) and is normally superficial to the iliac vein. It gives off the deep circumflex iliac artery and inferior epigastric artery, before becoming the common femoral artery (CFA) at the level of the inguinal ligament. The aorta and iliac arteries lie behind

the peritoneum, containing the bowel, which can make imaging of these vessels difficult due to overlying bowel gas. One branch of the CFA that can frequently be identified with ultrasound is the superficial epigastric artery.

The CFA divides into the deep femoral artery, also known as the profunda femoris artery, and the superficial femoral artery (SFA) at the level of the groin. The profunda femoris artery divides from the posterolateral aspect of the CFA running in a lateral course before curving to run deep under the SFA. It supplies blood to the thigh tissue and muscles. It also acts as an important collateral pathway in the presence of an SFA occlusion. The profunda femoris artery usually gives off the medial and lateral circumflex arteries just beyond its origin and there are also a number of perforating branches along its length. The SFA follows a medial course down the thigh, becoming the popliteal artery as it exits the adductor canal at the adductor hiatus above the knee. The SFA gives off relatively few major branches, although the descending genicular artery can act as an important collateral pathway. The popliteal artery then runs behind the knee, or popliteal fossa, and bifurcates below the knee into the anterior tibial (AT) artery and tibioperoneal trunk. The popliteal artery has a number of genicular and sural branches supplying blood to the knee joint and gastrocnemius and soleus muscles. The proximal AT artery runs in an anterolateral direction through the interosseous membrane to the anterolateral aspect of the upper calf. It then continues to run to the lower calf, becoming the dorsalis pedis artery over the dorsum of the foot. The tibioperoneal trunk can vary in length and bifurcates into the posterior tibial (PT) and peroneal arteries (Fig. 9.2B). The PT artery follows a medial course along the calf and runs behind the medial malleolus (or ankle bone) in its distal segment. The peroneal artery lies deeper than the PT artery against the border of the fibula and runs toward the lateral malleolus (outer aspect of the ankle) in its distal segment, dividing into

lateral malleolar, calcaneal, and perforating branches. It is important to note that the peroneal artery is often spared in the presence of tibial artery disease. This is why its identification can be useful if a distal bypass procedure is being considered.

The forefoot is mainly supplied by the dorsalis pedis artery and the medial and lateral plantar arteries, which are terminal branches of the PT artery (Fig. 9.2C). The lateral plantar artery runs toward the fifth metatarsal before turning medially forming the deep plantar arch

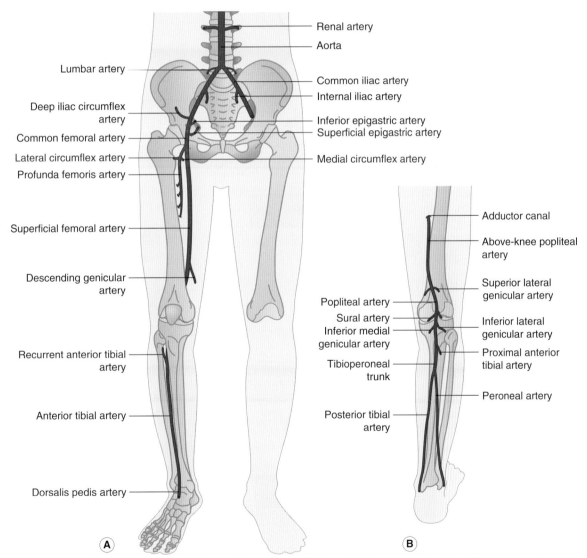

Fig. 9.2 (A) Arterial anatomy of the aortoiliac and lower-limb arteries from an anterior view. (B) Arterial anatomy of the lower limb from a posterior view.

Continued

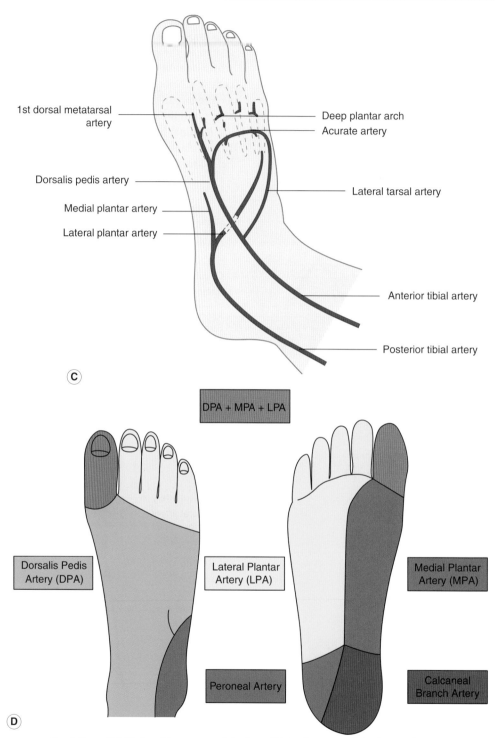

1st dorsal metatarsal artery

Deep plantar arch

Acurate artery

Dorsalis pedis artery

Lateral tarsal artery

Medial plantar artery

Lateral plantar artery

Anterior tibial artery

Posterior tibial artery

(C)

DPA + MPA + LPA

Dorsalis Pedis Artery (DPA)

Lateral Plantar Artery (LPA)

Medial Plantar Artery (MPA)

Peroneal Artery

Calcaneal Branch Artery

(D)

Fig. 9.2, cont'd (C) Arterial anatomy of the foot. (D) Angiosomes of the foot and ankle.

and anastomoses with the dorsalis pedis artery in the proximal inter-web space. The arcuate artery divides from the dorsalis pedis artery and runs laterally beneath the tendons and gives off dorsal metatarsal arteries. The first dorsal metatarsal artery is a continuation of the dorsalis pedis artery and supplies the great toe. Four plantar metatarsal arteries emanate from the plantar arch to supply the forefoot and toes. The presence of the plantar arch and other arterial interconnections can enable perfusion of the foot if one of the main tibial arteries is occluded. It is useful to have an understanding of the concept of angiosomes. The foot and ankle are composed of six distinct angiosomes that can be considered as three-dimensional blocks of tissue perfused and drained by specific tibial arteries and veins, respectively (Fig. 9.2D). Understanding angiosome and their source arteries can provide a basis for surgeons to plan arterial bypass reconstructions or local amputations.

There are a number of anatomical variations in the lower-limb arterial system that may occasionally be encountered during routine examinations. The most common variations are listed in Table 9.1.

Collateral Circulation and Pathways

Although symptoms are generally proportional to the extent of disease, it is sometimes surprising to find patients with arterial occlusions but relatively minor symptoms. Conversely, some patients with one or two stenoses can experience significant impairment to their lifestyle. This variability is mainly due to the quality of the collateral circulation. If an arterial segment is severely diseased or occluded, there are often alternative pathways that are able to carry blood flow around the diseased segment, referred to as collateral vessels. In this situation, reverse flow is observed in major branches of arteries just distal to an area of severe disease, where they help to resupply blood flow to the main vessel. One such example is flow reversal observed in the internal iliac artery, supplying blood to the external iliac artery in the presence of a CIA occlusion (Fig. 9.3). It should be noted that it is very difficult to follow collateral vessels for any length using the duplex scanner, especially in the pelvis. This is not really a problem, as it is the length and severity of the disease in the main vessels that the sonographer is attempting to document. However, the quality of the collateral circulation is very important, and this can be determined by assessing the patient clinically and measuring the ankle–brachial

TABLE 9.1 Anatomical Variations of the Lower-limb Arterial System

Artery	Variation
Common femoral artery bifurcation	The bifurcation can sometimes be very high; the proximal course of the profunda femoris artery can sometimes be variable and lies posterior and medial to the superficial femoral artery in a small number of cases. It can also give rise to additional branches proximally
Anterior tibial artery	High origin across the knee joint. It can be small or hypoplastic
Peroneal artery	Origin from anterior tibial artery rather than the tibioperoneal trunk

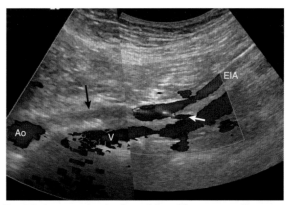

Fig. 9.3 An example of collateral flow. The common iliac artery is occluded *(black arrow)* at its origin from the distal aorta *(Ao)*. Reverse flow *(white arrow)*, seen as flow toward the probe, is demonstrated in the internal iliac artery, as it supplies flow to the external iliac artery *(EIA)*. The iliac vein *(V)* is seen in this image.

pressure index (ABPI). Common collateral pathways are summarized in Table 9.2.

SYMPTOMS OF LOWER-LIMB ARTERIAL DISEASE

Intermittent Claudication

Intermittent claudication is caused by arterial narrowing in the lower-limb arteries, and symptoms develop

TABLE 9.2   Common Collateral Pathways of the Lower-limb Arteries

Diseased Artery	Distal Normal Artery	Common Collateral Pathway
Common iliac artery	External iliac artery	Lumbar arteries communicating with the iliolumbar arteries of the ipsilateral internal iliac artery, which supply the external iliac artery via retrograde flow; there can also be communication between the contralateral internal iliac artery and ipsilateral internal iliac artery
External iliac artery	Common femoral artery	Ipsilateral internal iliac artery via pelvic connections to the deep iliac circumflex artery or inferior epigastric artery
Common femoral artery	Femoral bifurcation	Ipsilateral pelvic arteries filling the profunda femoris artery via the femoral circumflex arteries, which supply the superficial femoral artery via retrograde flow
Superficial femoral artery	Above-knee popliteal artery	Flow via profunda femoris artery (or branches of the proximal superficial femoral artery if patent) to the descending or superior genicular arteries, depending on the length of the superficial femoral artery occlusion
Superficial femoral artery	Below-knee popliteal artery	Profunda femoris artery branches to inferior genicular branches of the popliteal artery
Popliteal artery	Distal popliteal artery	Flow via the superior genicular arteries to inferior genicular arteries, depending on the level of the occlusion
Proximal tibial arteries	Distal tibial arteries	There are numerous arterial collateral connections in the calf, but they may not be large enough to carry sufficient flow to the foot

over a number of months or years. There is strong evidence that persons with claudication have a significantly higher mortality rate from cardiac disease than nonclaudicants (Aboyans et al. 2018). Claudication is typified by pain and cramping in the muscles of the leg while walking, which usually forces the patient to stop and rest for a few minutes in order to ease the symptoms. The severity of pain experienced and the distance a patient is able to walk can vary from day to day but, generally, walking briskly or on an incline will produce rapid onset of symptoms. The location of pain (i.e., calf, buttock, or thigh) is often associated with the distribution of disease. For instance, aortoiliac disease often produces thigh, buttock, and calf claudication whereas femoropopliteal disease is associated with calf pain. There are sometimes physical signs of deteriorating blood flow in the lower limb, such as hair loss from the calf and an absence of nail growth. Claudication only occurs during exercise because at rest, the muscle groups distal to a stenosis or occlusion remain adequately perfused with blood. However, during exercise, the metabolic demand of the muscles increases rapidly, and the stenosis or occlusion will limit the amount of additional blood flow that can reach the muscles causing claudication.

Many patients with intermittent claudication are treated by conservative methods. This includes reduction or elimination of risk factors associated with atherosclerosis, such as smoking. Patients are also advised to undertake a controlled exercise program to build up the collateral circulation around the diseased vessel, which may ease symptoms over time. If necessary, serial ABPI measurements or exercise tests can be performed to monitor the patient's progress in specialist or nurse-led claudication clinics. Interventional treatment is mainly by angioplasty, which involves the dilation of stenoses or occlusions with percutaneous balloon catheters. Arterial stents are sometimes used to prevent restenosis, although in-stent stenosis is known to occur in a proportion of cases due to the development of intimal hyperplasia (see Fig. 9.19). Surgical bypass is usually avoided, unless the patient is suffering from severe claudication, as there is a small potential risk of complications occurring during or after surgery, which in extreme cases could lead to amputation or even death.

Chronic Critical Lower-Limb Ischemia

Critical lower-limb ischemia occurs when blood flow beyond an arterial stenosis or occlusion is so low that

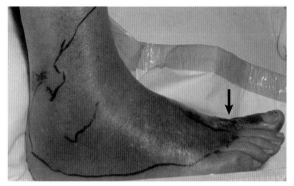

Fig. 9.4 The appearance of critical lower-limb ischemia with areas of necrosis (arrow) and infection.

| | | Ankle Systolic | |
Grade	ABI	Pressure (mmHg)	Toe Pressure, tcPO$_2$ (mmHg)
0	≥0.80	>100	≥60
1	0.6–0.79	70–100	40–59
2	0.4–0.59	50–70	30–39
3	≤0.39	<50	<30

TABLE 9.3 WIfI Scoring System for ABPI and Toe Pressure

Patients with diabetes should have TP measurements. If arterial calcification precludes reliable ABI or TP measurements, ischemia should be documented byTcPO2, SPP, or PVR. If TP and ABI measurements result in different grades, TP will be the primary determinant of ischemia grade.

PVR, pulse volume recording; *SPP*, skin perfusion pressure; *tcPO$_2$*, transcutaneous oximetry; *WIfI*, Wound, Ischemia, and foot Infection.
Mills et al. 2014.

the patient experiences pain in the leg or foot at rest because the metabolic requirements of the distal tissues cannot be maintained (see Fig. 9.4). This is frequently typified by severe rest pain at night, forcing the patient to sleep in a chair or to hang the leg in a dependent position over the side of the bed. This improves blood flow due to increased hydrostatic pressure. Several guideline and consensus documents have been published defining critical limb ischemia (CLI) and its management, such as the Trans-Atlantic Inter-Society Consensus for the management of peripheral arterial disease (TASC II) (Norgren et al. 2007). A more recent example is the Global Vascular Guidelines on the Management of Chronic Limb-Threatening Ischemia (CLTI), produced by the European Society for Vascular Surgery (Conte et al. 2019). The document makes the following recommendation for defining critical lower-limb ischemia:

CLTI should be defined to include a broader and more heterogeneous group of patients with varying degrees of ischemia that may delay wound healing and increase amputation risk. A diagnosis of CLTI requires objectively documented atherosclerotic PAD in association with ischemic rest pain or tissue loss (ulceration or gangrene).

It should be present for >2 weeks and be associated with one or more abnormal hemodynamic parameters. These parameters include an ankle-brachial index (ABI) <0.4 (using higher of the dorsalis pedis [DP] and posterior tibial [PT] arteries), absolute highest AP (ankle pressure) <50 mm Hg, absolute toe pressure <30 mm Hg.

The Society of Vascular Surgery Lower-Extremity Guidelines Committee has also developed a classification system for the threatened lower limb (Mills et al. 2013). Risk stratification is based on three major factors that impact amputation risk and clinical management known as the WIfI score. These are Wound, Ischemia, and foot Infection. Each of these factors is graded from 0 to 3, with 3 representing greater severity within each factor. The reader is directed to the guidelines cited above for an in-depth description of the WIfI scoring system. However, it is important to note that the ischemia grade is commonly assessed by ABPI or toe pressures. The grades are shown in Table 9.3.

The treatment of lower-limb ischemia includes angioplasty or arterial bypass grafting or endovascular procedures. Unfortunately, some patients are not suitable candidates for any form of limb salvage, and amputation is the inevitable outcome.

Acute Limb Ischemia

Acute limb ischemia, as the name suggests, is due to sudden arterial obstruction in the lower-limb arteries that may threaten limb viability. The duration of symptoms is less than 2 weeks, but patients can often present with symptoms of less than 12 hours. The position of the obstruction can vary. Main causes of acute ischemia are listed in Box 9.1. Acute thrombosis of an existing arterial lesion, a so-called acute-on-chronic occlusion, can occur when the blood flow across a diseased segment of an artery is so slow that it spontaneously thromboses. Long segments of an artery may occlude in this situation. Acute ischemia is more likely to occur if the collateral circulation around the disease is poorly developed. An embolus may be released from other areas of the body, such as the heart or from an aneurysm, which then travels distally down the leg, eventually obstructing

BOX 9.1   Cause of Acute Lower-limb Ischemia

- Thrombosis of an atherosclerotic artery
- Embolism from heart, aneurysm, plaque, or critical stenosis upstream (including cholesterol or athero-thrombotic emboli secondary to endovascular procedures)
- Thrombosed aneurysm with or without embolization
- Aortic/arterial dissection
- Arterial trauma
- Thrombosis of an arterial bypass graft
- Spontaneous thrombosis associated with a hypercoagulable state
- Popliteal entrapment with thrombosis
- Popliteal adventitial cyst with thrombosis

BOX 9.2   The Findings of Acute Limb Ischemia May Include the "6 Ps"

1. Pain
2. Pulselessness: check with Doppler measurements
3. Pallor: change in color is a common finding in acute limb ischemia. Venous filling may be slow or absent
4. Poikilothermia (perishing with cold)
5. Paresthesia: numbness occurs in more than half of patients
6. Paralysis is a sign of poor prognosis

the artery when the arterial diameter is less than that of the embolus. An embolus frequently obstructs bifurcations such as the common femoral bifurcation or distal popliteal artery and tibioperoneal trunk. Another example is obstruction of the aortic bifurcation by an embolus projecting down both CIA origins, referred to as a saddle embolus. The body has very little time to develop collateral circulation around embolic occlusions and the limb may be very ischemic.

The classic symptoms of acute ischemia are shown in Box 9.2. In this situation, emergency treatment by endovascular techniques, surgical embolectomy, bypass surgery, or thrombolysis should be performed, provided that the patient is fit enough for treatment. Left untreated, acute ischemia can lead to muscle death or necrosis. This can cause swelling of the calf muscle and eventually the sac, (fascia), surrounding the muscles will restrict any further swelling, leading to a pressure increase within the muscle compartments. This is known as compartment syndrome, and the acute increase in intramuscular

pressure can further exacerbate the muscle ischemia. If limb salvage is possible, surgical splitting of the fascia, called a fasciotomy, may be required to release the excess pressure.

Severe muscle ischemia can produce toxins that can lead to organ failure and eventual death. An urgent amputation is usually performed if there is no viable option to restore blood flow to the limb.

Microembolization into the foot is often called "trash foot" or "blue-toe syndrome." Localized tissue infarction occurs, leading to necrosis. It is not unusual for the patient to have a palpable ankle pulse. The outcome is often poor when a large area of tissue is affected and can result in local amputation of toes, forefoot, or leg.

DISEASE PATTERNS AND LOWER-LIMB WAVEFORM SHAPES

CAUTION

Remember, if the patient has just walked briskly from the waiting room to the examination table the shape of observed waveforms in normal arteries may demonstrate continuous forward flow, due to changes in peripheral resistance. The patient should be allowed to relax for several minutes before starting the examination.

It is important to have an understanding of the different patterns of disease that may be encountered during the examination as long segments of arteries are being interrogated (see Chapter 5). Common findings include isolated or multiple stenoses, occlusions, diffuse calcified wall disease, aneurysms, and, rarely, dissections. In addition, the ability to distinguish both visually and audibly between normal and abnormal Doppler waveforms is essential (Fig. 9.5). At rest, the normal spectral Doppler display recorded from a lower-limb extremity artery, excluding the aorta, which can have a biphasic pattern, is a triphasic flow pattern with a clear spectral window (see Fig. 9.5A). This characteristic pulsatile waveform shape is due to a combination of compliant distensible arterial walls and pulse wave reflections from the periphery. It may even be possible to see four phases in young healthy adults. The triphasic pattern is easily distinguished from the audio output. In elderly patients or patients with poor cardiac output, the waveform may be biphasic or even monophasic.

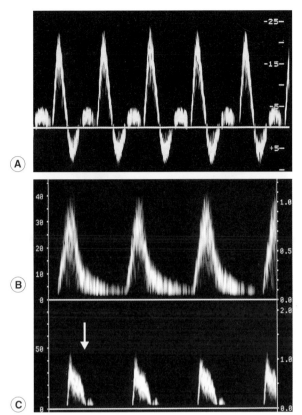

Fig. 9.5 Waveform shapes can reveal useful information about the condition of proximal and distal arteries. (A) A normal triphasic waveform recorded from the superficial femoral artery (SFA). (B) Damping of the common femoral artery waveform with an increased systolic acceleration time and loss of pulsatility indicates significant proximal disease. (C) A waveform recorded from the SFA just proximal to an occlusion. Note the high-resistance, low-volume waveform shape and characteristic shoulder on the systolic downstroke *(arrow)*, due to pulse wave reflection from distal disease.

Waveforms with an increased systolic rise time are characteristic of disease proximal to the point of measurement (Fig. 9.5B). For example, a study by Sensier et al. (1998) demonstrated that qualitative assessment of the CFA Doppler waveform has a sensitivity of 95%, a specificity of 80%, and an accuracy of 87% for the prediction of significant aortoiliac artery disease. This study therefore suggests that observation of the CFA waveform shape is a useful technique for the investigation of inflow disease. The presence of triphasic flow with a short systolic rise time is an indicator of normal inflow. However, care should be exercised when investigating younger patients who may have a very short

proximal iliac stenosis, as the arterial waveform shape may have recovered at the level of the CFA, appearing normal. Conversely, high-resistance, low-volume flow waveforms are indicative of severe disease distal to the point of measurement. One such example is the characteristic shoulder seen on the systolic downstroke of an SFA waveform recorded proximal to severe disease in the SFA (see Fig. 9.5C). This is due to a reflected wave from the disease or occlusion. Severe calcification of the arterial wall may also affect the shape of the recorded Doppler waveform due to changes in vessel compliance as the vessels become very rigid. This is commonly observed in the tibial vessels of diabetic patients, where the waveform shape may become monophasic with continuous forward flow throughout the cardiac cycle.

> **ADVICE**
>
> There are situations in which flow in nondiseased lower-limb arteries at rest may have reduced pulsatility or even be continuous. Examples include increased flow (hyperemia) due to limb-infected ulcers, cellulitis, or the presence of arteriovenous fistulas. Hyperemic flow will be demonstrated as continuous flow in one direction. In cases of hyperemia, blood flow velocities can be higher than normal.

ANKLE–BRACHIAL PRESSURE MEASUREMENTS AND EXERCISE TESTING

> **SOURCES OF ERROR**
>
> - Incompressibility of the calf vessels can be a problem, especially in patients with diabetes or significant renal disease, as medial calcification in the walls of the calf arteries can make them rigid and incompressible (Fig. 9.13B), leading to falsely elevated recordings. An example of such a measurement would be an ankle pressure of 280 mmHg and a brachial pressure of 120 mmHg (ankle–brachial pressure index [ABPI] = 2.3). An ABPI of >1.4 should be regarded as abnormal and further investigation may be required
> - Accidental probe movement during cuff inflation can give an impression that the signal has disappeared. Make sure that the probe is kept fixed over the point of measurement, particularly if the ankle and foot roll during cuff inflation. Hold the probe toward its tip with a finger resting on the skin for greater stability and control.

Before discussing the practical aspects of lower-limb scanning in detail, it is useful to discuss the role of simple hand held continuous-wave Doppler devices. The audio output of these devices can give a subjective impression of the quality of blood flow at specific sites, such as the ankle. Some hand-held Doppler devices also provide a visual trace of the Doppler waveform. However, for qualitative assessment, the measurement of the ABPI is a simple method of detecting and grading arterial disease (NICE CG 147, 2018). This is especially useful if the patient is presenting with leg ulceration and there is uncertainty whether this is primarily venous or arterial, as a normal ABPI would indicate a venous cause. The test normally takes 10 to 15 minutes and is performed as follows. Prior to the test the patient should be fully rested for at least 5 to 10 minutes and lying supine to remove the effect of hydrostatic pressure. A blood pressure cuff is then placed around the ankle. A high-frequency (8–10 MHz) continuous-wave Doppler probe is used to listen to the Doppler signals in the DP and PT arteries at the ankle, as shown in Fig. 9.6. To obtain an adequate audio signal, the probe normally needs to be angled to the skin surface. It is often a case of gently moving the position of the probe with slight adjustments in probe angle to obtain the strongest signal.

It is sometimes necessary to examine the peroneal artery, as it may be the only vessel supplying the foot in patients with severe arterial disease. The systolic blood pressure is measured at each of these points by briskly inflating the cuff to above the patient's systolic blood pressure, at which point the arterial flow signal disappears. The cuff should be inflated to at least 20 to 30 mmHg above the pressure that is required to occlude the artery. The cuff is then deflated steadily, and the pressure at which the arterial signal reappears, corresponding to the systolic pressure at the position of the cuff, is recorded. The systolic brachial pressure is then measured in a similar way from both arms, in case there is upper-extremity disease. The highest recorded AP is then divided by the highest brachial pressure to calculate the ABPI. This index is independent of the patient's systemic blood pressure and can be used to grade the severity of arterial disease, as shown in Table 9.4 (adapted from AbuRahma 2000). The index ranges between 1 and 1.4 in normal subjects due to amplification of the arterial pulse wave along the limb and reflected waves from the periphery. However, it is worth noting that many

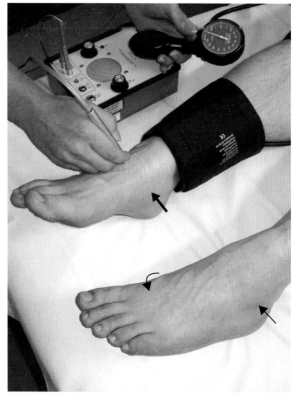

Fig. 9.6 Measurement of the ankle–brachial pressure index. Probe positions are shown to detect flow in the dorsalis pedis artery (probe) and the posterior tibial artery *(large arrow)*. The peroneal artery is located on the outer aspect of the ankle *(small arrow)*. The probe position has also been shown to detect flow from the plantar arch *(curved arrow)*.

TABLE 9.4	**Grading Arterial Disease Using the Ankle–Brachial Pressure Index (ABPI)**
ABPI	**Comment**
1–1.4	Normal
0.99–0.9	Mild disease "considered normal"
0.89–0.5	Claudication
0.49–0.3	Severe occlusive disease
<0.3	Ischemia and possible rest pain

scientific publications consider an index >0.9 to indicate a normal circulation.

Abnormal ABPI measurements can confirm the presence of arterial disease but do not give any indication of the position of the disease in the leg. Segmental pressures can help to isolate the diseased segment with the use of multiple pressure cuffs placed at the ankle, below the knee, above the knee, and at the top of the thigh. Significant pressure differences between cuffs would indicate disease between those segments. Some groups use pulse volume recording for identifying LLAD, which is a non-ultrasound technique and beyond the scope of this book.

PROBLEMS

There is no dorsalis pedis pulse:
- Make sure that the probe is not being pressed too hard onto the foot, as this can occlude the artery underneath
- Ensure that the foot is relaxed and not excessively plantar flexed (toes pointing down), as in some cases the artery can be stretched and temporally occluded in this position
- As a normal variation, the artery can be small or hypoplastic. Check the posterior tibial artery instead

Resting ABPI measurements may be normal in patients with mild to moderate claudication. However, ABPI measurements can be carried out before and after exercise on a treadmill to measure the patient's walking distance until the patient claudicates and to quantify the degree of pressure reduction following exercise. Exercise leads to an increase in blood flow to the muscles. In the presence of disease the resulting increased flow through a stenosis leads to higher velocities and a consequent increase in local pressure gradient, which will result in lower recorded pressure distally (see Chapter 5). Eventually a point will be reached at which the stenosis limits any further increase in flow and the patient experiences the onset of claudication in the muscle groups distal to the disease. Another alternative is to use commercially available foot flexion devices to exercise the calf muscles while the patient sits on the examination table. Exercise testing is also a particularly useful screening test, as some patients exhibiting symptoms of claudication may have other disorders producing their symptoms, such as spinal stenosis, sciatica, or musculoskeletal problems. In these cases, the postexercise pressures will be normal. Unfortunately, there is a wide range of exercise protocols used by vascular laboratories (e.g., speed 2–4 km/h, exercise duration 2–5 minutes, and treadmill incline 10%–12%). This can make comparisons of results among units difficult. However, individual patient's performance can be measured on sequential visits to monitor their treatment or progress.

The reader is also advised to understand the measurement of toe pressure measurements using toe cuffs and photoplethysmography sensors. There are a number of commercially available devices, some being part of a multitesting system, combining ABPI measurements and pulse volume recordings. Toe pressures can be useful if an ABPI measurement cannot be made due to incompressible calf arteries. A description of the test is beyond the scope of the book, and the reader is advised to consult specialist texts.

KEY POINTS

It is important to select the correct sized cuff for the ankle and arm. It should be long enough to ensure that 80% of the circumference of the upper arm or ankle can be covered by the bladder and the width is at least 40% of the limb circumference. Blood pressure will be overestimated if bladder is too short or too narrow (NICE CG 127. 2011).

It is important to monitor patients closely during exercise testing, as many with claudication have associated coronary artery disease. It is essential to have an emergency call system close at hand. In the absence of a treadmill it is possible to exercise the patient along the known length of a corridor.

In the presence of a severe stenosis or occlusion it is possible for the flow signal or pulse in the foot to be absent immediately after exercise. The flow signal will slowly recover to a preexercise level, which can be demonstrated with the hand-held Doppler.

PROBLEMS

If the leg is too swollen or too painful to measure blood pressure, a subjective audio assessment of the arterial waveform can be useful, as a triphasic waveform generally indicates normal arterial flow, whereas a damped monophasic waveform indicates the likelihood of significant disease. Be careful interpreting the signals in the presence of hyperemia, as flow may be monophasic in the absence of disease.

In patients with atrial fibrillation, the pressure measurement can vary. Take extra time and care when measuring the ABPI. The cuff may need to be inflated a few times to obtain a consistent reading. State any limitations in the report.

BOX 9.3   Scanning Objectives

The sonographer should be able to:
- Locate the site or sites of disease
- Detect lesions at multiple levels and, where possible, identify the most hemodynamically significant
- Differentiate stenoses from occlusions
- Grade the severity of stenoses
- Measure the length of occlusions
- Identify the presence and location of aneurysms
- Describe textural features of the disease such as excessive calcification (echogenic) or nonorganized thrombus (anechoic)
- Provide a concise report that can be interpreted by the relevant clinicians

---

PRACTICAL CONSIDERATIONS FOR LOWER-EXTREMITY DUPLEX SCANNING

The scanning objectives are shown in Box 9.3. The time allocated for the examination depends on the number of segments that need assessing. The femoropopliteal segment can normally be examined in both legs in half an hour. However, a bilateral aortoiliac to ankle scan may take up to an hour, depending on sonographer experience. There is usually no special preparation required before a lower-limb duplex scan. Nevertheless, some vascular units request patients to fast overnight before an examination of the aortoiliac arteries to improve imaging of this region. In our experience this is of little help, especially if patients require scans at short notice. Bowel preparations have proved useful, although in practice they can be difficult to administer to elderly or diabetic patients and are impractical in a single-visit clinic.

The patient should have an empty bladder before an aortoiliac scan as this improves the visualization of these segments and also causes less patient discomfort if transducer pressure has to be applied. The examination room should be at a comfortable ambient temperature (>20°C) to avoid peripheral vasoconstriction.

Scanner Setup

A peripheral arterial scanning option should be selected before starting the examination, but adjustment of the control settings will often be required in the presence of significant disease. When using a linear array transducer in B-mode, it is useful to use an extended field of view (trapezoid image). The color pulse repetition frequency (PRF) is usually set in the 2.5 to 3 kHz range or alternatively, the color scale set to 25 to 30 cm/s on the color bar for demonstrating moderately high-velocity flow. By using the correct settings normal arterial segments can be interrogated rapidly using color flow imaging. There should be color filling to the vessel walls. The color image normally demonstrates a pulsatile flow pattern with the color alternating between red and blue due to flow reversal during the diastolic phase (see Ch. 5). In instances of low flow distal to severe disease the PRF should be lowered and typically the color scale will need to be in the region of 10 cm/s. Ensure that wall filters are not set at a threshold that will prevent low-velocity flow being demonstrated.

STARTING THE SCAN

It is useful to start the assessment by examining the CFA at the groin, as the observed blood flow patterns at this level can reveal information about the condition of the aortoiliac arteries and also provide some clues to the condition of the SFA, as described earlier in the chapter (see Fig. 9.5). It is important to have a good understanding of the anatomy of the arteries and veins at the level of the groin and to be able to identify the major branches and junctions and their relationship to each other (see Fig. 9.7). A mid-frequency linear array transducer is the most suitable probe for scanning the femoral, popliteal, and calf arteries. A low-frequency, curvilinear array abdominal transducer is used for the aortoiliac segment. Low- or medium-frequency curvilinear transducers may be helpful in the thigh in larger patients. For the distal arteries in the calf and foot, a high-frequency linear array is beneficial. In addition, a "hockey stick" transducer provides the resolution and flexibility to investigate the distal PT, AT, DP, and plantar arteries. The investigation of each segment can be undertaken in any order, but examination of CFA flow is a good starting point. A combination of B-mode imaging, color flow imaging, and spectral Doppler recordings should be used throughout the examination. Color flow imaging is essential for identifying the aortoiliac and calf arteries. Spectral Doppler velocity measurements should be made at an angle of insonation of 60 degrees or less.

Assessment of the Aortoiliac Artery and CFA

The patient should be relaxed and lying in a supine position with the head supported by a pillow. The patient

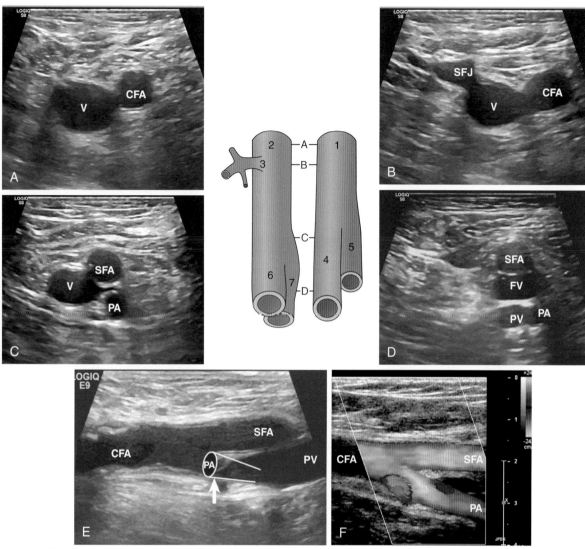

Fig. 9.7 The anatomy of the left femoral artery and vein at the groin, with corresponding transverse B-mode images at four different levels (A, B, C, D). Vessels shown on the diagram are: *1,* common femoral artery; *2,* common femoral vein; *3,* saphenofemoral junction; *4,* superficial femoral artery; *5,* profunda femoris artery; *6,* femoral vein; *7,* profunda vein. Vessels demonstrated on the images are the common femoral vein *(V),* common femoral artery *(CFA),* saphenofemoral junction *(SFJ),* superficial femoral artery *(SFA),* profunda femoris artery *(PA),* femoral vein *(FV),* and profunda vein *(PV).* Note that the femoral artery bifurcation is sometimes found above the level of the saphenofemoral junction. In addition, the superficial femoral artery tends to roll on top of the FV, as shown in the B-mode image. (E) In the B-mode longitudinal plane, it can be easy to mistake the PV for the artery. Although the image appears to demonstrate the profunda femoris artery, this is the PV and only the origin of the profunda femoris artery *(PA)* can be seen *(white arrow)* as the artery runs laterally, out of the image plane indicated by the partial cone. (F) In this example of the bifurcation, color flow imaging demonstrates that the probe has been correctly orientated to demonstrate the PA.

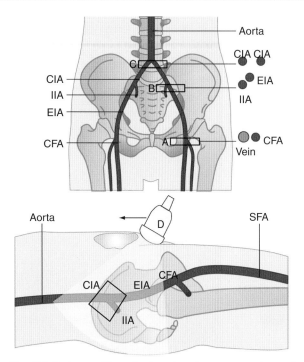

Fig. 9.8 Probe positions for imaging the common femoral artery *(CFA)* and aortoiliac arteries. *(A)* CFA transverse. *(B)* Origin of external and internal iliac arteries transverse. *(C)* Aortic bifurcation transverse. *(D)* Arteries in the longitudinal plane. Starting at the groin and pushing bowel gas upward with the transducer *(arrow)* can help visualization. Positioning the color box to the edge of the scan sector can improve the angle of insonation with spectral Doppler. *CIA*, Common iliac artery; *EIA*, external iliac artery; *IIA*, internal iliac artery; *SFA*, superficial femoral artery.

should be asked to relax the abdominal muscles and to rest the arms by the sides as this reduces tension in the abdominal muscles. Sometimes, rolling patients on to their side can improve visualization of the iliac arteries if obscuring bowel gas is present. The scanning positions for assessing the inflow arteries are shown in Fig. 9.8, and a color image of the arteries is shown in Fig. 9.9. The procedure for assessment is as follows:

1 Using a mid-frequency linear array transducer, the CFA is identified at the level of the groin in transverse section, where it lies lateral to the common femoral vein (Figs. 9.7 and 9.8A). The CFA is then followed proximally in longitudinal section until it runs deep under the inguinal ligament and can no longer be assessed with this probe. A low-frequency curvilinear transducer should then be selected. Using the probe to push any gas upward and driving the color

box toward the edge of the sector (field of view) can help in visualizing the aortoiliac region and in maintaining adequate spectral Doppler angles (see Fig. 9.8D).

2 The external iliac artery is then identified in longitudinal section and followed proximally toward its origin using color flow imaging. The artery is normally seen to lie above the iliac vein. Sometimes, tilting or rolling of the transducer and the use of oblique and coronal probe positions along the abdominal wall are useful in imaging around areas of bowel gas.

3 The common iliac bifurcation should be identified by locating the origin of the external iliac and internal iliac arteries. This can be achieved in the longitudinal plane, but transverse imaging is also helpful for confirmation if the image is adequate, as the internal iliac artery usually divides in a posteromedial direction (see Fig. 9.8B). This area serves as an important anatomical landmark for localizing areas of disease in the aortoiliac system. Sometimes it is not possible to identify the internal iliac artery, and the position of the common iliac bifurcation has to be inferred, as it usually lies in the deepest part of the pelvis as seen on the scan image, although the CIA is sometime fairly short and this is not always a reliable feature.

4 The CIA is then followed back to the aortic bifurcation in longitudinal section (Fig. 9.8D). At this point, it is useful to confirm the level of the aortic bifurcation in transverse plane (Fig. 9.8C). The origins of the CIA are assessed in the longitudinal plane. The aorta should also be examined in transverse and longitudinal planes to exclude an aortic aneurysm or stenosis (see Ch. 11).

Assessment of the Femoral and Popliteal Arteries

To start the examination, the patient should be lying reasonably flat with the leg rotated outward and the knee gently flexed and supported. The scanning positions for imaging the femoropopliteal arteries are shown in Fig. 9.10. The procedure for assessment is as follows:

1 The CFA is identified in transverse section with a mid-range linear array transducer at the groin and followed distally to demonstrate the femoral bifurcation (Figs. 9.7 and 9.10A). The CFA lies lateral to the common femoral vein.

2 Turning to a longitudinal plane, the femoral bifurcation is examined (Fig. 9.10B). The profunda

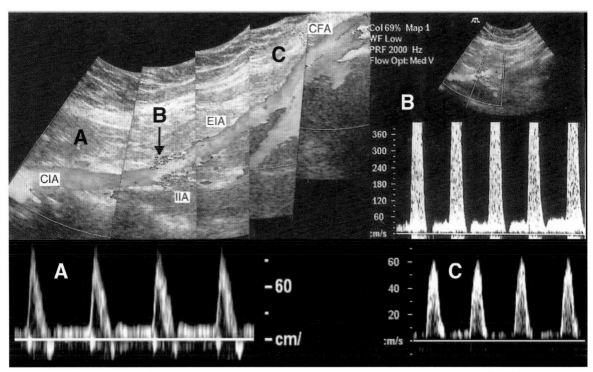

Fig. 9.9 *(Top right)* A color montage of the inflow arteries showing the common iliac artery *(CIA)*, external iliac *(EIA)* and internal iliac arteries *(IIA)*, and the common femoral artery *(CFA)*. Note the stenosis at the iliac artery bifurcation *(arrow)*, demonstrated by aliasing. (A to C) Spectral Doppler recordings are taken proximal to the stenosis *(point A)*, across the stenosis *(point B)*, and distal to the stenosis *(point C)*. High systolic velocity, aliasing, and spectral broadening at *point B* indicate a severe stenosis. There is an abnormal waveform distally at *point C* with increased systolic rise time and a loss of reverse flow.

femoris artery usually lies posterolateral to the SFA, requiring a slight outward turn of the transducer. The profunda femoris artery can often be followed for a considerable distance, particularly if the SFA is occluded and it is supplying a collateral pathway to the lower thigh. The origin of the SFA is usually located anteromedial to the profunda femoris artery, requiring a slight inward turn of the transducer.

3 The SFA is then followed distally along the medial aspect of the thigh in a longitudinal plane, where it will lie above the superficial femoral vein (Fig. 9.10C). If the image of the SFA is lost, it is easier to relocate in transverse section (Fig. 9.10D). In its distal segment the SFA runs deep and enters the adductor canal, becoming the popliteal artery at the adductor hiatus. It is usually possible to image the proximal popliteal artery to just above the knee level from this position

(Fig. 9.10E). A low-frequency transducer can help to image the artery in a large thigh. Using an anterior position at point (Fig. 9.10I) can also improve visualization in some cases.

4 The popliteal artery can be examined by rolling the patient onto the side. Alternatively, the patient can lie in a prone position, resting the foot on a pillow, although elderly patients may be unable to tolerate this position. It is also possible to image the popliteal artery with the legs hanging over the edge of the examination table and the feet resting on a stool. Whichever method is used, it is important not to overextend the knee joint, as this can make imaging difficult. Conversely, if the knee is too flexed, access to the popliteal fossa is difficult.

5 Starting in the middle of the popliteal fossa, the popliteal artery is located in transverse section and is seen deep to the popliteal vein (Fig. 9.10F). Turning

into a longitudinal plane, the popliteal artery is then followed proximally, above the popliteal fossa, to overlap the area previously examined from the lower medial thigh (Fig. 9.10G).

6 The popliteal artery is then examined longitudinally across and below the popliteal fossa, where it is possible to continue directly into the tibioperoneal trunk. The tibioperoneal trunk can be imaged from a number of positions.

Assessment of the Tibial Arteries

> ### PRACTICAL TIP
>
> Patients with critical leg ischemia often hang the leg in a dependent position and cannot tolerate lying flat for long periods of time. In this situation it is easier to scan the popliteal arteries and calf vessels with the leg dependent, as this will improve the detection of flow and also make the procedure more comfortable for the patient. The femoral vessels can be scanned with the end of the examination table tilted down.

The tibial arteries can be imaged from several different transducer positions, as demonstrated in Fig. 9.11, and a color montage of the proximal tibial arteries is shown in Fig. 9.12. It is often easier to locate the tibial arteries in the distal calf and follow them proximally to the top of the calf. However, for the purposes of this section, the description of the examination starts just below the knee. It should be noted that imaging of the distal tibial arteries at the ankle is often easier with a high-frequency linear array transducer.

Anterior Tibial Artery

1 With the leg rolled outward and the knee slightly flexed, the origin of the AT artery is imaged from a posteromedial position just below the knee, where it will be seen to drop immediately away from the popliteal artery (see Fig. 9.10H). Often it is only possible to see the first 1 to 2 cm of the AT from this position. The tibioperoneal trunk is usually seen as a direct continuation of the popliteal artery distal to the AT artery origin.

2 The proximal AT artery is then imaged from the anterolateral aspect of the upper calf, just below the knee, where it will be seen to rise toward the transducer in a curve, through the interosseous

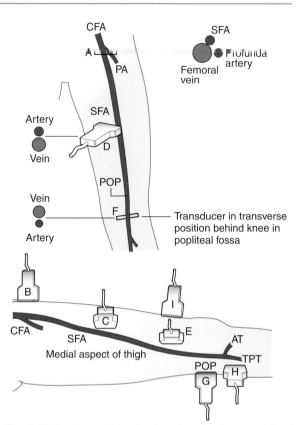

Fig. 9.10 Probe positions for imaging the femoropopliteal arteries. *(A)* Femoral artery bifurcation transverse. *(B)* Femoral bifurcation longitudinal. *(C)* Superficial femoral artery *(SFA)* longitudinal. *(D)* SFA transverse. *(E)* Proximal popliteal artery above-knee longitudinal. *(F)* Popliteal artery transverse. *(G)* Popliteal artery longitudinal, from the popliteal fossa. *(H)* Origin of the anterior tibial. Note that the distal SFA and proximal popliteal artery are sometimes easier to image by using a more anterior approach at point *I. CFA,* Common femoral artery; *PA,* profunda femoris artery; *POP,* popliteal artery; *TPT,* tibioperoneal trunk.

membrane. The membrane can be identified as a bright echogenic line running between the tibia and fibula in cross-section. The artery will lie on top of the membrane. The AT artery is then followed distally, along the anterolateral border of the calf, until it becomes the DP artery, over the top of the foot.

Posterior Tibial Artery

1 With the leg rolled outward and the knee flexed, the origin of the PT artery is imaged from a medial position, below the knee, where the tibioperoneal trunk divides into the PT artery and the peroneal artery.

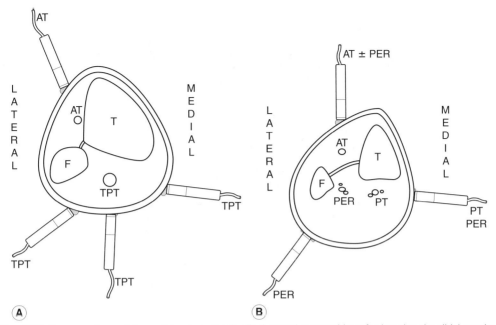

Fig. 9.11 Cross-sections of the calf to show longitudinal transducer positions for imaging the tibial arteries and veins in the calf. (A) Several positions can be used to image the vessels in the upper calf proximal to the bifurcation of the tibioperoneal trunk *(TPT)*. (B) Probe positions to image the posterior tibial *(PT)*, anterior tibial *(AT)*, and peroneal artery *(PER)* in the mid and lower calf. Note that it is possible to image two vessels from a similar position, as shown. *F,* Fibula; *T,* tibia.

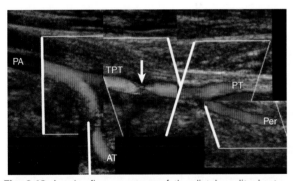

Fig. 9.12 A color flow montage of the distal popliteal artery *(PA)* and tibial artery origins, demonstrating the tibioperoneal trunk *(TPT)*, posterior tibial *(PT)*, anterior tibial *(AT)*, and peroneal artery *(Per)*. This image has been taken from medial posterior aspect of the upper calf. Note: an area of aliasing (arrow) may indicate a stenosis in the TPT.

The proximal PT artery will gently rise toward the transducer, and the associated paired veins act as useful landmarks. The origin of the peroneal artery is often visible from this plane and will lie posterior to the PT artery origin.

2 The PT artery is then followed along the medial aspect of the calf toward the inner ankle or medial malleolus. The PT artery lies superficial to the peroneal artery when imaged from the medial aspect of the calf.

3 The origin and a short segment of the PT artery can often be visualized from a posterolateral position below the knee, where it will be seen to run deep as it divides from the tibioperoneal trunk.

Peroneal Artery

Imaging of the peroneal artery may have to be performed from a number of different positions (see Fig. 9.11B). The optimum position varies from patient to patient.

• View 1 The peroneal artery can be followed from its origin along the calf using the same medial calf position as that described to image the PT artery. From this position, the peroneal artery will be seen lying deeper than the PT artery against the border of the fibula, surrounded by the larger peroneal veins. Slight anterior or posterior longitudinal tilting of the probe may be needed to follow the artery distally.

TABLE 9.5   Common Problems Encountered During Duplex Evaluation of the Lower-limb Arteries

Segment	Problem	Solutions
Aortoiliac arteries	Bowel gas obscuring part or all of the image	Try different probe positions (medial, lateral, or coronal positions); leave the segment and try again in a few minutes
Aortoiliac arteries	Tortuous arteries	Use the color display to follow the artery; considerable adjustment of the probe position is often needed
Femoropopliteal arteries	Severe calcification of the artery producing color image dropout	Try different transducer positions to work around the calcification
Femoropopliteal arteries	Obese patient with large thigh	When using a broad-band transducer, lower the color and spectral Doppler transmit frequencies for better penetration; consider switching to a low-frequency curved array transducer in very difficult situations
Tibial arteries	Large calf with gross edema	Start the scan at the ankle and work proximally; a low-frequency flat or curved array probe can be used to image these vessels proximally
Tibial arteries	Very low flow due to proximal occlusions, or difficulty locating the arteries	Lower the pulse repetition frequency and wall filters; place the leg in a dependent position to increase distal blood flow. Using calf augmentation can help identify the location of the major veins, which in turn helps to identify the location of adjacent arteries

- View 2 The peroneal artery can usually be followed distally from its origin using a posterolateral position, below the knee and along the calf.
- View 3 The peroneal artery can sometimes be imaged from the anterolateral aspect of the calf, where it will be seen lying deep to the AT artery. This is the most difficult position from which to obtain images of the peroneal artery.

Commonly Encountered Problems

There are a number of problems and pitfalls associated with lower-limb duplex scanning. Table 9.5 lists some of the more frequently encountered problems.

SCAN APPEARANCES

B-Mode Images

Normal Appearance

Like the carotid arteries, the lumen of a normal peripheral artery should appear clear, and the walls should be uniform along each arterial segment, although noise may cause speckle within the image of the vessel. Providing there is no disease proximal to the point of imaging, it should be possible to observer distention or "pulsing" of the arterial walls in time with each cardiac cycle if the

probe is held in a steady position for a few seconds. The intima-media layer of the arterial wall is sometimes seen in normal femoral and popliteal arteries. In practice, it is frequently difficult to image the vessels clearly in the aortoiliac segment, adductor canal region, and calf without the help of color flow imaging.

Abnormal Appearance

Areas of atheroma, particularly if they are calcified, may be seen within the vessel lumen. The atheroma may be extensive and diffusely distributed, especially in the SFA. Large plaques at the common femoral bifurcation are relatively easy to image, and these may extend into the proximal profunda artery or SFA. Localized plaques of the CFA often produce a "cauliflower" appearance and are normally located on the posterior wall (see Fig. 9.13A). Any plaques in the CFA should be highlighted on the scan report, as this is one of the main access points (catheter access) for radiological and endovascular intervention, and it is important that the clinician is aware of any disease or features that might make access difficult. Box 9.4 describes this in detail.

Calcification of the arterial walls, especially in diabetic patients, can produce strong ultrasound reflections. In particular, the walls of the calf arteries can appear

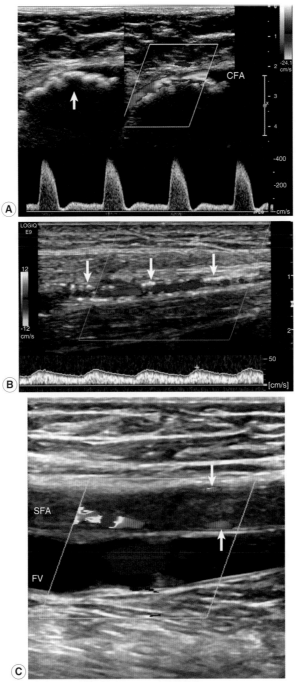

Fig. 9.13 (A) An extensive area of calcified atheroma *(arrow)* is present in the common femoral artery, leading to "drop-out" of the B-mode signal. A large acoustic shadow is present. The corresponding color flow image suggests significant narrowing and aliasing. (B) Calcified atheroma *(arrows)* is seen in the distal anterior tibial artery. There is a "beaded" appearance to the color flow display. The corresponding Doppler spectrum shows significant damping of flow. (C) An acute occlusion of the superficial femoral artery *(SFA)* shown is evidence by anechoic thrombus in the artery. In this example, there is evidence of some early recanalization as shown by color flow signals *(arrows)*. The femoral vein *(FV)* is posterior to the SFA.

prominent, and in some cases the vessel looks enlarged due to the extent of calcification (see Fig. 9.13B). When an arterial segment has been occluded for some time, the vessel may contract and appear as a small cord adjacent to the corresponding vein (see Fig. 9.16). This appearance is most frequently seen in the SFA and popliteal artery. If

there is difficulty in locating the artery, augmenting flow in the adjacent vein that runs parallel to the artery can aid identification. B-mode imaging in combination with color flow imaging is also very useful for identifying acute occlusions of the SFA or popliteal artery, where there may be fresh thrombus present in the vessel lumen. The lumen will appear clear or demonstrate minimal echoes on the image, because thrombus has a similar echogenicity to blood (Fig. 9.13C). However, color flow imaging reveals an absence of flow in the occluded segment of the vessel. The start of the occlusion can often be very abrupt, with little disease seen proximally. Sometimes there is visible pulsing lateral (to and fro) movement of the artery or even the thrombus due to the blood flow encountering the sudden obstruction.

Abnormal dilatations or arterial aneurysms should be measured using the B-mode image, as described in Chapter 11.

Color Flow Images
Abnormal Appearance
Utilizing the color controls as described in Chapter 7 and Appendix C, arterial stenoses will be demonstrated as areas of color flow disturbance or aliasing. Severe stenoses frequently produce a disturbed color flow pattern extending 3 to 4 vessel diameters beyond the lesion

---

BOX 9.4   Assessing Access to the CFA for Radiological or Endovascular Procedures

- If the CFA appears clear, ensure the Doppler waveform does not demonstrate turbulence or increased systolic rise time that could be associated with proximal disease.
- Assess the distribution of any plaques in CFA and their position, particularly if they are located on the anterior wall, as this may make arterial puncture more difficult and could disrupt the plaque. Grade any significant narrowing.
- Measure the diameter of the artery and where possible the residual lumen. Ensure there is not an aneurysm of the CFA or that there is no evidence of previous surgery or arterial reconstruction.
- Check the proximal SFA and profunda artery are patent.
- Check if the CFA bifurcation appears abnormally high, as this could result in a high puncture with risk of post-procedure bleeding.

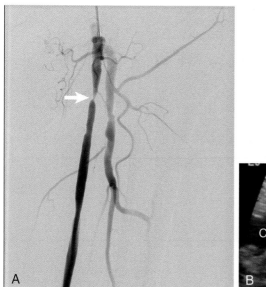

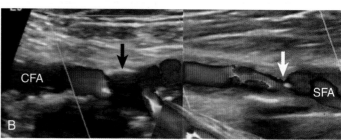

Fig. 9.14 (A) Angiography of the common femoral artery (CFA) bifurcation and superficial femoral artery (SFA) demonstrates some plaques and a severe stenosis (arrow) of the proximal SFA. (B) A color flow montage demonstrates calcified plaque at the CFA bifurcation with acoustic shadowing (black arrow) and corresponding severe stenosis of the proximal SFA (white arrow).

(Figs. 9.9, 9.14, and 9.15). Any areas of color flow disturbance should be investigated with angle-corrected spectral Doppler to estimate the degree of narrowing. In addition, the color flow image of flow in a nondiseased artery distal to severe proximal disease may demonstrate damped low-velocity flow, which will be seen as continuous flow in one direction.

Occlusions of lower-limb arteries most frequently occur in the SFA, popliteal artery, and tibial arteries. An occlusion is demonstrated by a total absence of color flow in the vessel. Occlusions can occur at the origins of arteries or in mid-segment. If an artery is occluded from its origin, at the level of a major bifurcation, flow will normally still be seen in the sister branch. For example, the profunda femoris artery is usually found to be patent when the SFA is occluded (Fig. 9.16). When an artery occludes in mid-segment, collateral vessels are normally seen dividing from the main trunk at the beginning of the occlusion. Similarly, collateral vessels resupply flow to the artery at the distal end of the occlusion (Fig. 9.17). Collateral vessels can follow tortuous routes as they divide from the main trunk, and they are sometimes only seen when the main artery is imaged in cross-section. It is therefore helpful to interrogate any suspected occlusion in both longitudinal and transverse imaging planes. The PRF often needs to be lowered (typically to 1 kHz or color scale in the region of 10 cm/s) distal to an occlusion in order to increase the sensitivity of the scanner to displaying lower flow velocities. The color flow image distal to an occlusion often demonstrates a continuous forward flow pattern with reduced pulsatility due to damping of the normal blood flow pattern. Blood flow in the main artery may also improve progressively over the first few centimeters distal to the occlusion as more collateral vessels join the main trunk. This effect can be observed on the color flow image. High-velocity flow in a collateral vessel can produce an area of marked color flow disturbance in the main artery at the point where the collateral joins (see Fig. 9.17). This can be misinterpreted as a stenosis. Spectral Doppler should be used to interrogate this area carefully. It is possible to misdiagnose a long stricture as an occlusion because of very slow flow through the stricture due to the development of good collateral flow around the diseased site. The color scale should be lowered to examine low-velocity flow across these lesions. In the calf arteries, diffuse calcification can cause a beading appearance of the color flow image (see Fig. 9.13B) due to difference

in attenuation caused by variable density of calcification distributed along the arterial wall.

Spectral Doppler
Abnormal Recordings and Grading of Stenosis

> ### REFERENCE VELOCITIES
>
> Data have been published for the average peak systolic velocity found in normal external iliac, superficial femoral, and popliteal arteries, which are 119, 90, and 68 cm/s, respectively (Jager et al. 1985), but resting velocities can vary with age and general health and it is important not to use these as a primary diagnostic tool.

Spectral Doppler should always be used to interrogate areas of color flow disturbance. The spectral Doppler sample volume can be increased in size to cover the lumen if there is difficulty in obtaining adequate signals. Measurements should be taken just proximal to, across, and just beyond the lesion. In the presence of a significant stenosis, there will be an increase in flow velocity across the lesion associated with spectral broadening and turbulence just distal to the lesion. As demonstrated previously (see Table 8.2), a concentric 50% diameter reduction of the arterial lumen will produce a 75% reduction in cross-sectional area, leading to significant velocity changes. However, as discussed in Chapter 8, many lesions are eccentric and the difference between diameter and area reduction is not constant. The main criterion used to grade the degree of narrowing in a lower-limb artery is the measurement of the peak systolic velocity (PSV) ratio. The PSV ratio is calculated by dividing the maximum PSV recorded across the stenosis (V_s) by the PSV recorded in a normal area of the artery just proximal to the stenosis (V_p), as demonstrated in Figs. 9.9 and 9.15. Different criteria have been published for defining a 50%, or greater, diameter reduction in the lower-limb arteries. Many of these were developed in the 1990s, but there has not been any major modification of these criteria since this period. Many vascular units use a PSV ratio of equal to or greater than 2 (≥ 2) (Cossman et al. 1989; Sensier et al. 1996), although a ratio of ≥ 2.5 is used by other centers (Legemate et al. 1991; Schlager et al. 2007). It is important to audit and evaluate the criterion used by your unit against other imaging techniques such as angiography or computed tomographic angiography (CTA) or magnetic resonance

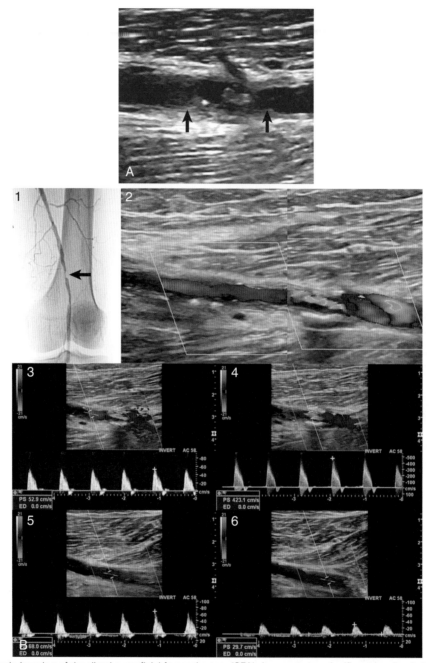

Fig. 9.15 (A) B-mode imaging of the distal superficial femoral artery (SFA) demonstrates significant localized plaque and narrowing (region between *arrows*). (B) This montage of images shows *(1)* an angiogram of the distal SFA confirming a tight stenosis, *(2)* duplex imaging with significant color flow disturbance and aliasing at the site of the stenosis, and *(3)* spectral Doppler recording just proximal to the stenosis with triphasic flow. The peak systolic velocity is 53 cm/s, *(4)* Doppler recordings across the stenosis at the point of maximum velocity (423 cm/s), *(5)* Doppler recordings just distal to the stenosis with a disturbed waveform, and *(6)* Doppler recordings taken 3 to 4 cm beyond the stenosis showing an overall reduction in velocity compared to the proximal waveform *(frame 3)* and biphasic flow. In this example the peak systolic velocity ratio will be calculated by dividing 423 cm/s by 53 cm/s = 8 times, confirming a severe hemodynamic stenosis.

angiography (MRA). Table 9.6 shows how the velocity ratio can be used to grade the severity of lower-limb disease using these criteria. Velocity ratios can still be used to grade stenoses in the presence of multisegment disease, although there is evidence that this is less reliable compared to the grading of a single lesion (Macharzina et al. 2015). However, in practice, flow distal to multiple lesions will normally be significantly affected as evidenced by abnormal waveforms. It is useful to indicate the length and position of diseased segments on a diagram. The grading of SFA disease by measuring maximum PSV across a stenosis has been described by Gao et al. (2018). They found cut-off thresholds for a 50% to 69% and 70% to 99% stenoses of ≥210 and ≥275 cm/s, respectively.

Assessment of aortoiliac lesions can be particularly difficult due to the high angle of insonation and potential velocity errors. A study by Coffi et al. (2001) comparing duplex velocity ratios to intra-arterial pressure measurements indicted that caution should be used in interpretation where velocity ratios are found to be between two and three times, indicating subcritical disease. Grading lesions at bifurcations can be technically challenging, especially if there is a natural diameter change between the proximal artery and the daughter artery and in the absence of any published data, the calculated ratio should be interpreted cautiously. This situation is encountered at the common femoral bifurcation. Another potentially confusing situation occurs when the aortoiliac and CFAs are clear but the SFA is occluded and the profunda femoris artery is severely stenosed. This can give rise to a monophasic waveform pattern in the CFA with a high end-diastolic velocity, although the systolic acceleration time remains short. A great deal of care should be used in interpreting flow patterns in this situation.

Finally, areas of aneurysmal dilation typically demonstrate a reduction in PSV, frequently associated with disturbed flow patterns.

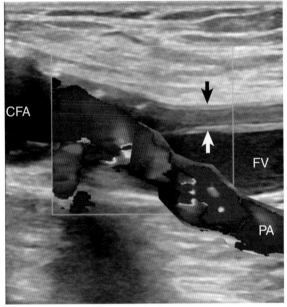

Fig. 9.16 A color flow montage of the common femoral artery *(CFA)* bifurcation demonstrating a superficial femoral artery origin occlusion (point between *arrows*). The occluded SFA appears small, and it is possible that this may be longstanding occlusion and possibly an acute thrombosis when it occurred, as intima detail can be seen in the SFA. The profunda femoris artery *(PA)* is patent with some disturbed flow due to diffuse plaques. The femoral vein *(FV)* is seen in this image.

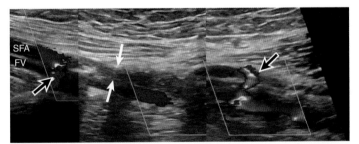

Fig. 9.17 A mid-superficial femoral artery *(SFA)* occlusion is demonstrated by an absence of color flow in the vessel (marked between the *white arrows*). Large collateral vessels are seen at both ends of the occlusion *(white outlined black arrows)*. Marked areas of flow disturbance and aliasing can occur at points where collateral vessels feed the main artery, due to the size of the collateral vessel and direction (angle) of flow with respect to the transducer. The femoral vein *(FV)* is seen in this image.

TABLE 9.6   Suggested Criteria for Grading Lower-limb Arterial Disease Using Velocity Ratios, Based on Several References

Diameter Reduction	Velocity Ratio (V_s/V_p)	Comments
0%–49%	<2	Waveform is triphasic, but mild spectral broadening and an increase in end-diastolic velocities are recorded as the degree of narrowing approaches 49%
50%–74%	≥2	Waveforms tend to become biphasic or monophasic; there is an increase in end-diastolic velocity; spectral broadening is present; flow disturbance and some damping are recorded distal to the stenosis
75%–99%	≥4	Waveform is usually monophasic with significant increase in end-diastolic velocity; marked turbulence and spectral broadening are demonstrated; flow is damped distal to the stenosis. If the stenosis is very short and in the absence of proximal disease, it is possible for biphasic flow to be recorded within the stenosis
Occluded	No flow detected	Doppler waveforms proximal to an occlusion often demonstrate a high-resistance flow pattern

Other methods of measurement have been used to grade LLAD, including pulsatility index, but these have tended to be used with continuous-wave Doppler and are probably less useful for duplex scanning where velocity changes can be measured directly.

Acute Limb Ischemia

Use of ultrasound in acute limb ischemia depends on the particular patient's presentation and pathway. If unilateral acute ischemia is suspected, initial examination of the CFA, popliteal, and distal tibial arteries can indicate at what level the occlusion lies. Distal to an acute occlusion, flow waveforms are very damped because collaterals haven't had time to develop. For a damped CFA waveform, comparison of the contralateral CFA waveform can help to indicate whether this results from an iliac artery occlusion or aortic occlusion; in the latter case both CFA waveforms will be damped. Once the level is identified, the location and length of the occlusion can be investigated to aid in planning for treatment and sites for interventional access.

An unusual cause of acute limb ischemia is due to extensive venous occlusion, termed phlegmasia cerulea dolens (see Ch. 14). It is an uncommon but potentially life-threatening complication of acute DVT characterized by marked swelling of the extremities with pain and cyanosis, which in turn may lead to arterial ischemia and ultimately cause gangrene with high amputation and mortality rates. In these cases, there is low-volume pulsatile arterial with pronounced reverse flow and indications of no net flow (to and fro waveform).

SPECIALIZED APPLICATIONS

Assessment of Tibial and Foot Arteries Including the Plantar Arch

Duplex scanning combined with continuous-wave Doppler recordings can be a useful method of assessing and mapping the foot circulation and also for locating target vessels prior to distal bypass surgery. In this way, it is possible to select a target vessel to position the distal anastomosis. This can be a challenging examination, particularly in the diabetic foot and presence of severe artery calcification. It should be undertaken by an operator with considerable experience. It is also useful to have an understanding of the concept of angiosomes, described earlier in the chapter, as blocks or regions of tissue supplied and drained by specific tibial arteries, as the site of ulcers or tissue necrosis can be directly related to disease in a specific tibial vessel (see Fig. 9.2D).

Imaging of the ankle and foot arteries may require a combination of mid- and high-frequency transducers, including a hockey stick transducer. This can be particularly useful for fitting into the contours around the ankle and toward the web spaces of the foot. For the PT artery, it is easiest to start the scan at the level of the medial malleolus and then follow it distally to the bifurcation into the medial and lateral plantar arteries. The DP can be imaged over the dorsum of the foot and then followed proximally and distally. Starting in cross-section with a high-frequency probe can be useful, especially if the arteries are calcified, as they will be prominent in the B-mode image. Assessing flow in the distal vessels of the foot in the region of the plantar arch can be achieved by scanning in cross-section and using a square color box in the region of the web spaces. The area just above the first web space is often the easiest area to detect flow. In the diabetic foot, significant disease is indicated if there is pulsatile (tri or biphasic) flow at the ankle but damped monophasic waveforms recorded from vessels in the arch region. An absence of forefoot flow in the presence of pulsatile flow recorded from patent distal tibial arteries could indicate a poor outcome in terms of healing of toe or foot ulcers due to the possibility of heavily diseased foot vessels.

For distal bypass there needs to be a low-resistance arterial pathway in the foot, distal to a graft, to ensure that the graft remains patent and the foot perfused. The three tibial arteries of the calf have connections to the plantar arch, but the PT and DP arteries usually contribute most flow to the arch via plantar arteries. The plantar arch supplies blood to the plantar metatarsal arteries and digital arteries of the toes. The patient should be assessed with the leg in a dependent position to maximize blood flow due to hydrostatic pressure and to make detection of arch signals easier. Using the duplex scanner, it is possible to assess the patency and quality of each of the tibial arteries to ankle level. A continuous-wave Doppler probe, or hockey stick transducer, is then used to assess the blood flow signal from the plantar arch. The probe position for recording flow at the plantar arch is demonstrated in Fig. 9.6. Once a plantar arch signal is detected, selective digital pressure is then applied to occlude the tibial artery at the ankle suggested by duplex scanning as a target vessel for distal bypass (see Fig. 9.18). A substantial reduction or cessation of flow at the plantar arch during compression would suggest that the arch is in continuation with the selected tibial artery. This type of assessment can be complex, as there may be more than one patent tibial artery supplying the plantar arch. The peroneal artery can also supply the distal AT artery or DP artery via branches, which in turn may supply the plantar arch.

ASSESSMENT OF ARTERIAL STENTS

Arterial stents are used to prevent restenosis of the artery following angioplasty. Stents are mainly deployed in the aortoiliac arteries and proximal CFA, although they are also used in the SFA and popliteal artery. Stents are available in different lengths and sizes, and multiple stents can be deployed if the disease is very extensive. They are usually visible on the B-mode image, producing a stronger reflection compared to the arterial wall. The cross-hatched, or lattice, metal structure can often be identified. It is sometimes possible to see nipping of the stent if the atheroma in the artery is very calcified or fibrous and has not been completely compressed to the vessel wall. Color flow imaging and spectral Doppler can be used to assess the flow across the stent (see Fig. 9.19). It is not uncommon to find some localized flow disturbance in the region of the stent due to the step between the arterial wall and proximal and distal ends of the stent. Stent stenosis is usually due to the development of neointimal hyperplasia (see Fig. 9.19B). Spectral Doppler should be used to grade the degree of any in-stent stenosis. Care should be taken when assessing velocity changes, as there is evidence that applying the same criteria for grading native lower-limb disease may lead to overestimation of the in-stent stenosis. A study by Baril et al. (2009) found that a PSV of 275 cm/s and PSV ratio of 3.5 was highly specific and predictive of characterizing an equal to or greater than 80% in-stent stenosis. Stents placed in arteries close to joints, such as the CFA or popliteal artery, can be stressed by joint movement and may kink, bend, or fracture. Some self-expanding stents constructed of Nitinol are designed to flex and can be deployed safely across these regions. Localized aneurysms can be excluded by inserting a covered stent across the aneurysm; this is discussed in Chapter 11.

ASSESSMENT OF COMPLICATIONS FOLLOWING CATHETER ACCESS

Ultrasound is useful for identifying suspected complications (iatrogenic) following catheter access. This includes failure of closure devices, used to seal the puncture in an artery following an angiogram or angioplasty. The majority of these involve the CFA and are related to false or pseudoaneurysms discussed in Chapter 11. There are instances where arteriovenous fistulas (AVF) can occur if the cannula has passed through a vein and artery resulting in low-resistance high-flow connection between the two. In rare cases, if there is vein lying above and below the artery it is possible for two fistulas to form if the cannula has passed through all three

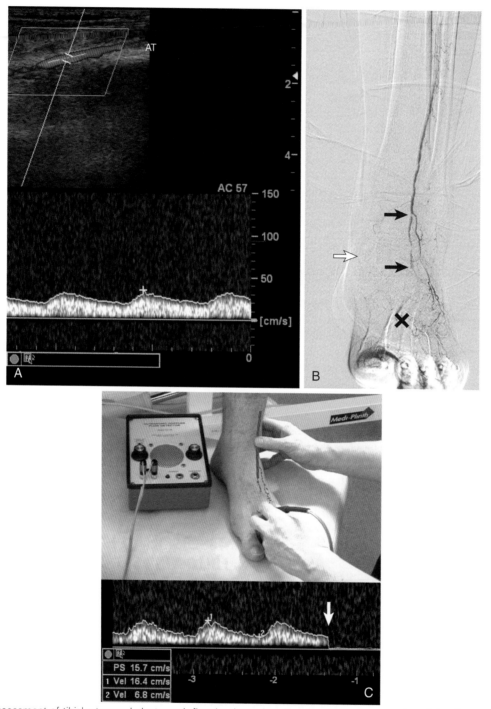

Fig. 9.18 Assessment of tibial artery and plantar arch flow by dependent Doppler. (A) Duplex scanning of the distal anterior tibial artery *(AT)* demonstrates a patent artery with damped flow. (B) An angiogram of the foot confirms a patent AT artery *(black arrow)*, but the dorsalis pedis artery is severely diseased with collateral branches feeding the region of the plantar arch (X). Note, the posterior tibial artery (position of *white arrow*) is occluded. (C) Doppler recordings from the pedal arch region demonstrate damped flow. Selective compression of the AT artery with digital pressure leads to abrupt cessation of flow in the plantar arch region *(arrow)* indicating that the AT is the dominant vessel feeding the arch, albeit via collateral vessels.

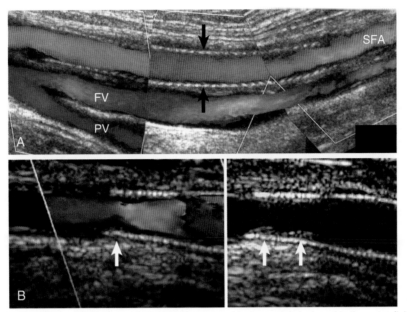

Fig. 9.19 (A) Color flow montage of a stent (areas between *black arrows*) deployed in the superficial femoral artery *(SFA)*. The femoral vein *(FV)* and profunda vein *(PV)* are seen in this image. (B) The proximal end of an SFA stent is shown in B-mode and color flow imaging demonstrating areas of hyperplasia *(arrows)* causing narrowing, demonstrated by the color flow image.

vessels. To investigate a suspected AVF, it is best to start in cross-section looking for any areas of high-velocity flow where the vein and artery are immediately adjacent to each other. Longitudinal imaging can be used to examine waveforms more closely as shown in Fig. 9.20. The arterial waveforms just proximal and distal to the AVF will exhibit different waveform shapes and a high-velocity jet, often with aliasing will be recorded across the AVF. Flow in the vein immediately adjacent to the fistula will be disturbed.

ASSEESMENT OF TRAUMA AND ARTERIAL TRAUMA

The use of ultrasound can be useful in instances of trauma, for instance, to detect flow at the ankle if there have been fractures or injuries to the leg and pulses are difficult to palpate or the lower leg very swollen. A simple hand held Doppler can be useful in the emergency room. Dissection of blood vessels, particularly the popliteal artery due to injuries of the knee, can result in acute ischemia (see Fig. 9.21). It can sometimes be possible to image the dissection flap and also observe poorly echogenic thrombus associated with the dissection.

OTHER ABNORMALITIES AND SYNDROMES

Lower-limb symptoms in younger patients are sometimes due to inflammatory or small-vessel disorders, such as Buerger's disease. Flow recordings are normal in the larger arteries proximally, but the distal vessels in the calf may demonstrate low-flow, high-resistance waveforms.

Popliteal Entrapment Syndrome

Popliteal entrapment syndrome (PES) is a rare condition mainly affecting younger active and athletic individuals. It describes a group of conditions where compression of the popliteal artery, veins, and nerves occurs singularly or in combination at the popliteal fossa by musculoskeletal structures. Popliteal artery entrapment syndrome (PAES) causes intermittent claudication or exertional leg pain that can lead to injury and occlusion of the artery and possible distal embolization due to arterial wall damage. In extreme cases, it can result in limb loss.

PAES can be anatomical or functional. It should be considered if other common causes of symptoms have been investigated and ruled out as shown in Box 9.5. In

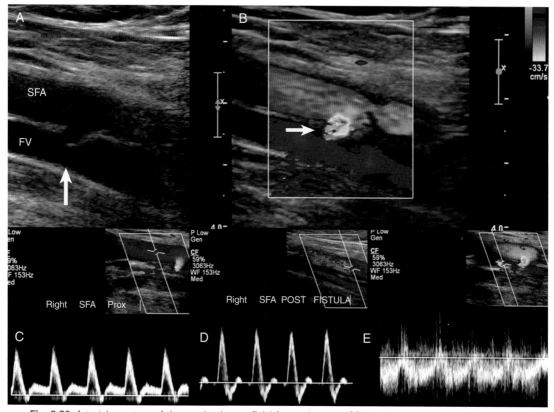

Fig. 9.20 Arterial puncture of the proximal superficial femoral artery *(SFA)* had resulted in an iatrogenic arteriovenous fistula between the artery and the femoral vein *(FV)* as the cannula has punctured the posterior wall of the artery. (A) The position of the fistula is shown by the arrow. (B) Color flow imaging demonstrates an area of aliasing due to high flow and velocity across the fistula *(arrow)*. (C) Doppler waveforms proximal to the fistula demonstrate high diastolic flow due to the low-resistance pathway across the fistula. (D) Waveforms distal to the fistula have a typical triphasic peripheral artery flow pattern. (E) Doppler recordings taken from the FV adjacent to the fistula have a pulsatile appearance.

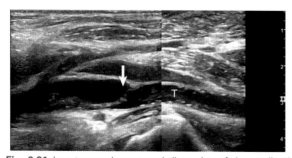

Fig. 9.21 Leg trauma has caused dissection of the popliteal artery with a large flap *(arrow)*. There is thrombus *(T)* in the popliteal artery distal to the flap.

> **BOX 9.5**　**Differential Diagnoses for Popliteal Artery Entrapment Syndrome**
>
> - Chronic exertional compartment syndrome
> - Cystic adventitial disease of the popliteal artery
> - Muscle strain or tears
> - Popliteal artery dissection
> - Fibular and tibial stress fractures
> - Nerve entrapment syndrome
> - Thrombosed popliteal artery aneurysm
> - Bakers cyst
> - Referred pain from lumbar disc herniation

the anatomical situation, the popliteal artery can follow an anomalous course across knee and is trapped by the heads of the gastrocnemius muscle during plantar flexion. The popliteal artery can also be trapped by fibrous bands arising from the popliteus muscle. In the functional situation, overdevelopment of muscles or high-performance exercise can lead to muscle hypertrophy. During activity, plantar flexion results in repeated

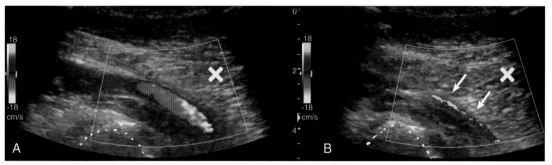

Fig. 9.22 Testing for popliteal entrapment syndrome. (A) The popliteal artery is widely patent at rest. The gastrocnemius muscle is shown by mark *X*. (B) During plantar flexion against counter pressure, the popliteal artery is virtually occluded *(arrows)* due to compression by the gastrocnemius muscle (X).

compression of the popliteal artery by gastrocnemius or soleus and/or popliteus muscles.

Exercise ABPIs are useful but can be equivocal, as any reduction in pressure may have recovered by the time the patient is placed on the examination table and the leg relaxed relieving any compression on the artery. When duplex scanning for PAES, it is useful to use an extended field of view when using a linear array transducer; a curvilinear transducer can also be useful for imaging in the region of the soleus muscle. There are two main methods to test for PAES using duplex. In the first, the patient should lie prone with the legs gently flexed and the feet hanging over the end of the examination table. The below-knee popliteal artery should be imaged at the level of the gastrocnemius muscle heads. The patient should point the foot down (plantar flex) against an increasing counterpressure, typically by having a colleague apply progressive pressure against the foot. In the second method, the patient performs a tip toe or heel-raising maneuver while imaging the artery. For both tests, the artery can be imaged in transverse and longitudinal section, but it is important in longitudinal section that the probe does not accidentally slide to the side of the artery as the muscles contract, giving the false impression of an occlusion. Narrowing or occlusion of the popliteal artery during these maneuvers may indicate PES (Fig. 9.22). However, there is evidence to suggest that significant compression of the popliteal artery can occur in normal volunteers during this investigation making diagnosis and management more difficult (Sinha et al. 2012).

Cystic Adventitial Disease of the Popliteal Artery

The etiology of adventitial cystic disease is uncertain and trauma, ganglion, systemic disorders, and

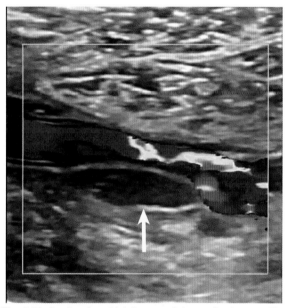

Fig. 9.23 Cystic adventitial disease of the popliteal artery. The hypoechoic cyst is shown by the *arrow* and is impinging into the arterial lumen.

embryonic development have been proposed. This rare disease is typically observed as a cystic swelling of the arterial wall, which impinges into the lumen of the popliteal artery, leading to eventual occlusion (see Fig. 9.23). The location of the lesion is often found across the knee joint. It should be considered as a potential cause of symptoms in the young patient, especially in the absence of any other pathology. Caliper-based diameter measurements, color flow, and spectral Doppler can all be used to assess the degree of stenosis. Treatment is by excision and local repair or arterial bypass.

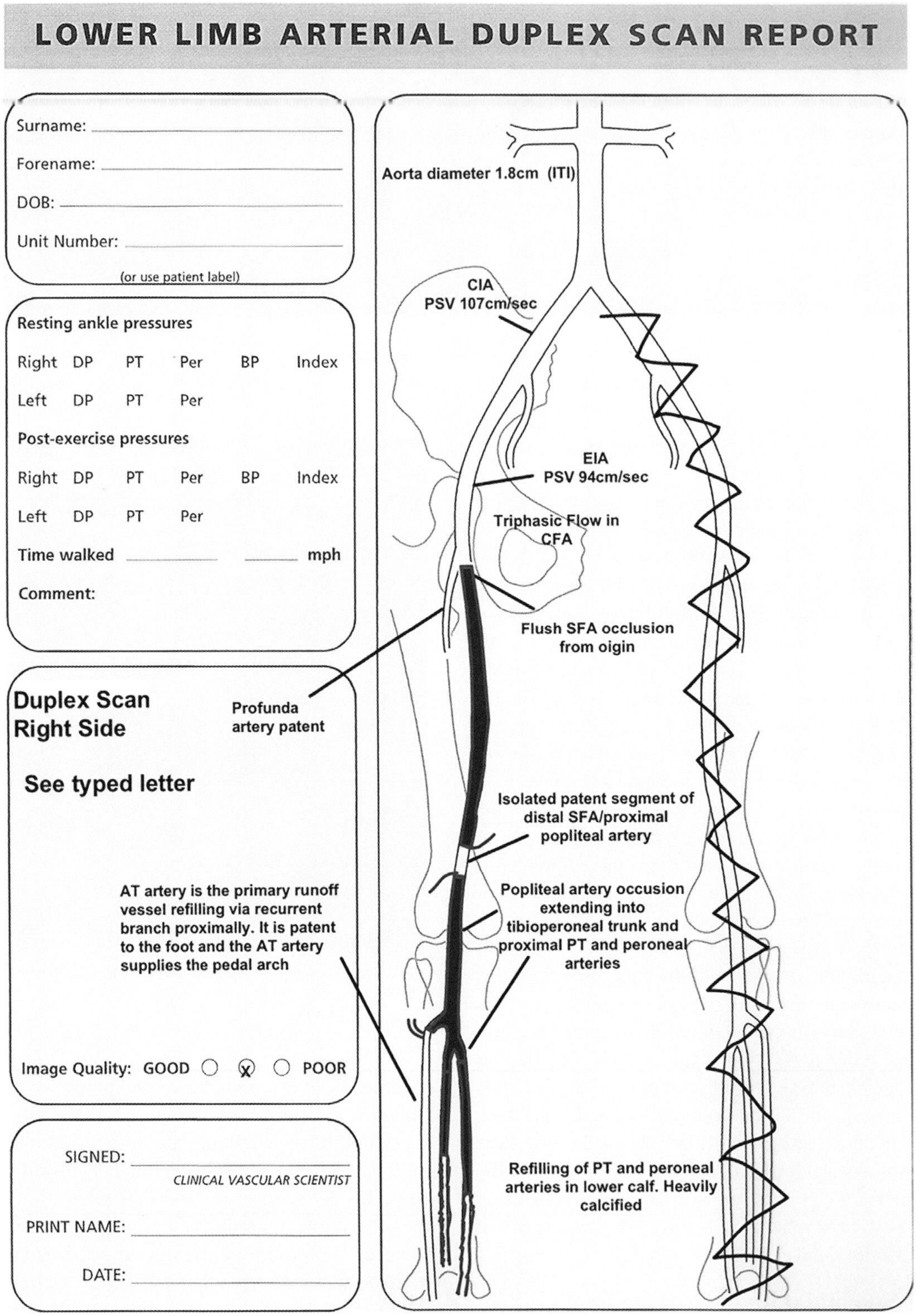

LOWER LIMB ARTERIAL DUPLEX SCAN REPORT

Surname: _____

Forename: _____

DOB: _____

Unit Number: _____

(or use patient label)

Resting ankle pressures

Right DP   PT   Per   BP   Index

Left   DP   PT   Per

Post-exercise pressures

Right DP   PT   Per   BP   Index

Left   DP   PT   Per

Time walked _____ _____ mph

Comment:

Duplex Scan
Right Side

See typed letter

AT artery is the primary runoff
vessel refilling via recurrent
branch proximally. It is patent
to the foot and the AT artery
supplies the pedal arch

Image Quality: GOOD ◯ ⊗ ◯ POOR

SIGNED: _____

CLINICAL VASCULAR SCIENTIST

PRINT NAME: _____

DATE: _____

Aorta diameter 1.8cm (ITI)

CIA
PSV 107cm/sec

EIA
PSV 94cm/sec

Triphasic Flow in
CFA

Flush SFA occlusion
from oigin

Profunda
artery patent

Isolated patent segment of
distal SFA/proximal
popliteal artery

Popliteal artery occusion
extending into
tibioperoneal trunk and
proximal PT and peroneal
arteries

Refilling of PT and peroneal
arteries in lower calf. Heavily
calcified

Fig. 9.24 The use of diagrams is an effective method of reporting lower-limb arterial scans. Areas of narrowing can be drawn on the map with corresponding velocity measurements. Occlusions are demonstrated by blocking out the appropriate regions. Comment can be added as appropriate. This example also includes a section for ankle–brachial pressure measurement.

REPORTING

In our experience, the use of diagrams demonstrating the position of disease and corresponding velocity measurements and ratios is the simplest method of reporting results, as shown in Fig. 9.24. Areas that were impossible to assess due to bowel gas or calcification can be hatched out on the diagram. Surgeons and physicians also find this method of reporting helpful when reviewing results in a busy outpatient clinic, as reading pages of text can be very time-consuming. Copies of the report can be sent to the radiology department with a request card if the patient requires an angiogram or angioplasty, thus allowing the radiologist to pre-plan puncture sites. In many situations an angioplasty can be performed without a diagnostic arteriogram.

10

Duplex Assessment of Upper-Limb Arterial Disease

INTRODUCTION

In contrast to lower-limb arteries, atherosclerotic disease in the upper extremities is less common and accounts for <10% of the average vascular laboratory workload. The most commonly affected sites are the brachiocephalic trunk, subclavian (SA), and axillary arteries. This is sometimes associated with extracranial carotid artery disease. Radiotherapy in this region can result in fibrosis and scarring and can also cause damage to the SA and axillary arteries. Compression of the SA in the area of the thoracic outlet, known as thoracic outlet syndrome (TOS), can produce significant upper-limb symptoms and in rare cases lead to SA aneurysms.

Acute obstruction of the axillary or brachial arteries may also occur due to embolization from the heart or SA aneurysms. In this situation, duplex scanning is useful for demonstrating the length and position of the occlusion. Pseudoaneurysms can occur following arterial access, mainly in the brachial or radial arteries. Microvascular disorders, such as Raynaud's phenomenon, can produce significant symptoms in the hands, which may be confused with atherosclerotic disease.

ANATOMY OF THE UPPER-EXTREMITY ARTERIES

The anatomy of the upper-extremity arteries is illustrated in Figs. 10.1 and 10.2. The left SA divides directly from the aortic arch, but the right SA originates from the brachiocephalic artery. The thoracic outlet is the point where the SA, subclavian vein, and brachial nerve plexus exit the chest. The SA runs between the anterior and middle scalene muscles and passes between the clavicle and first rib to become the axillary artery. The diameter of the SA ranges from 0.7 to 1.1 cm. The SA has a number of important branches, including the vertebral artery and internal thoracic artery (also referred

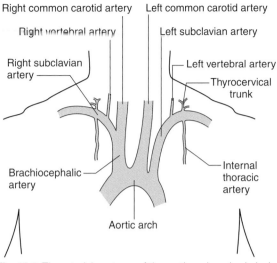

Fig. 10.1 The arterial anatomy of the aortic arch and subclavian artery.

to as the mammary artery), which is frequently used for coronary artery bypass surgery.

The axillary artery becomes the brachial artery as it crosses the lower margin of the tendon of the teres major muscle, at the top of the arm. The diameter of the axillary artery ranges between 0.6 and 0.8 cm. The brachial artery then runs distally on the medial or inner side of the arm in a groove between the triceps and biceps muscles. The deep brachial artery divides from the main trunk of the brachial artery in the upper arm and acts as an important collateral pathway around the elbow if the brachial artery is occluded distally. The brachial artery runs in a medial to lateral course over the inner aspect of the elbow (cubital fossa) and then divides, 1 to 2 cm below the elbow, into the radial and ulnar arteries. However, the bifurcation can be quite variable in position and can sometimes be seen in the upper arm. The ulnar artery dives deep beneath the flexor tendons in the upper forearm before becoming superficial in the mid-forearm. The radial artery runs along the lateral side of the forearm toward the thumb and is palpable at the wrist. The ulnar artery runs along the medial side of the forearm and is sometimes the dominant vessel of the forearm. The common interosseous artery is an important branch of the ulnar artery in the upper forearm as it can act as a collateral pathway if the radial and ulnar arteries are occluded. The hand is comprised of a complex vascular network formed from the branches and distal continuations of the radial and ulnar arteries.

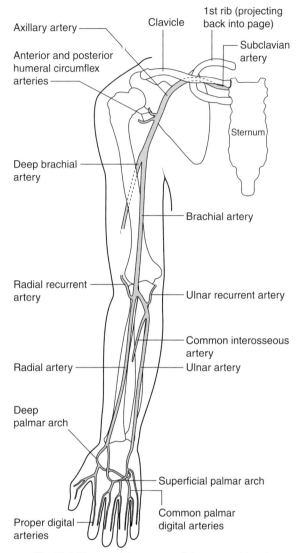

Fig. 10.2 The arterial anatomy of the arm and hand.

The radial artery supplies the deep palmar arch in the hand, and the ulnar artery supplies the superficial palmar arch. There are usually communicating arteries between the two systems. In some people only one of the wrist arteries will supply a palmar arch system. The fingers are supplied by the palmar digital arteries. There are a number of anatomical variations in the arm that are shown in Table 10.1. The arms normally develop good collateral circulation around diseased segments. The major collateral pathways of the arm are summarized in Table 10.2.

TABLE 10.1 Anatomical Variations of the Upper-limb Arteries

Artery	Variation
Left subclavian artery	Common origin with common carotid artery from aortic arch
Brachial artery	High bifurcation of brachial artery
Radial artery	High origin from axillary artery
Ulnar artery	High origin from axillary artery

TABLE 10.2 Major Collateral Pathways of the Upper Arm

Diseased Segment	Normal Distal Artery	Possible Pathways
Proximal subclavian artery	Distal subclavian artery	Vertebral artery, internal thoracic artery, and thyro-cervical trunk
Distal subclavian or proximal axillary artery	Distal axillary artery	Collateral flow to the circumflex humeral arteries
Brachial artery	Distal brachial artery or proximal radial and ulnar arteries	Deep brachial artery to the recurrent radial and ulnar arteries
Radial and ulnar arteries	Distal radial and ulnar arteries	Interosseous artery and branches of the recurrent radial and ulnar arteries

BOX 10.1 Common Causes of Symptoms Involving the Arterial and Microvascular Circulation of the Arms and Hands

- Atherosclerotic disease
- Acute obstruction due to emboli from the heart
- Aneurysms
- Fibrosis of the subclavian and axillary arteries due to radiotherapy
- Shoulder and arm dislocation
- Trauma or stab wounds
- Damage caused by arterial access and invasive blood pressure lines
- Thoracic outlet syndrome
- Raynaud's phenomenon
- CREST syndrome
- Reflex sympathetic dystrophy
- Vibration white-finger disease
- Takayasu's arteritis
- Giant cell arteritis

SYMPTOMS AND TREATMENT OF UPPER-LIMB ARTERIAL DISEASE

The main causes of upper-limb disorders are shown in Box 10.1. Many patients with chronic upper-limb arterial disease experience few symptoms because of the development of good collateral circulation in the arm. The presence of disease may only become apparent when cervical or supraclavicular bruits are detected, a difference between arm systolic blood pressure is recorded, or if there is a diminished brachial or radial artery pulse (Clark et al. 2012). However, some patients complain of aching and heaviness in the arm following a period of use or exercise. Vertebrobasilar symptoms can also be an indication of SA stenosis or occlusion, associated with reverse flow in the ipsilateral vertebral artery (subclavian steal). Disease of distal arteries including digital arteries of the fingers can occur in patients with diabetes and chronic kidney disease.

In asymptomatic disease, patients are normally treated using best medical therapy to reduce cardiovascular risk. Asymptomatic patients with subclavian stenosis can be considered for interventional treatment if they have an ipsilateral arteriovenous fistula for dialysis or an ipsilateral internal mammary artery graft to the coronary arteries. Symptomatic patients can be treated by angioplasty plus or minus stenting, provided that the lesion is suitable for dilation. Arterial bypass surgery is rarely performed in the upper extremities. Acute obstructions can produce marked distal ischemia, and the forearm and hand may be cold and painful. In many cases of acute ischemia, the condition of the arm and hand improves with appropriate anticoagulation. However, embolectomy, thrombolysis, or bypass surgery may be performed if there is persistent distal ischemia. Trauma, due to injury or stab wounds to the arm or shoulder, can result in arterial damage, requiring local repair or bypass surgery. SA or axillary artery aneurysms can be bypassed with grafts, although in some cases endovascular repair can be performed by deploying a covered stent across the aneurysm to exclude flow in the aneurysm sac. Occasionally, patients with vascular malformations will be encountered. These can be venous or arteriovenous malformations, ranging in size and distribution, and can affect the fingers, hand, or arm or multiple sites.

PRACTICAL CONSIDERATIONS AND PATIENT POSITIONING FOR DUPLEX ASSESSMENT OF UPPER-EXTREMITY ARTERIAL DISEASE

OBJECTIVES OF AN UPPER-LIMB ARTERIAL SCAN

- Locate, identify, and grade the severity of atherosclerotic disease
- Identify the level of acute occlusions due to embolus or thrombus and assess the impairment to distal circulation
- Identify dilations and aneurysms, including false aneurysms caused by arterial cannulation
- Assess for arterial thoracic outlet syndrome
- Half an hour should be sufficient for most upper-limb examinations.

There is no special preparation required prior to the scan, although the patient will have to expose the shoulder and upper arm for scanning of the distal SA and axillary arteries. The examination room should be at a comfortable ambient temperature (>20°C) to prevent vasoconstriction of the distal arteries. It is possible to scan the arm vessels with the patient in a sitting position or lying supine. When scanning the patient in a supine position, the head can be supported on a pillow for comfort and the SA and proximal axillary artery scanned with the operator sitting at the side of the patient or at the end of the examination couch behind the patient, similar to a carotid scan. To image the distal axillary and brachial arteries, the patient should be examined from the side of the examination table and the arm should be abducted, externally rotated, and resting on an arm board or a suitable rest (see Fig. 10.3). The distal brachial, radial, and ulnar arteries are imaged with the hand in a palm-up position (supination), resting on a support. Scanning the patient in the sitting position is particularly useful for thoracic outlet examinations, as this enables full freedom of arm movement during provocation

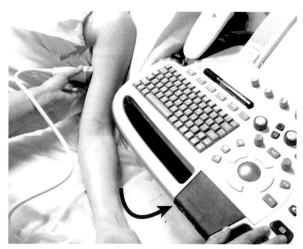

Fig. 10.3 Scanning position for imaging the distal axillary, brachial, radial, and ulnar arteries. To image the mid-axillary artery from the axilla *(blue arrow)*, the arm can be abducted *(direction of curved black arrow)*.

maneuvers. The scanner should be configured for a peripheral arterial examination, and in the absence of a specific upper-limb preset, a lower-limb arterial preset would be an appropriate alternative. The color scale is set for detecting medium- to high-velocity pulsatile flow in the SA and axillary artery, typically between 20 and 30 cm/s. For the radial and ulnar arteries, the scale often needs to be lowered to 15 to 20 cm/s.

SCANNING TECHNIQUES

A mid-frequency linear array transducer is the most suitable probe for scanning the SA and axillary arteries. A high-frequency linear array transducer produces the best images of the brachial, radial, and ulnar arteries, particularly as the radial and ulnar arteries are very superficial at the wrist. A hockey-stick probe can be useful at this level. Imaging of the digital arteries is easier with a hockey-stick probe. In addition, a mid-frequency curvilinear array transducer can be useful for imaging the proximal SA at the level of the supraclavicular fossa, as it fits more easily into the contour of this region. The transducer positions for imaging the upper-extremity arteries are shown in Fig. 10.4. A color flow montage of the upper-extremity arteries is shown in Fig. 10.5.

Subclavian and Axillary Arteries

The SA is initially located in a transverse plane in the supraclavicular fossa, where it will lie superior to the subclavian vein. The transducer is turned to image the artery in longitudinal section and followed proximally. On the right side, it can often be possible to image and investigate flow in the distal brachiocephalic artery. The

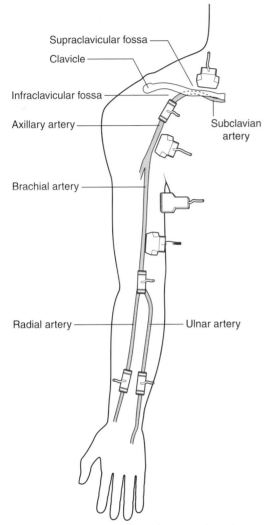

Supraclavicular fossa

Clavicle

Infraclavicular fossa

Axillary artery

Subclavian artery

Brachial artery

Radial artery

Ulnar artery

Fig. 10.4 Transducer positions for scanning the upper-extremity arteries.

left SA origin is normally difficult to image with a standard linear array transducer, as the vessel arises from the aortic arch. It can sometimes be tracked toward its origin with a low-frequency phased array or mid-frequency curvilinear transducer. This type of transducer can also be useful for imaging the proximal and mid-section of the brachiocephalic artery, as it has a small footprint that allows access to the limited imaging window. Sometimes the origin of the right SA can be difficult to image, especially if the patient has a large or short neck or if there is significant respiratory movement. Extra gel may be needed to fill the depression of the supraclavicular fossa to enable good contact with a linear array transducer. The SA should then be followed distally in longitudinal section, where it will disappear underneath the clavicle. There will be a large acoustic shadow below the clavicle (see Fig. 10.5). A mirroring artifact of the SA is often seen due to the chest wall beneath the artery (see Fig. 4.23).

The SA reappears from underneath the clavicle and is followed distally, where it becomes the axillary artery. Two positions may be used to image the length of the axillary artery. The first is the anterior approach, in which the axillary artery will be seen to run deep beneath the shoulder muscles. A low-frequency curvilinear transducer can sometimes be useful for following the distal axillary artery from this position as the axillary artery can lie quite deep in the image at this point. The second approach images the axillary artery from the axilla (armpit), with the arm abducted, where it can be followed distally to the brachial artery (Fig. 10.3).

It is worth noting that the proximal segment of the internal thoracic artery, a branch of the SA, can often be imaged from the supraclavicular fossa. This artery is frequently used in coronary bypass surgery and is surgically grafted to the heart. It divides at a 90° angle from the inferior aspect of the SA to run down the chest wall. Beyond its origin it runs behind the upper ribs and is only visible in the spaces between them. It is possible to confirm graft patency by identifying flow in the

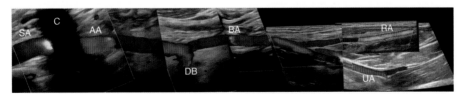

Fig. 10.5 A color flow montage of the left upper-extremity arteries demonstrating the subclavian artery (*SA*), axillary artery (*AA*), brachial artery (*BA*), deep brachial artery (*DB*), radial artery (*RA*), and ulnar artery (*UA*). A large acoustic shadow is seen due to the clavicle (*C*).

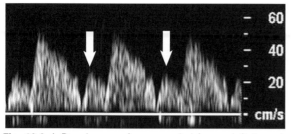

Fig. 10.6 A Doppler waveform recorded from a left thoracic artery grafted to a coronary artery following heart bypass surgery. The systolic phase is shown by the *arrows*.

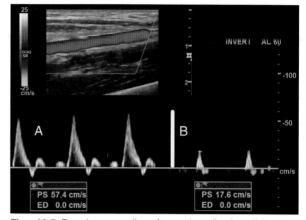

Fig. 10.7 Doppler recording from the distal radial artery demonstrating the effect of temperature on flow. *(A)* indicates strong triphasic flow recorded in a very warm room. *(B)* Shows a reduction in flow with increased peripheral resistance after the hand was cooled, and room temperature reduced.

proximal thoracic artery just beyond its origin. The flow pattern in the artery supplying the heart will exhibit an unusual waveform shape, as most of the flow occurs in the diastolic phase of the cardiac cycle (see Fig. 10.6).

Brachial Artery

The brachial artery is followed as a continuation of the axillary artery along the inner aspect of the arm to the elbow, where it curves around to the cubital fossa and lies in a superficial position. The distal brachial artery is scanned across the elbow to the point where it divides in the upper forearm into the radial and ulnar arteries. The level of the brachial artery bifurcation does vary and can be high in the arm and is easier to locate in transverse plane.

Radial and Ulnar Arteries

CAUTION

Cold examination rooms or cold ultrasound gel applied to the hand can cause significant peripheral vasoconstriction leading to high-resistance flow signals in the radial ulnar and digital vessels that may not be detected with a default upper-limb scanner setting (see Fig 10.7). The color scale may have to be reduced to 8 to 10 cm/s. There can also be a cyclical appearance from low to high resistance flow over a period of about 20 seconds (Fig. 10.8).

The bifurcation of the brachial artery into the radial and ulnar arteries is easier to locate in a transverse plane. The two arteries are then followed distally to the wrist in a longitudinal plane. In its proximal segment, the ulnar artery runs in deep below the muscles and flexor tendons before becoming more superficial in the mid-forearm.

It is often easier to locate the radial and ulnar arteries at the wrist and then to follow them back to the elbow.

Palmar Arch and Digital Arteries

Duplex scanning can be used to image the palmar arch and digital vessels, although continuous-wave (CW) Doppler can be considerably quicker and easier to use for the detection of arterial signals, especially in the digital arteries. It is recommended to use a CW probe having a minimum frequency of at least 8 MHz. However, high-frequency hockey-stick transducers can provide detailed B-mode and color images of the digital arteries and are easier to manipulate than standard transducers for this assessment. With the hand palm up, apply the probe at an approximate 45° angle to each side of the fingers to locate the digital arteries.

The radial artery is sometimes harvested to be used as a graft for coronary artery bypass surgery. It can also be used for maxillofacial reconstructive surgery. To ensure that the ulnar artery will maintain perfusion to the hand, it is possible to listen to arterial flow signals in the hand with CW Doppler and then manually compress the radial artery. If the arterial signal from the hand is severely diminished or disappears, removal of the radial artery could result in hand ischemia. Alternatively, an Allen's test can be performed. The hand is clenched tight and then the radial and ulnar arteries are simultaneously compressed at the wrist with finger and thumb pressure to occlude them. The hand is then opened while maintaining pressure on each artery. At this point, pressure on the radial artery is released. Rapid "pinking" or reperfusion of the hand confirms flow continuity into the hand. However, if the hand remains blanched for more than 10 to 20 seconds, this indicates limited or poor perfusion from the radial artery. The test is then repeated with pressure being released from the ulnar artery to assess its contribution.

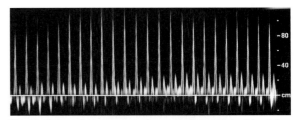

Fig. 10.8 A cyclical change in the appearance of the blood flow patterns in the radial and ulnar arteries can be observed, relating to factors such as the control of body temperature.

PROBLEMS

- The proximity of major veins and arteries in the region of supraclavicular fossa can present a confusing display, and venous signals may appear pulsatile due to the proximity of the right side of the heart.
- There may be mirroring artifact of the subclavian due to the chest wall (see Fig. 4.23).
- Imaging of the axillary artery can be difficult where the artery runs deep under the shoulder muscles. Scanning from the axilla or selecting a lower-frequency probe may help.
- With B-mode imaging, it can be initially difficult to differentiate the brachial artery from adjacent brachial and basilic veins in the upper arm. Transverse color flow imaging can help identify the artery and the veins should be compressible with moderate transducer pressure.

ULTRASOUND APPEARANCE

Normal Appearance

The normal appearance of upper-extremity arteries is the same as that described for the duplex scanning of lower-limb arteries (see Ch. 9). The spectral Doppler waveform is normally triphasic at rest but becomes hyperemic with high diastolic flow following exercise. Changes in external temperature can have marked effects on the observed flow patterns in the distal arteries (Fig. 10.7). There is a cyclical effect on the appearance of the flow patterns in the distal arteries toward the wrist and hand related to factors such as body temperature control. This cyclical effect can cause the waveform shape to change from high-resistance flow to hyperemic flow within the space of a minute (Fig. 10.8). Peripheral vasodilation will cause a reduction in peripheral resistance and an increase in flow. In this situation, the waveform in the radial and ulnar arteries can become hyperemic and reverse flow may be absent. Vasoconstriction increases peripheral resistance, causing a reduction in flow, and

the waveform can become multiphasic. The average peak systolic velocity in the SA has been reported in the region of 70 to 120 cm/s, but this will vary with age (Talbot 2012). It is often assumed that the radial artery is the dominant vessel in the forearm because it is easier to palpate at the wrist, but in some cases there is higher flow in the ulnar artery.

Abnormal Appearance

Any atheroma is normally visible in the arm arteries due to their superficial position except for the proximal SA. Sometimes areas of micro-calcification can be seen in the mid to distal radial and ulnar arteries, but the arteries usually remain widely patent. In the absence of any specific criteria for grading upper-limb disease, we would advocate the same criteria as for grading lower-limb disease. Therefore, a doubling of the peak systolic velocity across a stenosis compared with the proximal normal adjacent segment indicates a >50% diameter reduction (Fig. 10.9). However, many upper-limb lesions are located at the origin to the SA, making proximal measurements from the aortic arch or brachiocephalic artery unreliable or impossible due to vessel depth, size, and geometry. In this situation the diagnosis is usually made by indirect signs, such as high-velocity jets, turbulence, or poststenotic damping (Figs. 10.10 and 10.11). Mousa et al. (2017) found that a peak systolic velocity of 240 cm/s has good sensitivity for detecting a >70% SA stenosis. In addition, the ipsilateral vertebral artery should be examined for evidence of subclavian steal (see Ch. 8). It can also be difficult to visibly identify plaques at the origin to the SA. Occlusions of the proximal SA can be difficult to differentiate from severe stenoses, particularly on the left side and any uncertainty should be highlighted in the report. If there is suspicion of extensive arch disease, CTA or MRA will provide more detail. Dissection of the radial, brachial, or axillary arteries can

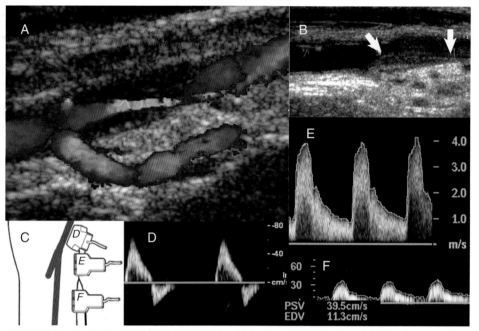

Fig. 10.9 A high-grade stenosis of the proximal brachial artery. (A) Color flow imaging demonstrates the severe stenosis. The proximal deep brachial artery is seen in this image. (B) B-mode imaging demonstrates mainly low echogenicity atheroma *(arrows)*. (C) A diagram showing the transducer positions of recorded Doppler waveforms, *(D)* proximal to the stenosis, *(E)* across the stenosis and *(F)* distal to the stenosis. The corresponding Doppler waveforms are shown in parts D, E, and F. Note the damped monophasic flow seen in F.

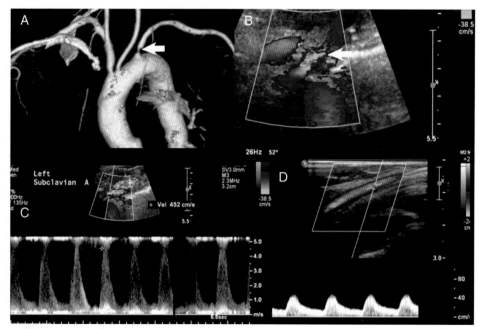

Fig. 10.10 A severe stenosis of the left subclavian artery. (A) MRI scan demonstrating the stenosis *(arrow)*. (B) Color flow image demonstrating the stenosis *(arrow)*. (C) Doppler recordings across the stenosis indicate an abnormally high velocity of 452 cm/s. (D) There is marked damping of the brachial artery waveform distally, indicating the hemodynamic significance of the stenosis.

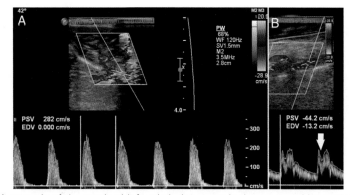

Fig. 10.11 (A) A stenosis of the proximal left subclavian artery is demonstrated by marked color flow disturbance and aliasing. High peak systolic velocity (282 cm/s) is recorded in the region of the stenosis. (B) Doppler waveforms from the ipsilateral vertebral artery demonstrate a systolic dip *(arrow)* due to the proximal subclavian artery stenosis (see Ch. 8). This figure represents the real-life difficulty when attempting to image and grade subclavian artery disease, as this stenosis was difficult to image in B-mode. The presence of a color bruit and mirroring artifact due to the chest wall makes positioning of the sample volume and angle correction difficult. A low-frequency curvilinear or phased array transducer may have helped.

occur due to trauma of the vessel wall following catheter access. It may be possible to see flaps, dual lumens, or acute obstruction.

Acute occlusions of upper-extremity arteries are frequently caused by embolization from the heart and occur most commonly in the brachial, radial, and ulnar arteries. The arterial lumen may appear relatively clear, but there will be an absence of flow in the vessel, as demonstrated by color flow imaging (Fig. 10.12). Requests can be made for repeat scanning of acute occlusions following anticoagulation therapy, as there can be no, partial, or full recanalization of affected vessels. Some acute occlusions occur as a result of embolization from the SA due to damage caused by TOS.

The SA and axillary artery are also sites of large-vessel arteritis (see Ch. 8). Lesions are characterized by enlargement of the media layer that has uniform echogenicity around the circumference of the vessel. Investigation of the arm arteries for arteritis occurs for patients with upper-limb symptoms (for example, poor radial pulses) and as part of protocols for investigation of giant cell arteritis.

Large arteriovenous malformations will be immediately obvious with color flow imaging as a region of high vascularity. Spectral Doppler will demonstrate low-resistance, high-volume flow waveforms within the malformation and often the artery proximal to the malformation. In venous malformations, multiple dark spaces may be seen in the mass that is often soft and

collapses with transducer pressure. A low color flow scale is required to demonstrate flow in these lesions.

THORACIC OUTLET SYNDROME

The vascular laboratory is frequently asked to assess patients with suspected TOS. The thoracic outlet is defined by an area through which the subclavian vein, SA, and brachial plexus all emerge as a neurovascular bundle. Anatomically, the outlet is defined superiorly and inferiorly by the clavicle and first rib, respectively; this area is called the costoclavicular space. The SA and brachial plexus leave the chest and pass between the anterior and middle scalene muscles over the first rib and underneath the clavicle (Fig. 10.13). This is a compact anatomical area, and compression on the nerves or arteries by a number of mechanisms can produce sensory symptoms in both the hand and arm. Compression can occur in three main areas. The first is at the point where the SA passes between the scalene muscles and can be caused by muscle hypertrophy or fibrous bands or may be due to the presence of an additional accessory rib originating from the seventh thoracic vertebra, termed a cervical rib (Fig. 10.14). Accessory ribs occur in less than 1% of the population (Makhoul & Machleder 1992). The second area of compression occurs as the artery runs between the first rib and clavicle. Fibrous bands or fibrosis due to injuries in this region, such as fractures of the clavicle, can also cause compression.

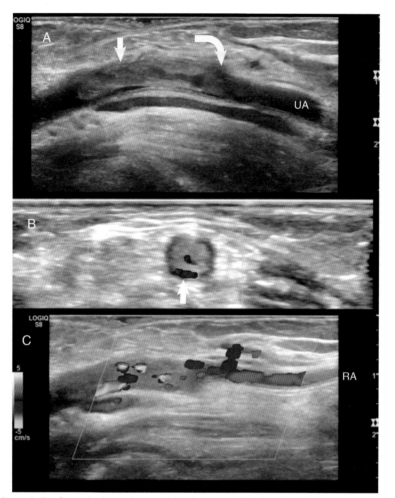

Fig. 10.12 An embolus from the heart has acutely obstructed the distal brachial artery and bifurcation. (A) B-mode imaging shows the embolus *(straight arrow)* in the artery. The origin of the ulnar artery *(UA)* is visible *(curved arrow)*. (B) A transverse image following initial anticoagulation shows an eccentric area of flow *(arrow)*. (C) This longitudinal image shows an improving situation a day later, with some areas of recanalization. The radial artery *(RA)* is patent.

The third, less common area of compression occurs in the subcoracoid region, where the axillary artery runs under the pectoralis minor muscle and close to the coracoid process of the scapula.

Typically, the vessels and nerves are compressed when the arm is placed in specific positions. The symptoms include intermittent pain, numbness, and tingling, "pins and needles" in the hand, hand weakness, sensory changes, and other neurological disorders on the ipsilateral side. It can be difficult to distinguish these from other causes such as disc disorders or complex regional pain syndrome. TOS can be purely neurogenic, due to

compression of the brachial plexus alone (this accounts for approximately 90%–95% of cases). Neurogenic TOS often produces abnormal nerve conduction recordings and can be associated with muscle weakness and wasting in the lower arm or hand.

Arterial and venous TOS is less common and accounts for less than 10% of cases, although there is sometimes a combination of neurogenic and vascular compression. Aneurysmal dilations of the SA are sometimes seen just distal to the point of compression due to poststenotic dilation. These aneurysms can be the source of distal emboli in the fingers, which can

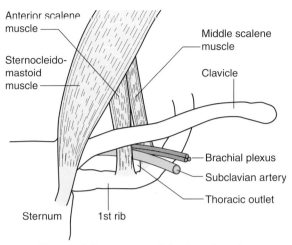

Fig. 10.13 The anatomy of the thoracic outlet.

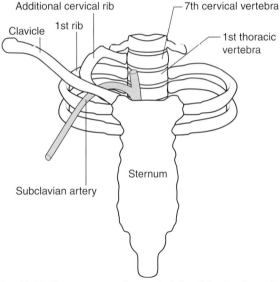

Fig. 10.14 The presence of a cervical rib originating from the seventh thoracic vertebra can cause compression of the brachial nerve plexus and subclavian artery.

be the initial presentation of a patient with TOS. There is still considerable debate about the assessment and treatment of TOS, which often involves surgical resection of a cervical rib and sometimes the first rib, with the division of any fibrous bands to relieve the compression (Illig et al. 2016). Although the majority of patients who have undergone surgery show improvement in symptoms, a few show no signs of improvement and may return to the vascular laboratory for further assessment.

Maneuvers for Assessing TOS

CW Doppler recording of the radial artery signal, performed with the arm in a range of positions, can be a useful prelude to the duplex examination. There are a range of provocation maneuvers that can be used (Fig. 10.15). Unfortunately, testing can be associated with false-positive and false-negative responses, and findings should be interpreted with caution. Like popliteal entrapment syndrome, compression of the SA has been demonstrated in asymptomatic healthy volunteers. The maneuvers may need to be repeated a number of times to obtain consistent readings. It should be noted that there appears to be considerable variability in the descriptions of these tests for thoracic TOS in medical literature.

Adson's Test

The patient is seated, and the arm abducted 30° at the shoulder, and the arm then maximally extended or pulled down. Then the patient is asked to extend their neck and rotate their head toward the side being tested and instructed to take a deep breath and hold it. The radial artery can be palpated during the test to see if it disappears during the maneuver.

Roos Test

In this test, the patient raises their arms to 90° of abduction in the frontal plane of the body with the arms fully externally rotated so the palms of the hands are pointing forward and the elbows at 90° of flexion (surrender position). The patient then opens and closes their hands for 2 to 3 minutes.

Hyperabduction Test

The patient should be sitting comfortably, and the arm should then be slowly extended outward (abducted). With the arm fully abducted, the forearm is rotated so that the palm faces upward and the elbow downward (external rotation). The arm should be raised and lowered in this position and the patient's head turned away from the side under investigation. This test can indicate compression between the clavicle and first rib or coracoid region.

Costoclavicular Maneuver

The patient is asked to push the chest outward while forcing the shoulders backward with deep inhalation, the so-called military position, as this may reveal arterial compression between the clavicle and first rib.

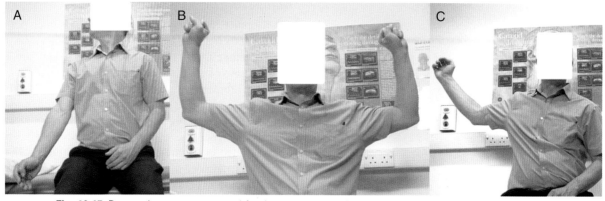

Fig. 10.15 Provocation maneuvers used for the assessment of thoracic outlet syndrome. (A) Adson's test. (B) Roos test. (C) Hyperabduction test.

Deep Inspiration Maneuver

During deep inspiration the patient is asked to extend the neck and rotate the head to the affected side and then to the other side while the pulse is checked at the wrist. A positive test indicates possible compression between the scalene muscles or the presence of a cervical rib.

Finally, the patient should also be asked to place the arm in any position that provokes symptoms, such as raising it above the head. In some cases, this will lead to a positive result even though the maneuvers above may have been negative. Any change to, or loss of, the Doppler signal during these maneuvers suggests compression of the SA. The patient should also be asked to indicate any symptoms that occur during arm maneuvers, as a normal Doppler signal in the presence of symptoms may indicate a nonvascular cause for the complaint.

Duplex Assessment of TOS

It is generally easier to image the arteries with the patient in a sitting position so that provocation tests can be performed. The SA is initially imaged from the supraclavicular and infraclavicular positions. The flow velocities are recorded and any abnormalities, such as tortuosity or aneurysmal dilations, noted. The SA can then be imaged using any of the provocation maneuvers that were found to reduce or obliterate the radial artery signal with CW. It is easiest to image the SA adjacent to the clavicle in the infraclavicular area (see Fig. 16.3) with the patient's arm in resting position. Then ask the patient to slowly undertake the appropriate provocation maneuver while observing the color flow display. It will be necessary to make slight adjustments to the probe

position if the arm is abducted due to movement of the shoulder. Any changes in the flow pattern or areas of significant velocity increase in the SA during provocation tests should be recorded. Typically, most high-velocity jets are recorded in the region of the clavicle (Fig. 10.16). There are no clearly defined criteria as to the point at which TOS is indicated, but a doubling of the peak systolic velocity at one location is indicative of a hemodynamic effect. Patients with severe vascular symptoms show complete occlusion of the SA during provocation maneuvers, posing less of a diagnostic dilemma. Many clinicians request examination of both arms, as both sides could be positive but only one symptomatic, and this may suggest that treatment of the symptomatic side may be less beneficial.

ANEURYSMS

Aneurysms involving the upper extremities are rare and are most frequently seen in the SA, associated with TOS (Fig. 10.17). False aneurysms or pseudoaneurysms are most commonly seen in the radial, brachial, or axillary artery following arterial puncture for catheter access. It is important to remember that some false aneurysms can originate from the posterior wall of the artery if the catheter has punctured both walls. Localized swelling following arterial puncture can be due to hematoma, and ultrasound can confirm or exclude a false aneurysm (Fig. 10.18). Some patients present to the clinic with visible pulsatile swelling in the supraclavicular fossa, which is usually on the right side of the neck. This is invariably due to tortuosity of the distal brachiocephalic artery, proximal common

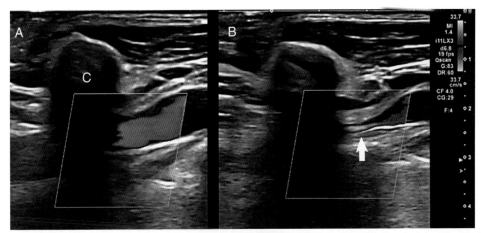

Fig. 10.16 (A) A color flow image of the subclavian artery as it passes underneath the clavicle *(C)* with the arm at rest and the artery widely patent. (B) Following arm abduction, there is marked compression of the subclavian artery associated with color aliasing *(arrow)*, indicating thoracic outlet syndrome. Note the large acoustic shadow below the clavicle.

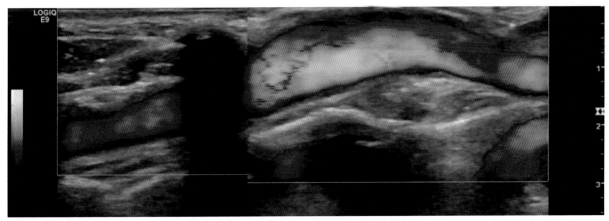

Fig. 10.17 A power Doppler image of a distal subclavian and proximal axillary artery aneurysm that has developed in a patient with thoracic outlet syndrome.

carotid artery, and proximal SA (see Ch. 8). Occasionally, pulsatile swellings are seen in the area of the radial or ulnar artery at the wrist, and this can be due to a ganglion lying adjacent to the artery and distorting its path.

OTHER DISORDERS OF THE UPPER-EXTREMITY CIRCULATION

Some hand and arm symptoms are due to microvascular or neurological disorders. Duplex scanning can exclude large-vessel disease, but patients suffering from these types of abnormalities are best evaluated in specialist microvascular units.

Raynaud's phenomenon can be a primary disorder related to vasospasm in the fingers or a rarer and more serious secondary disorder associated with connective tissue diseases such as scleroderma or CREST syndrome (Calcinosis, Raynaud's phenomenon, Esophageal dysfunction, Sclerodactyly, Telangiectasia). Primary Raynaud's phenomenon produces symptoms of digital ischemia in response to changes in ambient temperature and emotional state. This is observed as color changes of the fingers, causing blanching, or bluish discoloration due to cold. The blanching is followed by a period of rubor (redness) caused by hyperemia as the fingers warm. These signs may be mistaken for the presence

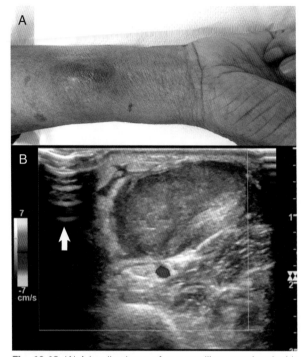

Fig. 10.18 (A) A localized area of arm swelling associated with tenderness is seen following radial artery catheterization that could indicate a false aneurysm. (B) A transverse duplex image demonstrated a large area of hematoma overlying the artery coded red. No false aneurysm was identified, and the hematoma is reasonably echogenic with no anechoic spaces. Note the difficulty of imaging in the arm and in areas of localized swelling with a flat linear probe, as it is easy to lose contact with the skin *(region with arrow)* due to the acute curvature of the arm or swelling.

of atherosclerotic occlusive disease, but pencil Doppler recordings will detect pulsatile flow signals in the radial and ulnar arteries, and the brachial systolic pressure should be equal in both arms. Secondary Raynaud's

causes more persistent symptoms and in extreme cases can result in amputation of one or more fingers.

Vibration white-finger disease is a disorder caused by the use of drills and other vibrating machinery over a long period of time, leading to damage to the nerves and microvascular circulation in the fingers and hand. It can result in blanching of some or all of the fingers, loss of sensation, and loss of dexterity. Again, Doppler signals may be normal to wrist level. However, Doppler recordings may demonstrate high-resistance flow patterns in the digital arteries due to the increased resistance to flow caused by the damaged arterioles and capillary beds. If the damage is severe, no flow may be detected with Doppler interrogation.

Reflex sympathetic dystrophy (RSD) is a poorly understood condition that usually occurs after local trauma, sometimes minor, to the hand or arm and results in severe pain, sensitivity, and restricted movement of the affected area. Patients often report pain that is out of proportion to the severity of the injury, which might be a simple sprain or bruise. The condition can persist for many months, and intensive treatment is sometimes required to restore full use to the limb. This condition can affect young adults and children. The hand or arm may feel cold to the touch and appear discolored or cyanosed. However, Doppler recordings usually demonstrate pulsatile arterial signals in the brachial, radial, and ulnar arteries. RSD can also affect the lower extremities.

REPORTING

The simplest form of reporting upper-extremity investigations is with the use of diagrams and images, similar to the method used for lower-limb investigation (see Fig. 9.24) This can be associated with a brief report. In the case of TOS, a written report may suffice with appropriate images.

11

Duplex Assessment of Aneurysms and Endovascular Repair

INTRODUCTION

True aneurysms are abnormal dilations of arteries. The term ectasia is often used to describe a moderate dilation of arteries. The abdominal aorta is one of the commonest sites for aneurysms to occur. Men aged 65 years and over are the most common group to be affected by abdominal aortic aneurysms (AAA). In the UK, the prevalence of AAA in this group is 1 in every 100 men (Earnshaw & Lees 2017). The main risk of AAA is rupture, which is fatal in most cases. Ultrasound can detect almost all AAA and when screening is combined with elective surgery the mortality associated with the disease is almost halved (Thompson et al. 2012). Consequently populations screening programs have been introduced in several

countries. In the United States, the US Preventive Services Task Force 2019 (Statement 2019) recommends one-time screening with abdominal ultrasonography for all men aged 65 to 75 years who have ever smoked. In the UK, the four nations offer screening to all men in their 65th year. A similar program operates in Sweden.

Ultrasound is an ideal modality for AAA screening as it is a cheap, simple, noninvasive, and easy to perform. Ultrasound surveillance can be used to monitor detected aneurysms for growth and ongoing management. However, if surgical intervention is being considered, other imaging techniques, such as computed tomography (CT) and magnetic resonance imaging (MRI), are required to demonstrate the relationship of an aneurysm to major branches and other structures and organs within the body. In the past, treatment of AAA was by open surgery, but nowadays many patients are treated by the less invasive technique of endovascular aortic aneurysm repair (EVAR), where a stent graft is inserted via the femoral arteries. Endovascular repair can also be used to treat aneurysms in other areas of the body. This chapter concentrates on ultrasound scanning of aortic aneurysms and surveillance of EVAR procedures but also considers the assessment of aneurysms in other areas of the peripheral circulation.

DEFINITION OF AN ANEURYSM

It is suggested that an aneurysm is a permanent localized dilation of an artery having at least a 50% increase in diameter compared to the normal expected diameter (Johnston et al. 1991). Ectasia is characterized by a diameter increase <50% of the normal expected diameter. It is important to note that there is a range of normal (non-aneurysm) diameters for specific arteries in the population. Globally, there is also variation between clinicians as to what size an aneurysm should be repaired.

ANATOMY OF THE ABDOMINAL AORTA

The abdominal aorta commences at the level of the diaphragm and lies just in front of the spine. It descends slightly to the left of the midline to the level of the fourth lumbar vertebra, where it divides into the left and right common iliac arteries (Fig. 11.1). It is approximately 13 to 14 cm in length. It tapers slightly as it descends, owing to the large branches it gives off. Major branches of the aorta that can be identified with ultrasound include the celiac axis and superior mesenteric artery (SMA) (see Ch. 12). These can act as important reference points when determining the upper limit of an aneurysm. Visualization of the inferior mesenteric artery is variable. The vena cava lies to the right of the aorta and may assume a variety of shapes, especially in the presence of an aneurysm, and commonly appears "flattened" when compared to the circular shape of the aorta.

PATHOLOGY OF AAA

The mechanism of aneurysm development is uncertain but may involve a multifactorial process leading to the destruction of aortic wall connective tissue. There may also be a genetic component. Nonmodifiable risk factors include age, male gender, and family history. The prevalence of aortic aneurysms is five to six times greater in men than women and population screening for women is not considered cost-effective, although selectively targeting women who smoke may be of benefit. In addition, there seems to be a strong familial link, with siblings of aneurysm patients having a higher risk of developing an aneurysm compared with

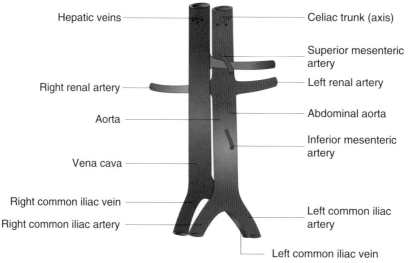

Hepatic veins — Celiac trunk (axis)

Superior mesenteric artery

Right renal artery — Left renal artery

Aorta — Abdominal aorta

Inferior mesenteric artery

Vena cava —

Right common iliac vein — Left common iliac artery

Right common iliac artery —

Left common iliac vein

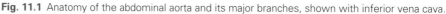

Fig. 11.1 Anatomy of the abdominal aorta and its major branches, shown with inferior vena cava.

the general population. Modifiable risk factors include smoking, hypertension, and cardiovascular disease. Best medical therapy and advice can be provided to try and slow aneurysm growth. The lumen of an aneurysm is often lined with large amounts of thrombus that can be a potential source of emboli. This is also why arteriograms, which only demonstrate the flow lumen, are not accurate for estimating the true diameter of an aneurysm, as the flow lumen can be significantly smaller than the diameter of the entire vessel. Aortic aneurysms can also extend into the iliac arteries. Some aortic aneurysms are involved in an inflammatory process, with marked periaortic fibrosis surrounding the aorta making surgical resection difficult (see Fig. 11.10). Aneurysms can also be caused by a variety of infections, such as bacterial endocarditis, and are termed *mycotic aneurysms*. These can occur anywhere in the body.

Popliteal aneurysms may be the source of distal emboli. They can also occlude, leading to symptoms of acute lower-limb ischemia. This should always be considered as a potential cause of the acutely ischemic leg, especially in patients with no other obvious risk factors.

False aneurysms occur predominantly in the femoral artery following puncture of the arterial wall for catheter access. In this situation, blood continues to flow backward and forward through the puncture site into a false flow cavity outside the artery.

ANEURYSM SHAPES AND TYPES

Aneurysms vary considerably in shape and size (Fig. 11.2). Most aneurysms are fusiform in shape, and there is uniform dilation across the entire cross-section of the vessel. Saccular aneurysms exhibit a typical localized bulging of the wall. Dissecting aneurysms occur due to a disruption of the intimal lining of the vessel, allowing blood to enter the subintimal space. This can result in the stripping of the intima, and sometimes of the media, from the artery wall. If the aorta partially dissects, large amounts of thrombus may be seen in the subintimal space (Fig. 11.2F). If there is a full dissection, a false flow lumen is created and the dissected layer of intima may be seen flapping freely in time with arterial pulsation (Fig. 11.2G). Some aortic dissections are not associated with aneurysms and can start in the chest, extending through the aorta into the iliac arteries. It is possible for aortic branches, such as renal arteries, to be supplied via either lumen. Occasionally, two aneurysmal dilations may be seen along the length of the abdominal aorta, separated by a normal segment of the aorta, which gives rise to a classic "dumbbell" shape when viewed in longitudinal section (Fig. 11.2H). As the aorta dilates, it also tends to increase in length, producing tortuosity that often shifts the aorta to the left of the midline or deflects it in an anterior direction.

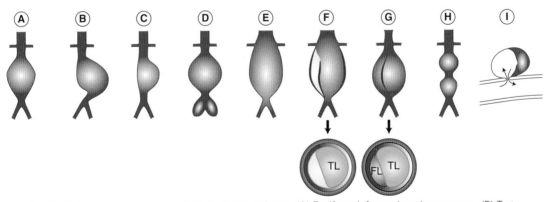

Fig. 11.2 Aneurysms are very variable in shape and type. (A) Fusiform infrarenal aortic aneurysm. (B) Tortuous elongated aortic aneurysm with the sac shifted to the left of the midline. (C) Saccular aortic aneurysm. (D) Infrarenal aortic aneurysm extending into the iliac arteries. (E) Suprarenal aortic aneurysm involving the renal arteries. (F) Dissecting aortic aneurysm with a tear between the intima and media allowing blood into the subintimal space. (G) Dissecting aortic aneurysm in which the intima has fully dissected, creating a false flow lumen. (H) Double aneurysm of the aorta producing a "dumb-bell" appearance. (I) False aneurysm of the common femoral artery following arterial puncture. *FL,* False lumen; *TL,* true lumen.

AORTIC ANEURYSMS: GROWTH, SYMPTOMS, AND TREATMENT

The typical size of the abdominal aorta varies between 1.2 and 2.5 cm in diameter (Fig. 11.3). Aortas measuring between 2.6 and 2.9 cm in diameter are not classified as aneurysms but are sometimes referred to as sub-aneurysmal dilatations. An AAA is generally defined as an aorta having a diameter of equal to or greater than 3 cm. Some vascular units monitor patients with sub-aneurysmal aortas (2.5–2.9 cm), especially if the patient is below the age of 70. As the aorta increases in size, there is a potential for rupture due to increased tension in the arterial wall. The RESCAN collaborators (2013) demonstrated that a male patient with a 3-cm AAA had a mean growth rate of 1.28 mm a year. For aneurysms 5 cm in diameter, the mean estimated growth rate was 3.61 mm per year. Growth rates do vary between individuals, and there is also some evidence that patients with diabetes may exhibit slower growth rates.

Clinically, there are usually no symptoms associated with the development of an aortic aneurysm, and many are discovered incidentally during routine examination of the abdomen or as an incidental finding through abdominal imaging. Occasionally, patients present with symptoms of renal hydronephrosis. This is caused by compression of a ureter leading from one of the kidneys by the aneurysm sac and most frequently occurs on the left side. The symptoms associated with aneurysm leakage or rupture include back or abdominal pain and acute shock. Ultrasound can be used to confirm the diagnosis in the emergency room, although the symptoms are usually so acute that emergency surgery is required. However, an emergency room scan that excludes an aneurysm can be useful, and many emergency physicians have been trained to undertake rapid AAA scanning. The mortality

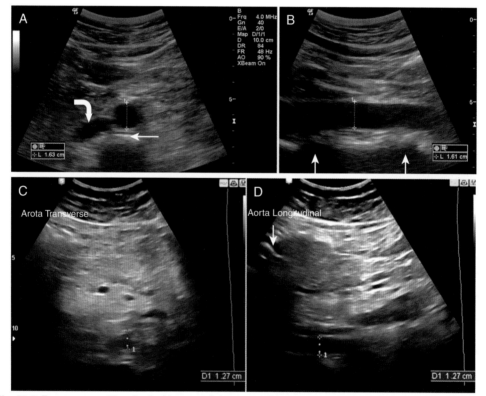

Fig. 11.3 Transverse and longitudinal images of the aorta without an aneurysm, showing how the quality of images can vary. (A) A transverse image of the abdominal aorta. The inferior vena cava *(curved arrow)* is seen to the right of the aorta, and the anterior border of a lumbar vertebra is shown by the *straight arrow* (note that the probe orientation means that the right side of the patient is on the left of the image). (B) A longitudinal image of the same aorta with lumbar vertebrae marked with *arrows*. (C) A transverse image of the aorta in a patient with high body mass index. (D) A longitudinal image of the same aorta with an area of bowel gas *(arrow)* creating shadowing, obscuring a view of the proximal abdominal aorta.

rate for acute rupture of an aortic aneurysm is high, 65% to 85% (Kniemeyer et al. 2000; Lindholt et al. 2012), and many patients do not reach hospital alive.

The risk of aortic aneurysm rupture increases with size. Data from the English national AAA screening program found the risk of rupture for men in surveillance with 3- to 5.4-cm aortic diameter was <0.5% per annum (Oliver-Williams et al. 2019). However, larger aneurysms are associated with a higher rate of rupture. For instance, the average risk of rupture in male patients with a 7- to 8-cm diameter AAA is estimated to be 20% to 40% per year (Brewster et al. 2003).

Clearly, there are benefits in detecting aneurysms at an early stage so that the patient can be entered into a surveillance program and elective repair performed if the aneurysm reaches the appropriate threshold. Trials have shown no survival benefit for offering elective open repair of aneurysms measuring less than 5.5 cm in diameter compared to ultrasound surveillance (The UK Small Aneurysm Trial Participants 2007). Although aortic aneurysms are much more prevalent in men, there is concern that women with AAA may have higher rupture rates, although definitive evidence is currently lacking.

Surgical Techniques for Aortic Aneurysm Repair

Open Repair

Open repair of aortic aneurysms was described over 50 years ago. The procedure involves a large incision in the abdomen and mobilization of the intestines to expose the aorta. Fortunately, most abdominal aneurysms (approximately 90%) start below the level of the renal arteries (infrarenal aneurysms). This means that surgical clamps, to control the aneurysm, can be positioned below the renal arteries, ensuring that the kidneys are perfused during the operation. Aortic aneurysms that extend above the renal arteries (suprarenal aneurysms) carry a higher rate of perioperative and postoperative complications, as the aorta must be clamped above the level of the renal arteries and reimplantation of the renal arteries is necessary. Patients can suffer from renal failure following this procedure; it is important that the surgeon be aware of the upper extent of the AAA and level of the proximal neck before surgery is performed. Aortic aneurysms are repaired using straight tube grafts unless the aneurysm extends into the iliac arteries, where a bifurcating graft is used. The graft is sutured into position and the sac closed around the graft. Postoperatively, patients normally spend a day or two in intensive care

and usually leave hospital 7 to 10 days after surgery. The elective mortality rate for open repair is in the region of 3% to 4%. However, surgically unfit patients carry a risk of much higher morbidity and mortality rates.

Endovascular Repair

Endovascular repair of aortic aneurysms was described in the early 1990s. There have been major technical developments in this field since that time, with many different devices available to treat AAAs including aortas with challenging anatomy and shape and AAA associated with complex iliac artery aneurysms. The prosthetic stent graft is introduced through an arteriotomy made in the femoral artery and deployed in the aorta to exclude flow into the aneurysm sac. The grafts are made of a synthetic material such as Dacron and polytetrafluoroethylene (PTFE) and are supported on an expandable metal framework, or skeleton, of nitinol or stainless steel to prevent kinks and twisting.

The majority of endovascular grafts are bifurcating devices (Fig. 11.4). These are modular systems with the graft supplied in separate parts. In an uncomplicated repair the main component consists of the main body, one complete limb, and the short stump of the second limb. The remaining modular limb is delivered separately via an arteriotomy in the contralateral common femoral artery. The grafts are prepacked on to the delivery catheter

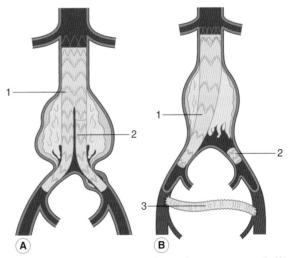

Fig. 11.4 Examples of endovascular aortic aneurysm repair. (A) A bifurcating device: *(1)* main body, *(2)* modular limb. (B) An aorto-uni-iliac device: *(1)* and crossover graft *(3)*. Note the left common iliac artery has been occluded with a covered stopper *(2)*. (Courtesy of WL Gore & Associates.)

during the manufacturing process and retained in place by an outer sheath until deployed in the aorta. During the procedure the femoral artery Is surgically exposed, and the catheter containing the main graft is inserted over a guide wire and positioned with the aid of fluoroscopy so that the top of the graft lies just below the renal arteries in the proximal neck. Many of these devices have uncovered metal stents that extend across the renal arteries (suprarenal fixation) to hold the device in place.

The graft is deployed by slowly withdrawing the outer covering sheath. If needed, a soft balloon is inflated to ensure the graft is fully expanded in the proximal neck, just above the sac. Some grafts have hooks at the top that anchor into the aortic wall for further security. The modular limb is then delivered on a separate catheter via the contralateral femoral artery. Under radiographic control it is positioned so that it fits into the stunted limb of the main body and then is fully expanded, using a balloon if necessary, to make a seal. The distal end is then anchored in the common iliac artery (CIA). In some cases, an aortic uni-iliac device can be inserted if one of the iliac arteries is diseased, occluded, or excessively aneurysmal (Fig. 11.4B).

As the devices are modular, it is possible to add extensions to the limbs to exclude long iliac artery aneurysms. Postoperative recovery is usually very quick, with some patients going home within 1 to 2 days. Advances in EVAR technology have enabled the treatment of complex aneurysms extending above the renal arteries by fenestrated endovascular aneurysm repair (FEVAR). The stent graft has holes or fenestrations positioned at the origin of the renal arteries to maintain renal perfusion. Stents can be placed across the fenestration into the renal arteries. These devices have scallops to allow for perfusion of the mesenteric artery. EVAR can also be combined with thoracic endovascular aneurysm repair. More complex treatments involve the use of adjunctive procedures with the use of "chimney" and "snorkel" techniques. This is beyond the scope of this book, and the reader is advised to consult specialist texts. Not all aneurysms are suitable for endovascular repair. This can be due to aneurysm tortuosity, excessive proximal neck diameter, limited proximal neck length, severe iliac artery disease, and marked iliac artery tortuosity. The Endovascular Aneurysm Repair Trial 1 (EVAR 2005) reported a two-thirds reduction in 30-day postoperative mortality compared to open repair. Although endovascular repair appears much less traumatic for the patient, the EVAR 1 trial also found that, by 4 years, 40% of patients who had undergone

endovascular repair had suffered a complication and that 20% had required reintervention, including the correction of endoleak. For this reason it has been recommended that patients should undergo lifelong surveillance to detect endoleaks or other graft-related complications. There is also evidence that EVAR may have an inferior survival benefit in the long term (>10 years) compared to open repair (Patel et al. 2016). An endoleak occurs when blood leaks into the aneurysm sac from an inadequate seal between the graft and aorta or from another source, such as a lumbar or inferior mesenteric artery. In this situation the aneurysm sac can continue to expand and, in some cases, rupture (van Marrewijk et al. 2002; Deery et al. 2018). The rupture rate in the EVAR 1 trial was 1%. However, there is evidence to suggest that some types of endoleak (type 2) are benign and can be safely left alone unless there is progressive sac expansion. The different types of endoleak and their ultrasound appearances and management are discussed later in this chapter.

PRACTICAL CONSIDERATIONS FOR DUPLEX SCANNING OF THE AORTA AND AORTIC ANEURYSMS

WHAT INFORMATION CAN BE PROVIDED?

- The maximum diameter of the aorta
- Any relevant aneurysm features such as shape position and tortuosity
- Any features that could raise concern such as a "bleb" or an obvious area of wall ulceration
- Is there evidence that the aneurysm involves the proximal abdominal aorta (suprarenal aneurysm) or a suspicion of thoracic aortic aneurysm?
- Does the aneurysm extend across the iliac bifurcation into the common iliac arteries?
- Is there an isolated iliac artery aneurysm separate to the AAA?
- Indications of thrombus load or mobile areas of thrombus
- Any dissection flaps
- Incidental findings

It is important to note any limitations of the scan and to state clearly what measurements were made and from what positions. Ensure the report is easy to understand and clearly states the maximum diameter of the aorta as ambiguous reporting can lead to the overall length of an aneurysm being mistakenly interpreted as its diameter.

The purpose of the scan is to determine if there is an aneurysm involving the aorta or peripheral arterial system, identify key features, or to monitor aneurysm size by surveillance. A screening scan can be performed in 5 minutes, but more detailed scan may take 10 to 15 minutes.

No special preparation is required, although some units use a bowel preparation to improve visualization of the aorta; for screening scans this is rarely necessary, nor is it practical. The patient should be lying supine with the head supported on a pillow and the arms resting by the sides as this helps to relax the abdominal muscles. Sometimes the patient may have to roll on their side to improve visualization, as this may shift obscuring bowel or gas. The scanner should be configured for an aortic investigation but, in the absence of a specific preset, a general abdominal examination setup should be selected. Ensure that the image depth setting is not too shallow or too deep. A depth setting of 8 to 12 cm is usually sufficient for the average-sized patient. A low-frequency curvilinear array transducer is the most suitable probe for this investigation. The image gain, focus position, and dynamic range can be adjusted to optimize the image. It is useful if there is the ability to adjust the imaging frequency as a lower frequency can be selected to image patients with high BMI. Harmonic imaging and compound imaging are normally switched on.

SCANNING TECHNIQUE

For screening scans, the key measurement is the maximum diameter of the aorta. However, the following description is for a comprehensive investigation of the aorta. The shape of the aneurysm and features such as tortuosity or dissection should be documented. The scanning technique for imaging the aorta is demonstrated in Fig. 11.5. The procedure is as follows:

1 The aorta is usually easiest to identify by starting with the transducer in a transverse image plane, approximately 2 to 3 cm above the umbilicus. The depth settings should be adjusted so that the anterior border of the lumbar spine is visible in the lower part of the image, and in most cases, it should be possible to identify the inferior vena cava. The aorta is then imaged throughout its visible length and, if possible, from the upper abdomen above the celiac axis, or SMA, to and across the aortic bifurcation into the proximal CIAs. Bowel gas in the transverse colon can obscure the view of the proximal aorta (Fig. 11.3D).

2 The abdominal aorta is then imaged in a longitudinal or sagittal plane, from the midline along its length to the aortic bifurcation.

3 The aorta can be imaged from a coronal scan plane throughout its length longitudinally if an accurate measurement of the lateral diameter of the aorta (side to side) is required.

4 It is good practice to assess the proximal iliac arteries in transverse and longitudinal scan planes (see Ch. 9) to exclude an isolated iliac artery aneurysm or to define the lower limit of an aneurysm if it extends into the iliac arteries (see Fig. 11.23).

ULTRASOUND APPEARANCE

No Aneurysm

The aorta should measure less than 3 cm at its maximum diameter (Fig. 11.3) and there can be slight tapering of the aorta from top to bottom. In the longitudinal plane, the aorta is sometimes seen to curve gently in a

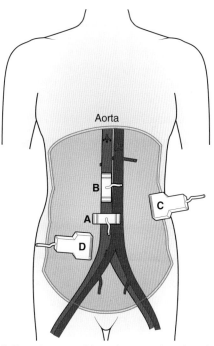

Fig. 11.5 Transducer positions for scanning the abdominal aorta. *(A)* Transverse. *(B)* Sagittal or longitudinal. *(C)* Coronal. The coronal view is used for measuring the lateral diameter of the aorta (i.e., side to side). *(D)* Right oblique position for imaging both common iliac artery origins in the same image. Examples of the images obtained from these positions are shown in Fig. 11.6.

slight convex direction as it lies on the lumbar spine. Although a diameter of <3 cm excludes an AAA, some departments consider the aorta to be sub-aneurysmal if it measures between 2.6 and 2.9 cm.

Aneurysm Detected

The aorta appears abnormally enlarged measuring ≥3 cm in diameter (Fig. 11.6). The shape of the aneurysm can vary (Fig. 11.2). Marked kinking of the posterior wall can occur due to elongation of the aorta, which can be mistaken as an atherosclerotic stenosis (Fig. 11.7). If the aneurysm deflects in an anterior direction, it can be very difficult to demonstrate the level of the renal arteries, and the proximal segment of the abdominal aorta may become tortuous, which is sometimes described as a "swan neck" appearance. Saccular bulges are sometimes seen, and it is important to scrutinize these carefully, as they can be part of a much larger AAA where the majority of the sac contains thrombus and can be easily missed. A localized bulge or "bleb" can also be associated with infection or wall ulceration and erosion (Fig. 11.8). Any concerns should be brought to the attention of a clinician.

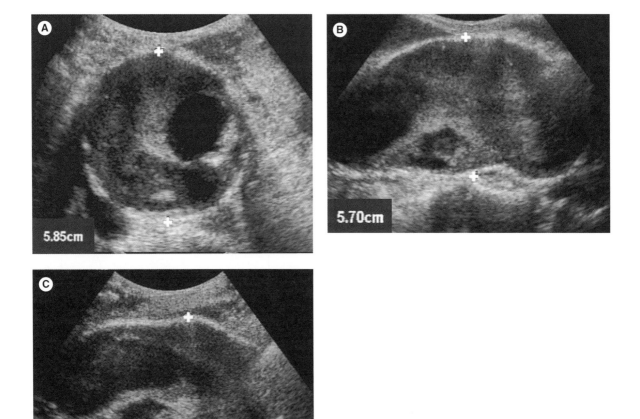

Fig. 11.6 A large abdominal aortic aneurysm is shown from three different imaging planes demonstrated in Fig. 11.5. (A) Transverse image. (B) A sagittal image. (C) Image from the coronal position. Note that in this example there is some variation in the diameter measurements between imaging planes. Generally, the largest diameter should be quoted unless there is a large discrepancy, for instance due to obliquity.

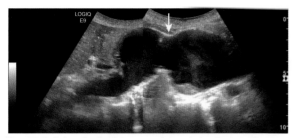

Fig. 11.7 A longitudinal image of an abdominal aortic aneurysm demonstrating tortuosity of the proximal section. This has given rise to a dumb-bell appearance with a narrower section *(arrow)* between the two main areas of dilatation.

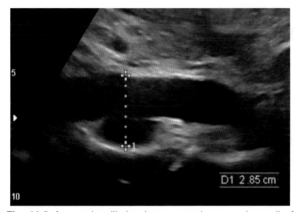

Fig. 11.8 A saccular dilation is seen at the posterior wall of the aorta. Although the diameter of the aorta including the dilation is less than 3 cm and does not represent an aneurysm, this localized dilation could represent an ulcer or wall erosion. Ideally the appearance should be discussed with a clinician. It would also be important to scan the aorta in cross-section to ensure there is not a large area of thrombus associated with the dilatation outside this longitudinal imaging plane.

Thrombus may be imaged as concentric layers with differing degrees of echogenicity depending on the age and organization. Sometimes localized liquefaction of the thrombus can occur, which appears as hypoechoic areas within the thrombus (see Fig. 11.14). This appearance can be confused with a dissection, although there is usually a thick layer of thrombus separating the liquefied region and the flow lumen. A dissection may be undetected, as blood that has leaked into the wall may be mistaken for mural thrombus. In a full dissection, flow will be observed in the false flow lumen, which is separated from the true lumen by a flap of intima and, sometimes, media (Fig. 11.9). Sometimes just a calcified or fibrosed flap is imaged projecting into the lumen

(Fig. 11.9C). Inflammatory aneurysms demonstrate a hypoechoic area of ill-defined fibrosis around the aorta on the B-mode image, but this appearance can be confused with the presence of periaortic lymph nodes (Fig. 11.10). The ultrasound diagnosis of a leaking aneurysm is extremely difficult, although it is sometimes possible to identify areas of fresh blood or hematoma as hypoechoic areas associated with the aneurysm in the retroperitoneal space. This type of assessment should be carried out by an experienced sonographer; however, other imaging techniques, such as CT and MRI, are better suited for excluding leaking aneurysms.

MEASURING AORTIC DIAMETER; WHICH TECHNIQUE?

There are three main methods of measuring maximum aortic diameter, but each will provide a different diameter for a given aorta as shown in Fig. 11.11 (Hartshorne et al. 2011; Long et al. 2012; Borgbjerg et al. 2018).

- Outer anterior wall to outer posterior wall (OTO) will provide the largest diameter measurement, but defining the outer posterior wall of the aorta can be difficult, as the boundary can merge with tissues between aortic wall and lumbar spine (Fig. 11.12).
- Inner anterior wall to inner posterior wall (ITI) will result in the smallest diameter measurement, but evidence suggests the inner walls can be more consistently defined to enable placement of measurement calipers and improve reproducibility. This method is used by national AAA screening programs in the UK.
- Outer anterior wall to inner posterior wall (OTI), sometimes referred as the leading edge to leading edge method, will provide an intermediate measurement between OTO and ITI. It is the technique used in the Swedish AAA screening program.

There is generally a 2- to 3-mm diameter difference when the same aorta is measured by the ITI or OTO method. Despite this, data from the English AAA screening program indicate men are still safe to remain in AAA surveillance with aortas measuring up to 5.4 cm in diameter using the ITI method.

It is also important to emphasize that due to the pulsatile nature of blood flow, aortic diameter can vary through the cardiac cycle, and it is advised to freeze the image at peak systole when the aorta is maximally distended to improve reproducibility between surveillance

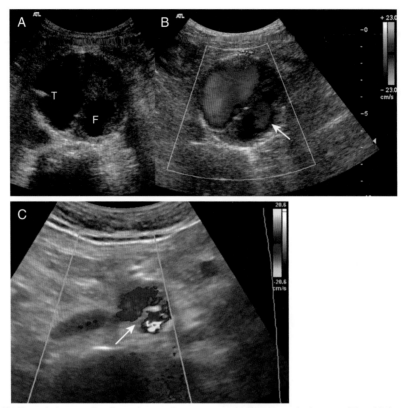

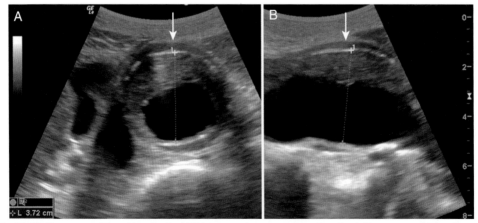

Fig. 11.9 (A) B-mode image of a dissecting aortic aneurysm. In this example the true *(T)* and false *(F)* lumens are seen. (B) Color flow imaging demonstrates flow in the false flow lumen *(arrow)*. (C) This image gives the appearance of a dissection with a suggestion of two flow lumens, but there was a single lumen with a large projecting fibrous flap *(arrow)*.

Fig. 11.10 Transverse (A) and longitudinal (B) images of an aneurysm showing inflammatory thickening, particularly of the anterior wall *(arrow)*. The diameter of the aneurysm can be measured including and excluding the inflammatory component and both clearly quoted to avoid ambiguity.

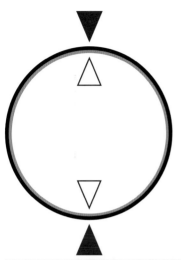

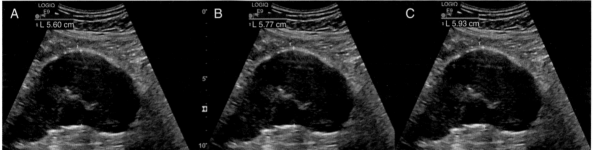

Fig. 11.11 Measurement of aortic diameter can be made using three methods (see text). *(Top image)* Schematic transverse image of the abdominal aorta. The *inner red circle* represents the tunica intima and media and the *outer black circle* represents the tunica adventitia. The three principal methods of caliper placement in ultrasound assessment of maximum abdominal aortic diameter are inner wall to inner wall (ITI, *black outline arrow heads*), outer anterior wall to inner posterior wall (OTI, *downward solid arrowhead to downward outline arrowhead*), and outer anterior wall to outer posterior wall (OTO, *solid black arrowheads*). The *bottom row* shows a captured image of an abdominal aortic aneurysm showing measurement by ITI method (A), OTI method (leading edge to leading edge) (B), and OTO method (C). Note the difference in diameter measurement between each method.

scans. Scrolling through the cineloop can help to identify this point.

MEASUREMENTS

It is important to make accurate diameter measurements of the aorta, especially when a patient is in a surveillance program. In the UK screening programs, the largest diameter, in either the transverse or longitudinal scan plane, is reported and recorded. As with most measurement techniques, there will be some intra- and interobserver error (Long et al. 2012). The UK Small Aneurysm Trial Participants (1998) showed that the

error between operators (interobserver) was in the region of 0.2 cm for aneurysms measuring 4 to 5.5 cm in diameter. This section explains how to make diameter measurements of the aorta and identifies the potential pitfalls that may be involved. It should be noted that some of these measurements may not be necessary for screening scans.

Aorta Diameter
Transverse Scanning Plane
The maximum diameter of the aorta can be measured in the anteroposterior (AP) direction by the methods described earlier (Figs. 11.3, 11.6, and 11.11). However,

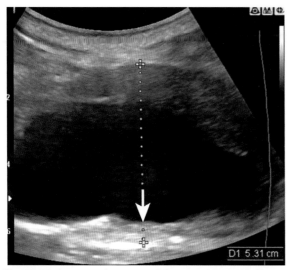

Fig. 11.12 Accurate placement of the measurement caliper at the posterior wall can sometimes be difficult, as there may be poor differentiation between outer aortic wall and the tissue between the wall, and lumbar spine *(arrow)*. In this example the measurement caliper has been incorrectly placed toward the border of the lumbar spine with overestimation of aortic diameter.

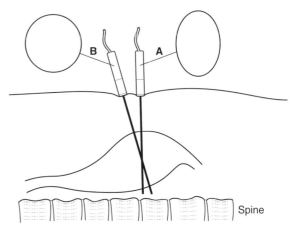

Fig. 11.13 The anteroposterior diameter of a tortuous aorta may be overestimated because of measurement in the wrong scan plane. In this example, the aorta is deflecting in an anterior direction. Scanning in a transverse plane along line *A* will result in an oblique image of the aorta, and the anteroposterior diameter will be overestimated. The transducer should be tilted to obtain the correct line of measurement along line *B*.

such as CT scanning are more appropriate for this measurement.

if an aneurysm is present, overestimation of its size can occur due to obliquity if the direction of the aorta is not perpendicular to the point where it runs through the transverse scan plane (Fig. 11.13). Measurements of the lateral diameter of the aneurysm (i.e., from left to right side walls) in a transverse scan plane are prone to error, as the lateral vessel walls are parallel to the ultrasound beam, which therefore produces a very poor image (see Ch. 2). The thickness of any thrombus can also be measured in the AP plane. It is sometimes possible to assess whether the aneurysm starts below the level of the renal arteries by measuring the diameter of the aorta at this level with the aid of color flow imaging. With the transducer in a transverse plane, positioned at the upper abdomen, the right renal artery is normally seen dividing from the aorta at a 10 o'clock position and the left renal artery from a 4 o'clock position (see Figs. 12.9 and 12.10). The left renal vein can be another landmark to indicate this position. In practice the renal arteries or veins can be very difficult to image in the presence of an aneurysm, especially if the aneurysm is tortuous or projecting upward or kinked, and other imaging modalities

Longitudinal Scan Plane, From Sagittal and Coronal Positions

To find the maximum diameter of the aorta in the longitudinal plane, the transducer should be swept laterally (side to side) across the image of the aorta until the widest point can be seen (Fig. 11.6B). Whenever possible, the probe should be manipulated so that the image of the aorta is perpendicular to the direction of the imaging beams in the center of the image sector as this will provide the strongest reflection and back-scatter from the aortic walls. It is also important to avoid oblique lines of measurement as this can lead to overestimation of diameter (Fig. 11.14). The coronal imaging plane can be used for measuring the lateral diameter (side to side) of the aneurysm, as some aneurysms are larger in the lateral than in the AP dimension. The length of the aneurysm sac should also be measured in the longitudinal scan plane. The presence and thickness of thrombus can sometimes be difficult to assess on a poor B-mode image. Color flow imaging can be useful for demonstrating the lumen, which may be small in the presence of a large thrombus load.

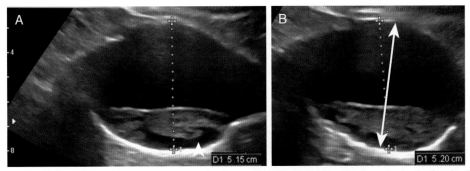

Fig. 11.14 Oblique lines of measurement can lead to overestimation of aortic diameter in the longitudinal plane. (A) The aorta is orientated perpendicular to the image axis with the correct line of measurement. (B) The aorta runs in a slightly diagonal path across the image with an oblique line of measurement *(green dotted line)*. To avoid an oblique measurement, the diameter should be measured along the position of the *white arrowed line*. Although in this illustration there is only minor difference between (A) and (B) diameters, in more extreme cases it can lead to >2 mm overestimation of aortic diameter. In this example there are some anechoic areas in the sac which could represent areas of liquefaction *(arrowhead)*.

AORTIC ANEURYSM SCREENING PROGRAMS

Abdominal aortic aneurysm (AAA) screening can be performed using portable ultrasound scanners. These scans can be performed in the community or at centralized locations dependent on local requirements. Table 11.1 shows the protocol used by the four nations in the UK AAA screening programs. In addition to aortic diameter, some departments also review AAA growth rates as shown in Table 11.2.

Limitations, errors, and comparative imaging

The main limitation of aortic scanning is poor visualization due to bowel gas or high body mass index. Imaging in patients who have had major abdominal surgery or mesh repairs of abdominal wall hernias can be challenging. Any limitations or doubts should be documented. A major pitfall is to set the image depth too deep when scanning thin patients and misinterpret the lumbar spine as the aorta (Fig. 11.15). It is also important to highlight any incidental findings, such as large cysts or masses to the referring clinician, even if they cannot be categorized, for further investigation.

Comment

There are often discrepancies between the reported diameter of a given aneurysm measured by computed tomography (CT) scanning and ultrasound. CT scanning normally reports a larger diameter, and this is particularly true for the ITI method of diameter measurement.

TABLE 11.1 Screening and Surveillance for Abdominal Aortic Aneurysms

Aorta Diameter (cm)	Follow-up and Comments
<2.9	No further follow-up
≥3–4.4	Yearly
≥4.5–5.4	3-monthly
≥5.5	Refer to vascular service

TABLE 11.2 Abdominal Aortic Aneurysm Growth Rates

AAA Growth Rates	Action
>5 mm in 6 months	Refer to vascular surgeon
>1 cm in 1 year	Refer to vascular surgeon

SURVEILLANCE OF ENDOVASCULAR ANEURYSM REPAIR

Rationale

Duplex ultrasound has been shown to be a useful method for the detection of endoleaks following endovascular repair (McCafferty et al. 2002). Ultrasound can be used in conjunction with CT scanning in the surveillance program (Sandford et al. 2006; Gray et al. 2012) (Fig. 11.16) or as the primary method of surveillance. Apart from cost-effectiveness and convenience, another major advantage of ultrasound is that the patient is exposed to fewer CT scans and associated contrast injections over the surveillance period, especially as a single abdominal CT scan is roughly equivalent to the radiation dose of 100–200 chest X-rays.

Technique

A minimum of 15 minutes should be allowed for the scan. It is important to know how to optimize

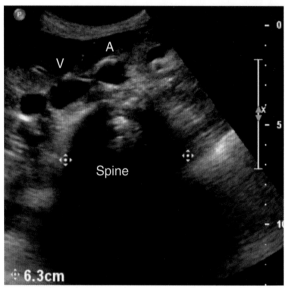

Fig. 11.15 In this image, the scanning depth has been set too deep in a thin patient, and the lumbar spine (S) has been mistaken for an aneurysm. The aorta (A) is of normal diameter. The vena cava (V) can be seen to the right of the aorta.

the scanner controls so that the system is sensitive to detecting low-velocity flow. This can be achieved by reducing the pulse repetition frequency or color scale to 1–1.5 kHz or 10–15 cm/s, respectively, and increasing color sensitivity. The wall filter should be set to a minimum level to avoid filtering out low-velocity leaks. The write zoom can be used to image the area of interest to maintain frame rate. This can produce a noisy color image, but without appropriate optimization it is possible, in our experience, to miss endoleaks.

Scanning Technique for a Bifurcating Device

1 It is easiest to start the scan by imaging the aorta in transverse section in the middle of the sac using B-mode imaging alone. At this level, if a bifurcating device has been deployed, it is usual to see the two limbs of the graft, which usually lie adjacent to each other (see Fig. 11.17B). In some circumstances they can be seen to spiral around each other as the probe is moved in a superior or inferior direction. If poor images are obtained, the patient may need to be rolled onto the side into a lateral decubitus position.
2 The graft is then followed proximally through the sac in transverse section. The bifurcation of the graft should be clearly seen, and it is usually possible to see the upper extent of the main body of the graft and sometimes the aorta at the level of the renal arteries (Fig. 11.17A).

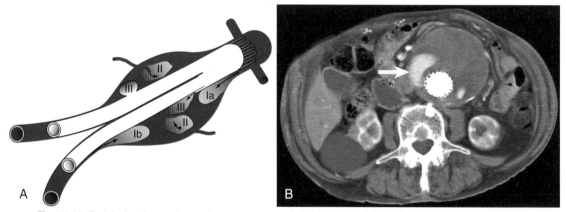

Fig. 11.16 Endoleaks after endovascular aneurysm repair. (A) Diagram of the different types of endoleak that can occur following endovascular repair of an aortic aneurysm (see text for description). Type *Ia* and *Ib*, failure of proximal or distal anastomotic seals, respectively. Type *II*, perfusion of the sac via patent lumbar or inferior mesenteric arteries. Type *III*, failure of the modular limb seal or perforation and tears in the graft material. Type *IV*, endoleak cannot be demonstrated in this diagram. (B) CT scan demonstrating a large endoleak (arrow) adjacent to the main body of the graft.

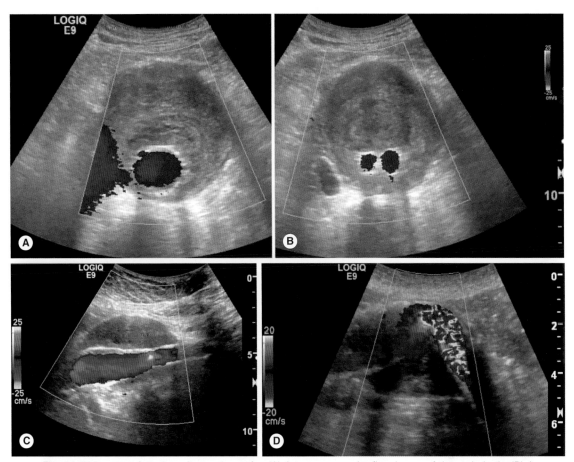

Fig. 11.17 Images of aortic endovascular grafts. (A) A transverse color flow image of the main body. (B) A transverse color flow image showing both graft limbs. (C) Longitudinal color flow image. In this example of a bifurcating device, only one limb is visible, as the two limbs were lying side by side, and a slight rotation of the probe is needed to image the other limb. (D) A kink has developed between the main body and limb resulting in flow disturbance. This was found to be related to limb retraction from its distal attachment site.

3 Next, the aneurysm and graft are followed distally to the aortic bifurcation, where the two graft limbs should be seen to run down the CIAs. Generally, the quality of the image tends to become poorer at the level of the aortic bifurcation. Anechoic areas in the aneurysm sac should be noted, as these could represent areas of blood flow, and should be scrutinized carefully with color flow imaging.

4 The aorta is then scanned in transverse section using color flow imaging. There should be color filling of the graft but no flow visible in the sac outside the device (Fig. 11.17). When using color flow imaging in the transverse plane, the transducer should be tilted with respect to the graft and aneurysm sac, as this

will improve color filling by creating a Doppler angle (Fig. 11.18). The maximum diameter of the aneurysm sac should be recorded so that any changes in size can be assessed on serial scans. A progressively expanding sac could indicate an undetected endoleak or endotension. A variety of scan planes, including a coronal plane, may be required to obtain the maximum diameter. Some units also measure proximal neck diameter to monitor any increase in size due to progression of aneurysmal disease.

5 Color flow imaging in longitudinal section using sagittal and coronal planes is used to examine flow through the device and to identify any areas of flow disturbance or stenosis that could be caused by

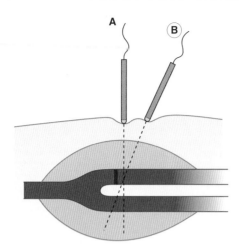

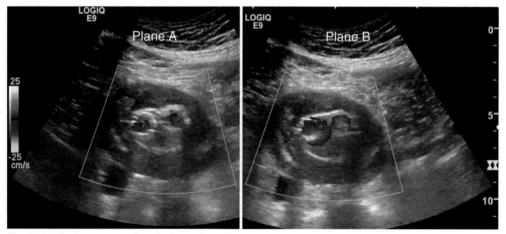

Fig. 11.18 To demonstrate flow in the graft or detect an endoleak with color flow imaging in the transverse plane, it is usually necessary to tilt the transducer from position *(A)* to *(B)*, so that an angle of insonation of <90° is created relative to the device and sac. Optimum imaging *(plane B)* does not demonstrate any evidence of endoleak.

kinking of the graft, especially of the limbs as they run into the CIAs or at the distal attachment sites (Fig. 11.17C and D). Spectral Doppler can then be used to assess the flow in the graft limbs and any abnormal areas demonstrated on the color flow image. The sac should also be examined for endoleaks in the longitudinal orientation, as this may help to identify leaks or the source of leaks not seen in the transverse plane.

Types of Endoleak

Endoleaks have been categorized into the following types (Veith et al. 2002) and are demonstrated in Fig.

11.16A. The ultrasound appearance of various endoleaks is shown in Fig. 11.19. Remember that it may be possible for a patient to have more than one type of endoleak.

Type Ia and Ib. Attachment site leaks. These occur at the proximal (Ia) or distal attachment sites (Ib) when there is an inadequate seal between the device and the aortic or iliac artery wall, respectively. Color flow imaging demonstrates evidence of flow, often in the form of a jet at the point of the leak, filling part of the aneurysm sac (Fig. 11.19A and B). The amount of flow in the sac can vary and, in some cases, a large proportion of the sac may be perfused. There may be an outflow artery patent such as the IMA.

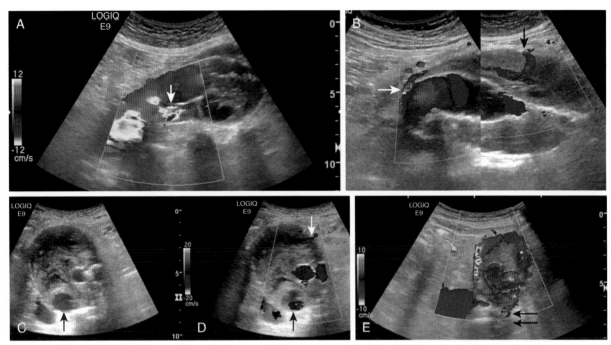

Fig. 11.19 Color flow and B-mode images of different types of endoleak. (A) Longitudinal image showing a type Ia endoleak *(arrow)* from the proximal end of the graft into the sac due to graft migration. (B) A type Ia endoleak due to an inadequate seal at the proximal attachment zone *(white arrow)*. The leak runs through the anterior sac and has an exit via the inferior mesenteric artery *(black arrow)*. (C) A transverse B-mode image shows an anechoic area at the bottom of the sac which is suspicious for an endoleak *(arrow)*. (D) Color flow imaging confirms a type II endoleak *(black arrow)* that was supplied from the inferior mesenteric artery *(white arrow)* via a tortuous route across the sac. (E) A transverse color flow image of a large type II endoleak is seen from a lumbar artery *(black arrows)*.

Type II. Collateral endoleaks involve some filling of the sac via lumbar vessels or the inferior mesenteric artery or accessory renal arteries (Fig. 11.19D and E). Any leak into the sac can sometimes have an outflow via another branch of the aorta (Fig. 11.20B).

Type III. Leaks between the modular limb and main body of the graft or tears in the graft fabric. These types of leaks are rare.

Type IV. Thought to occur due to graft porosity or "sweating" of graft material, leading to progressive increase in sac size within the first month. It is not possible to image this type of leak in real time, but serial surveillance scans may show a progressive increase in the diameter of the aneurysm sac. This type of leak is thought to be less common in the new generation of grafts.

Endotension has been classed as a fifth type of leak. This is described as a persistent or recurrent pressurization of the sac without a visualized endoleak. This can

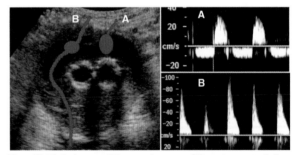

Fig. 11.20 It is possible to observe different spectral flow patterns associated with endoleaks. In example *(A)*, the superimposed drawing shows a blind ending in the sac and a reverberant waveform similar to the type observed with false aneurysms (A). In example *(B)*, there are separate entry and exit points and the Doppler waveform demonstrates net flow from a lumbar artery to the inferior mesenteric artery (B).

lead to expansion of the sac and potential rupture. The causes of endotension are uncertain, but it has been suggested that the sac is pressurized by mechanisms

TABLE 11.3 Other Endovascular Aortic Aneurysm Repair Device Complications

Complication	Comment
Graft limb occlusion or stenosis	Easy to assess with ultrasound
Thrombus along the graft wall	Mural thrombus can sometime be seen, typically along the posterior wall. It seems to occur due to flow dynamics in the main body of the graft. Thrombus can be monitored for any increase in amount.
Kinking of graft limbs	This can cause a stenosis with reduced flow distally. Kinking can occur if there is distal graft retraction with the risk of seal failure at the distal attachment site.
Graft migration	Difficult to assess with ultrasound unless there has been a significant migration (Fig. 11.19A).
Stent strut failure	Assessed with plane X-ray

such as excessive pulsation of the graft, osmosis into the sac, or transmission of pressure through the thrombus. In practice, some cases of endotension could be due to a very small, undetected endoleak.

Current practice suggests that type I and III endoleaks should be investigated carefully with other imaging modalities. They may require intervention such as a stent cuff extension to occlude the leak, as these types of endoleak are more closely associated with increasing sac size and potential rupture. In contrast, most type II leaks are simply monitored unless there is a significant or persistent increase in sac size. Other device complications are shown in Table 11.3, but not all of these can be detected with ultrasound.

Doppler Flow Patterns and Endoleaks

It is possible to observe different spectral Doppler waveform patterns associated with endoleaks (Beeman et al. 2010).

First, to and fro or reverberant spectral waveforms, similar to the type seen in false aneurysm (Fig. 11.20A), are usually observed when there is a blind ending in the aneurysm sac, i.e., there is only one point of communication with no outflow. This pattern is often recorded in type II branch leaks but can occur in type I and III leaks. Close inspection of the color flow image may show forward and reverse flow across the entry point to the leak in the systolic and diastolic phases, respectively.

Second, it is possible for a separate entry point and an exit point to exist so that there is net flow across the sac. Color flow and spectral Doppler can be used to determine the flow direction; for example, if it is from inferior mesenteric artery to lumbar artery or vice versa (Fig. 11.20B).

In addition, with type II endoleaks the timing of the systolic phase observed on the color flow image may be slightly out of phase with the systolic pulse in the graft, lagging slightly behind the graft pulse, as the blood may have had further to travel to arrive at the position of the leak (Fig. 11.21).

Ultrasound Contrast Studies for Endoleak

The use of ultrasound contrast agents can be used to enhance the accuracy of ultrasound in the detection of endoleaks and has been shown to compliment CT imaging. In some cases, it can provide more information about the source of the leak, as the contrast scan is a dynamic real-time technique, whereas the CT scan captures images at a point in time (Millen et al. 2013). It can also be used for patients who are allergic to iodinated contrast agents used in CT imaging, claustrophobic patients who are unable to tolerate a CT scanner, or patients with renal impairment. At the current time, SonoVue is the most commonly used contrast agent. It consists of sulfur hexafluoride microbubbles stabilized in a phospholipid shell. It is mixed with saline prior to injection. A feature of the microbubbles is nonlinear oscillation within the path of an ultrasound beam (see Ch. 2). Pulse inversion/phase inversion techniques can be used to extract the signal produced by the contrast agent providing a clear definition of areas with blood flow perfusion. A low mechanical index (<0.3) is used for this type of study to avoid destroying or collapsing the bubbles. This is the reason the B-mode image can appear dark during contrast studies. It is also possible to use high MI pulses (flash pulse) to destroy the bubbles and then study the reperfusion of the graft limbs and any endoleaks. To perform a contrast scan, the scanner should have a contrast-specific function/preset. The manufacturer's instructions should be followed for

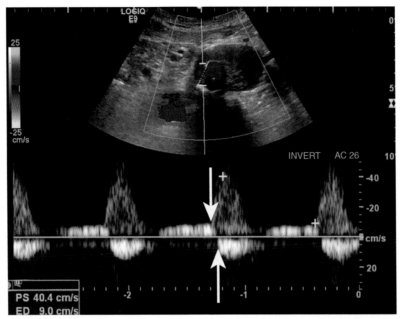

Fig. 11.21 The spectral Doppler sample volume has been widened to capture flow in the graft and a type II endoleak. In this example the onset of systole appears to differ between flow in the graft (waveform above baseline, *downward facing arrow*) and the endoleak (waveform below the baseline, *upward facing arrow*).

preparing and injecting the contrast solution. Contrast agents are contraindicated in some patients.

Performing the Contrast Scan for Endoleaks

It is important to perform a conventional scan of the aorta and endovascular graft before the contrast agent is injected. This is to enable the sonographer to identify the position of the graft within the sac and to identify any areas in the sac that could be associated with an endoleak, such as anechoic regions. It is also important to review any CT images and reports as this may provide some information on the position of the suspected endoleak. When preparation is complete, it is recommended to start the scan in transverse plane. Once the contrast bolus is injected a timer on the scanner can be started to measure the time since the injection. Within 5 to 10 seconds the contrast should be evident in the graft. It is important to observe any areas within the sac where there is rapid contrast filling. Some endoleaks exhibit very slow flow and it can be more than 10 to 20 seconds before these become evident (Fig. 11.22). Such slow and delayed leaks are unlikely to be type 1 leaks. Any identified endoleaks can also be imaged in longitudinal section as this can reveal more information about the source. When required, the microbubbles can be

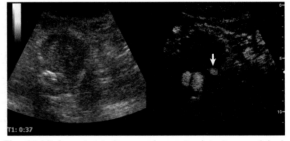

Fig. 11.22 A contrast ultrasound scan to detect an endoleak. On the left side, only the B-mode image is shown. On the right side, the contrast image displays the presence of contrast within the aneurysm sac. The two graft limbs are clearly visible along with the endoleak shown by the *arrow*. This was a low-flow type II endoleak. This image has been captured 37 seconds after contrast injection (timer shown). Note that strong reflections from the aortic wall are evident in the contrast image *(right)* but are also evident on the noncontrast image *(left)* and do not represent flow.

destroyed by a flash pulse to observe the contrast reperfusion of the endoleak as this can add information about the timing of the leak, for example, to help identify if reperfusion is rapid or slow. The contrast is normally stable within the circulation for up to 4 to 5 minutes, but the microbubbles will naturally collapse and fracture over time leading to a decrease in signal intensity. A second bolus may need to be given in some studies. Calcification in the aortic sac, or adjacent to the inner wall, can mimic a contrast endoleak, leading to a false-positive result. However, such areas should have been identified when scanning prior to the contrast injection.

Long-Term Surveillance

In the absence of any significant complications, many aneurysm sacs slowly shrink in size and may disappear altogether. Some remain a similar size to the original AAA. It is less common to see an increase in sac size when there is no obvious cause. If a number of sonographers are involved in the surveillance program, it is important that they all follow the same protocol for measuring the maximum diameter of the sac size, using sagittal and coronal planes, otherwise significant discrepancies may be recorded between sequential scans.

Surveillance of Aneurysms Excluded by Covered Stents and Plugs

Flow can be excluded in aneurysms involving other areas of the arterial circulation by inserting a covered stent across the region of the aneurysm. The proximal and distal ends of the stent are positioned above and below the aneurysm. These types of stents are commonly used in the iliac arteries to exclude true aneurysms. They can also be used to exclude flow into false aneurysms following vessel perforation or rupture during angioplasty. They are occasionally used in the subclavian arteries.

The stent is usually visible on the ultrasound image. Flow should be assessed across the stent and then the aneurysm should be scanned, using low-flow settings, to detect any possible filling of the aneurysm sac. Sometimes a vascular plug is used to occlude an artery or aneurysm as part of the treatment process. An example is the occlusion of the internal iliac artery to prevent backflow and endoleak during EVAR if aneurysmal disease of the CIA precludes graft placement proximal to the IIA origin. In this case the limb seal would be in the external iliac artery.

OTHER TRUE ANEURYSMS

Common Iliac Aneurysms

The diameter of the CIA typically ranges between 1.1 and 1.4 cm (Johnston et al. 1991). There is global variation as to what diameter constitutes an iliac aneurysm

and what surveillance intervals should be implemented (Williams et al. 2014). Generally, a CIA measuring 1.5 cm in diameter appears to be a threshold for ongoing surveillance. Iliac artery aneurysms usually occur as an extension of, or in association with, aortic aneurysms (Fig. 11.23). Isolated iliac aneurysms are relatively rare, but rupture can be fatal, and elective repair may be considered for aneurysms measuring 3.5 cm or larger (Santelli et al. 2000; Williams et al. 2014). The technique for scanning the iliac arteries is described in Chapter 9. The measurement of iliac aneurysms is more accurate in a longitudinal plane, as it is difficult to avoid oblique planes if imaging in transverse section. Iliac aneurysms are clinically difficult to diagnose, and ultrasound, CT, and MRI are the methods used for diagnosis.

Popliteal Aneurysms

Patients with an aortic aneurysm have a higher incidence of popliteal aneurysms compared to patients without such aneurysms. Popliteal aneurysms are bilateral in about half of patients, and for this reason it is worth scanning the opposite artery when a popliteal aneurysm is detected. The normal diameter of the popliteal artery ranges between 0.4 and 0.9 cm, and

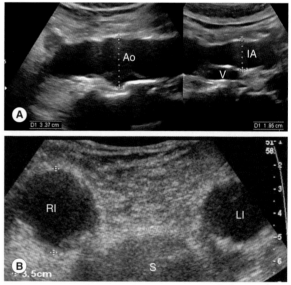

Fig. 11.23 (A) A longitudinal image of a small aortic aneurysm *(Ao)* and iliac artery *(IA)* aneurysm. Note the left common iliac vein *(V)* is seen posterior to the IA and sometimes the two can appear to merge together, giving the impression of a larger IA aneurysm. (B) Transverse image of large right *(RI)* and left *(LI)* aneurysms. The spine *(S)* is visible.

a popliteal aneurysm is frequently classified as a vessel diameter of equal to or greater than 1.5 cm (Fig 11.24), although some clinicians will consider a diameter between 1 and 1.5 cm abnormal. The complications associated with popliteal aneurysms include embolization, acute occlusion, or, occasionally, rupture. The symptoms of popliteal aneurysms can include pain or a feeling of fullness in the popliteal fossa. Sometimes patients present with a deep-vein thrombosis due to compression of the popliteal vein by the aneurysm. Ultrasound is the primary technique for the diagnosis of popliteal aneurysms.

Scanning of Popliteal Aneurysms

Using a mid-frequency linear array transducer, the popliteal artery is examined in transverse and longitudinal planes from the popliteal fossa and from the medial aspect of the lower thigh in the adductor canal, as some aneurysms can be located above the knee. Remember that the diameter of a normal popliteal will vary slightly along its length, being larger proximally. B-mode imaging is used to assess the diameter and length of the aneurysms and amount of thrombus within the aneurysm. Color flow imaging is used to demonstrate the size of the flow lumen if the B-mode imaging is poor. It is also useful to assess the patency of the tibial vessels during ongoing surveillance scans, as a newly identified occlusion could indicate active embolization from the aneurysm. Occluded popliteal aneurysms are demonstrated by an absence of color flow in the lumen. The popliteal

vein should also be assessed for patency. A major diagnostic pitfall is the misdiagnosis of a Baker's cyst as an occluded popliteal aneurysm. Baker's cysts have a typical appearance of a neck trailing from the main body of the cyst to the joint capsule, and they have a hypoechoic appearance due to the synovial fluid inside (see Ch. 14).

Femoral Artery Aneurysms

True femoral artery aneurysms occur less frequently and are usually associated with aneurysmal disease elsewhere. Approximately 2% to 3% of patients with an aortic aneurysm have femoral artery aneurysms. Common femoral artery diameters of greater than 1.5 cm are considered abnormal, but there is little consensus as to what diameter they should be repaired. Aneurysmal dilations can occur where graft anastomoses have been performed.

FALSE ANEURYSMS

False aneurysms, also known as pseudoaneurysms, primarily occur following arterial puncture for catheter access, due to poor control of arterial bleeding at the end of the procedure. This is usually due to insufficient pressure being applied over the puncture site or pressure being applied for too short a time, or failure of a closure device. They may also occur following trauma. Blood flows backward and forward through a hole in the arterial wall into the surrounding tissue, forming a flow cavity in the tissue adjacent to the artery (Fig. 11.25). The false

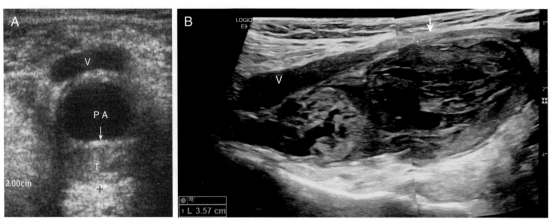

Fig. 11.24 (A) A transverse image of a popliteal artery *(PA)* aneurysm containing thrombus *(T)* below the *arrow*. The popliteal vein *(V)* is compressed in this example. (B) A longitudinal panoramic image of a large popliteal aneurysm containing significant amounts of thrombus. The popliteal vein *(V)* is seen superficial to the artery and appears to be compressed at the widest point of the aneurysm *(arrow)*.

lumen often contains thrombus, which may be layered. False aneurysms can increase in size over time and may have multiple chambers. Color flow imaging should be used to confirm flow in the false lumen. The color flow image typically demonstrates a high-velocity jet originating from the defect in the artery wall, which is associated with a swirling pattern inside the false lumen, similar to the yin–yang sign. Spectral Doppler usually demonstrates strong forward and reverse flow components within the arterial jet as flow enters the false aneurysm during systole and exits during diastole (Fig. 11.25C). The audible Doppler signal is very characteristic, with high-frequency Doppler shifts heard in the forward phase.

The common femoral artery is the main vessel in which false aneurysms occur, as it is the commonest site for catheter access. Femoral artery false aneurysms may be very large, and bleeding into the retroperitoneal cavity can be a serious complication, leading to shock and death.

Scanning False Femoral Aneurysms

The patient should lie as flat as possible. The procedure should be started by scanning the common femoral artery in transverse section. A mid-frequency linear array transducer will usually provide an adequate image. However, in some cases an abdominal curved array transducer may be required, especially if the patient is obese or if the puncture has been very high. In addition, areas of hematoma lying over the vessel, associated with the puncture site, can make the imaging difficult. The common femoral artery should be identified and scanned along its length in transverse section using color flow imaging. The proximal few centimeters of the superficial femoral artery and profunda femoris artery should also be examined, as low punctures can result in false aneurysms of these vessels. In rare instances the false aneurysm may originate from the posterior wall of the artery if the cannula has passed through both artery

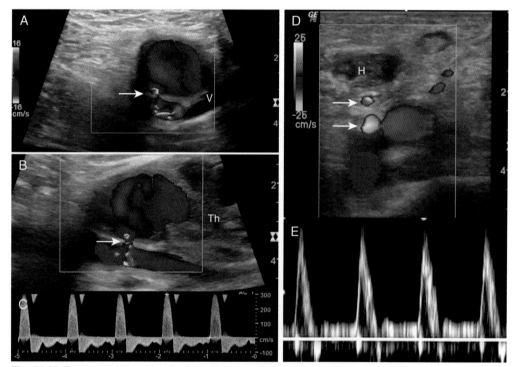

Fig. 11.25 Transverse (A) and longitudinal (B) image of a false femoral artery aneurysm and corresponding spectral Doppler waveform (C) from the communicating jet (*arrow* in the images). Note, there is compression of the vein *(V)* in the transverse image and large amount of thrombus *(Th)* in the longitudinal image. (D) A transverse image of femoral artery showing an area of hematoma (H) following catheter puncture. There are flow signals close to the hematoma (*arrows*) giving the potential impression of small false aneurysm, but these were branches of the femoral artery with evidence of net forward flow, shown in (E), rather than a false aneurysm type waveform.

walls. A potentially confusing situation can occur if the superficial epigastric artery, a superficial branch of the common femoral artery, or another vessel run close to an area of hematoma or swelling, as this might be mistaken for a small leak. Spectral Doppler recordings taken from the superficial epigastric artery or other arteries will demonstrate a peripheral arterial-type waveform with overall flow in the forward direction as opposed to the high forward and reverse flow components seen in the necks of false aneurysms (Fig. 11.25C). If there is any doubt, alternate imaging or a follow-up scan may be needed.

The report of the test should include the overall dimensions of the false aneurysm, the diameter of the false flow lumen, and, if possible, an estimation of the size of the neck or communication to the artery.

Treatment of False Femoral Aneurysms

Traditionally, false aneurysms were repaired surgically. Ultrasound compression of pseudoaneurysms has also been demonstrated as a safe and effective technique for thrombosing false aneurysms. However, more recently, ultrasound-guided thrombin injection into the false lumen has proved to be a highly effective method of treating false aneurysms and is considerably easier and less time-consuming, offering higher success rates than compression (Krueger et al. 2005; Webber et al. 2007). Blood in the false lumen clots within 1 to 2 seconds of the injection, and this can be observed on the ultrasound image. The injection should be away from the point of communication between the artery, to avoid any thrombin entering the systemic circulation.

12

Vascular Ultrasound of Abdominal Aortic Branches

INTRODUCTION

Doppler investigation of abdominal vessels often forms part of an abdominal ultrasound study. Texts on abdominal ultrasound include details of Doppler investigations, although this is not their main emphasis. For those centers or units whose main interest is vascular ultrasound, there is an increasing requirement to investigate the major aortic branches, particularly the renal vessels, because:

- The staff have skills and equipment to conduct high-quality Doppler studies of renal and other visceral vessels
- Many patients have coexisting arterial disease of leg, carotid, and renal arteries
- Renal and mesenteric arteries are frequently involved in aortic aneurysms; noninvasive examination of the flow in these is useful pre- and postoperatively and can complement computed tomography (CT) investigation.

This chapter mainly covers investigation of renal arteries and the renal circulation, which, from our experience, is by far the most commonly requested investigation of abdominal vasculature in a vascular laboratory. There is a brief overview of Doppler investigation of

renal transplants and of the celiac axis (CA) and mesenteric arteries. Hepatic arteries, portal vein hemodynamics, and liver transplants are not included.

DOPPLER INVESTIGATION OF NATIVE KIDNEYS

Doppler ultrasound of the renal circulation is usually for:
- Investigation of renal artery stenosis (RAS)
- Assessment of acute and chronic changes to the circulation
- Investigation of viability—is there any flow in the kidney, for example, following surgery or stenting of abdominal aortic aneurysm?
- Investigation of renal vein thrombosis.

RENAL VASCULAR ANATOMY, HEMODYNAMICS, AND DOPPLER APPEARANCE

The kidneys are supplied most commonly by a single renal artery from the aorta, which arises within 3 cm distal to the superior mesenteric artery (SMA). The renal artery divides, usually at the level of the renal hilum into five segmental arteries. These further branch into

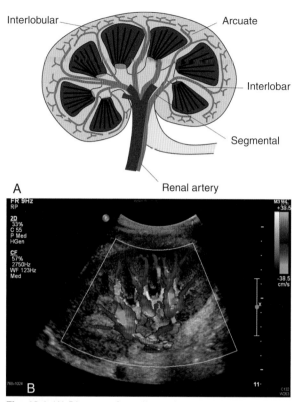

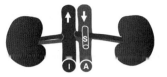

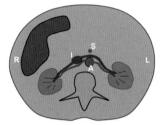

Fig. 12.2 The most common renovascular anatomy. The right renal artery passes deep to the inferior vena cava *(I)*. The left renal vein passes between the superior mesenteric artery *(S)* and the aorta *(A)*.

Fig. 12.1 (A) Diagram of renal vasculature indicating the main intrarenal arteries. Intrarenal veins are omitted for clarity. (B) A color flow ultrasound image shows several interlobar arteries and veins.

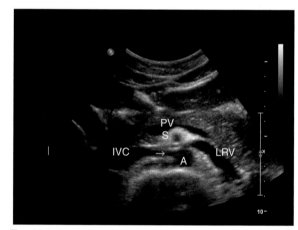

Fig. 12.3 Transverse image from an anterior approach of the right renal artery *(arrowed)* arising from the aorta *(A)*. Also imaged are the inferior vena cava *(IVC)*, superior mesenteric artery *(S)*, left renal vein *(LRV)*, and portal vein *(PV)*.

interlobar arteries which in turn lead to arcuate arteries at the cortex/medulla border (Fig. 12.1). In the cortex, these branch into interlobular arteries from which arise the afferent arterioles to the glomeruli where filtration occurs as part of the renal process. There are no major arterial collateral paths. Venous drainage is similar in pattern, draining to the renal vein that leaves the kidney through the hilum.

Multiple renal arteries have been reported in 20% to 38% of individuals. The most common variant is a single polar artery proximal or distal to the main renal artery, but three or four arteries are not uncommon. This poses challenges for ultrasound investigation and is sometimes used to question the role of ultrasound in the investigation of RAS.

The right renal artery usually passes under the inferior vena cava and posterior to the renal vein. The left renal vein passes between the aorta and SMA with the left renal artery posterior to it (Figs. 12.2 and 12.3).

The rapid subdivision from renal artery to over 1 million afferent arterioles within a few centimeters means that there is a high density of medium-sized arteries and veins in the kidney, with a corresponding vivid appearance on color flow imaging. In good health, kidneys receive approximately 20% of resting blood flow, approximately 1000 to 1200 mL/min. Flow is fairly constant, with a slight rise following a high-protein meal. The high flow and low resistance lead to flow waveforms with high diastolic flow. Resistive index (RI) at interlobar artery level is in the range 0.55 to 0.7, rising slightly

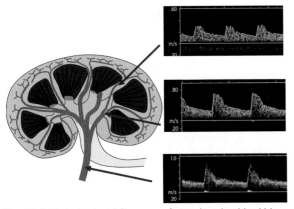

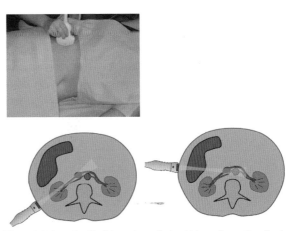

Fig. 12.4 Typical arterial flow waveforms in a healthy kidney. Velocities decrease as arteries subdivide into smaller branches. Flow waveforms become more damped toward the cortex.

Fig. 12.5 Longitudinal imaging of the kidney from the flank. Different approaches may be necessary to image the kidney *(lower left)* and the proximal renal artery *(lower right)*.

with age. Flow waveforms are slightly more pulsatile in the proximal renal artery and progressively dampen as blood flows to the smaller arteries within the kidney (see Fig. 12.4). Because of this natural change, intrarenal flow RIs should be measured at interlobar artery level to ensure consistency. Blood velocities diminish rapidly as the arteries subdivide. For those with experience of imaging carotid arteries, the flow waveforms and velocities in the renal artery are similar to those in the internal carotid artery. This is a useful aide-mémoire when considering velocity increases to indicate RAS.

SCANNING THE RENAL VASCULATURE

It is imperative to use low-frequency transducers to image the renal arteries. High velocities in deep abdominal arteries produce problems of aliasing and pulse repetition frequency (PRF) limits. Using low color and spectral Doppler transmit frequencies results in low Doppler frequencies, leading to a better chance of unambiguous velocity measurement. Low frequencies also penetrate better and give improved color and spectral sensitivity at large depths. Low-frequency curvilinear arrays (typically 1–4 MHz operating at 2 MHz for Doppler modes) can be used, but it is sometimes advantageous to use low-frequency phased array transducers that have good color flow and Doppler sensitivity and are useful when access is limited, for example, when the ribs overlie the kidney. However, the phased array B-mode imaging is markedly inferior to its curvilinear counterpart. For imaging intrarenally, higher transmit frequencies give higher Doppler frequencies and

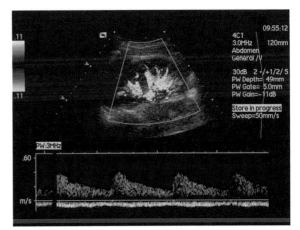

Fig. 12.6 Longitudinal image of the kidney from a flank coronal approach. The color image shows several intrarenal arteries and veins. The sonogram shows low-resistance arterial flow and venous flow with slight fluctuations from vessels at the interlobar level. Note the strength of the venous flow signal in the sonogram; at low-velocity scales, low velocities in intrarenal veins make a large contribution to the color or power Doppler image.

improved visualization of the flow waveform for lower velocities in the smaller arteries.

If possible, the patient should be examined in a fasting state. The intrarenal vessels are best imaged by ultrasound from the flank (Figs. 12.5 and 12.6). The patient lies in the left (for the right kidney) and right (for the left) decubitus position and the kidneys are imaged with the transducer placed below the ribs. In longitudinal view the large intrarenal arteries in the mid-pole flow toward the transducer, giving good color and spectral Doppler images (Fig. 12.6) adequate for flow waveform analysis. By angling the probe, changing focal position, and reducing transmit frequency, the renal artery can be followed to the origin from the aorta. If images are clear, this view may include both renal arteries, the classic "banana peel" image (Fig. 12.7), more commonly reproduced in textbooks than in everyday scanning. If there are clear views and if the beam/vessel angle correction is acceptable, then it is worthwhile obtaining velocities from the opposite renal artery origin, since this may be the clearer view than when scanning from the opposite flank. This scanning approach may also reveal the presence of multiple renal arteries (Fig. 12.7D and E).

The probe can be turned in the transverse plane, which often allows the entire length of the renal artery and vein to be viewed in one plane (Fig. 12.8). There is no standard optimum approach to use from the flank, and sometimes the best image of the renal arteries can be obtained from a more anterior approach.

The proximal renal arteries are also usually imaged successfully from an anterior approach. Scanning transversely, the renal arteries are seen in B-mode. From a midline approach the renal arteries are almost perpendicular to the ultrasound beam—good for B-mode images but unsuitable for Doppler imaging (Fig. 12.9). By moving the transducer slightly to the left the beam can image "down" the right renal artery with Doppler angles suitable for velocity measurement. Similarly, Doppler images of the left renal artery are best if the probe is translated slightly to the right of the midline. Angle correction is usually required for peak systolic velocity (PSV) measurement in this view (Fig. 12.10). Examination of the renal arteries should also include imaging of the aorta, both to exclude unsuspected aortic aneurysm and to measure aortic flow velocities for comparison.

Renal vein flows are seen in the same images as those from arteries. Intrarenal venous velocities are lower than arterial velocities, but veins are larger and at low scales/PRFs can dominate the color image. Renal veins show pulsations dependent on proximal pressure changes from the right heart and from breathing (Fig. 12.11). If venous blood pressure is high, then pulsations in the renal vein may be strong with reverse flow (Fig. 12.12). If arterial flow is difficult to identify, venous fluctuations may mask the arterial signal. This can cause confusion for inexperienced operators.

ABNORMAL RESULTS

High-Resistance Flow Waveforms

Many studies have used Doppler ultrasound measurement of intrarenal flow waveforms to assess renal blood flow (RBF) and function in acute kidney injury (AKI) and in chronic kidney disease (CKD). Broadly, AKI is a sudden decrease in kidney function over 7 days or less, and CKD is an abnormal function that persists for over 90 days. An overview of this complex topic is given in a consensus document (Chawla 2017).

In deteriorating renal function, renal flow waveforms exhibit reduced diastolic flow and alterations to the systolic peak that result in an increase in RI. The term RI is an oversimplification of the changes that RI signify (O'Neill 2014). Increased RI in kidneys has been shown to be indicative of systemic vascular disease and vascular risk factors in addition to intrarenal changes (Heine et al. 2007). Nevertheless, RI has been shown to be a reliable indication of change in renal function and of prognosis.

In recent years there has been interest in using RI as a measure of reversibility of AKI. Several studies have shown that high RIs (typically ≥0.8) are predictive of persistent AKI while lower values were associated with transient AKI. These have been summarized in a review that also examines possible causes of changes in the circulation (Ninet et al. 2015).

For CKD, elevated intrarenal RIs have been associated with diabetic nephropathy (Platt et al. 1994) and a range of other chronic changes leading to glomerular sclerosis, tubulointerstitial changes, and arteriolosclerosis (Mostbeck et al. 1991; Ikee et al. 2005). High RIs (≥0.8) have been shown to be associated with impaired renal function and a poor prognosis (Radermacher et al. 2002). RIs of 1 are associated with severely impaired renal function (Fig. 12.13B).

Renal Vein Thrombosis

Renal vein thrombosis is evident as absent venous signals and pulsatile arterial flow with reverse flow in diastole matching inflow in systole with no net flow (Fig. 12.14). Thrombus may be evident in the renal vein or inferior vena cava.

Renal Artery Stenosis

RAS can, if severe enough, reduce flow and blood pressure to the kidney and cause impairment of renal

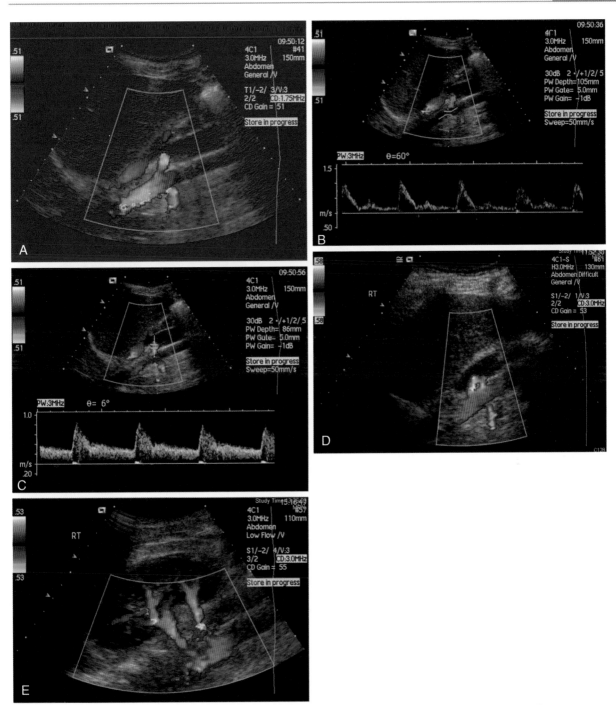

Fig. 12.7 (A) Right *(red)* and left *(blue)* proximal renal arteries arising from the aorta from a flank view. Flow waveforms from (B) the aorta and (C) proximal renal arteries. Note the low angle correction required for the renal artery sonogram. In practice, angle correction need not be made if beam/flow angles are low, since velocities will be minimally affected between 0° and 20°. The flank approach offers the best views to detect multiple renal arteries (D and E).

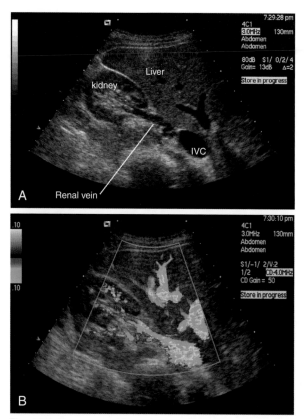

Fig. 12.8 Transverse oblique image of the kidney and renal vein in B-mode (A) and with color flow imaging (B). *IVC*, Inferior vena cava.

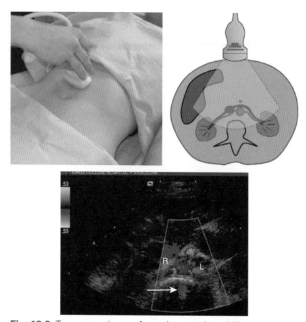

Fig. 12.9 Transverse image from the anterior midline approach. The right *(R)* and left *(L)* renal arteries are at a poor angle for spectral Doppler insonation with angle close to 90°, as evidenced by the change in color in the left renal artery. The color arrowed is a mirror artifact from ultrasound reflected from the spine surface which insonates flow in the aorta.

function. RAS can lead to renovascular hypertension, the cause of approximately 2% to 4% cases of hypertension in adults. However, hypertension is itself a risk factor for atherosclerotic disease of the renal arteries as it is for other arteries, and the presence of a stenosis in a hypertensive patient does not necessarily mean that RAS is causative.

There are two distinct types of RAS referred for imaging:

1 Atheromatous RAS usually affects the renal artery ostium and proximal renal artery. It can lead to hypertension and eventually renal failure. Stenosis is more resistant to angioplasty; if required, intervention is usually by stenting.

2 Dysplasia usually affects the mid and distal renal artery and occurs in younger patients and more frequently in women. It causes hypertension with no or little loss of renal function. Dysplasia responds well to angioplasty.

The role of intervention in atheromatous RAS is complex and controversial. For hypertension, nephrologists in this hospital ask for angioplasty and stenting in only a small number of patients with resistant hypertension. They are more willing to use intervention to preserve renal function in chronic renal failure where RAS is the suspected cause in order to postpone the need for dialysis.

Indications for investigation for RAS are given in Box 12.1.

Criteria for Renal Artery Stenosis

If images are clear, then direct measurements of velocities in the RA are the most reliable indication of the presence and severity of a RAS. Imaging of the intrarenal flow waveforms is often more easily accomplished, and the downstream changes to flow waveforms have been proposed as an indication of RAS. However, this indirect method is less sensitive to detection of RAS. Since early studies were published, ultrasound technology has improved so that color flow and spectral Doppler sensitivity usually enable clear direct imaging of abdominal arteries, even in large patients.

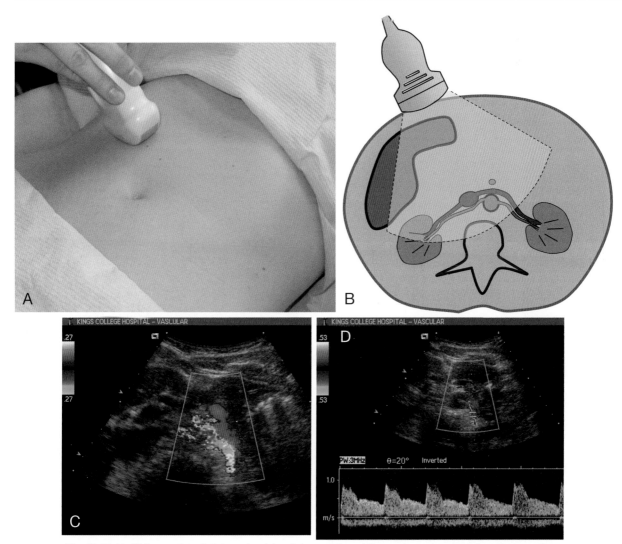

Fig. 12.10 (A–D) By moving slightly to the right of the anterior midline, color and spectral Doppler beam/flow angles in the left renal artery are lower with improved signals and an acceptable angle correction.

In the direct method the arteries are imaged as described earlier from the aorta to the hilum. The anterior (Fig. 12.15) and flank (Fig. 12.16) approaches should be used; the approach for optimum images is unpredictable. If the color scale is set correctly for the artery, typically 40 to 60 cm/s, a stenosis will show as an area of aliasing, possibly with multicolored bleeding into the surrounding area of tissue if the stenosis is severe enough to cause a bruit. Good color flow penetration and color and spectral Doppler sensitivity are essential.

If a flank approach is used, then little or no angle correction may be required if the renal artery keeps to within a few degrees of the ultrasound beam, since angle corrections between 0° and 20° make negligible differences to the measured velocity. However, renal arteries may be tortuous, and angle correction is then required.

The degree of narrowing is determined by the highest PSV in the stenosis. In studies comparing Doppler with angiographic measurement of RAS, PSVs of 180 and 200 cm/s have been reported to be indicative of a 60% stenosis. This is similar to values for internal carotid

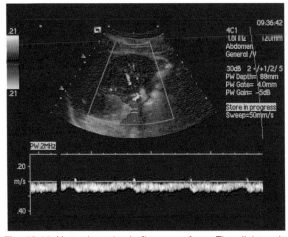

Fig. 12.11 Normal renal vein flow waveform. The slight variation in renal vein velocity is caused by subtle changes in venous pressure, which demonstrate that there is no major obstruction to flow between the measurement site and the right heart.

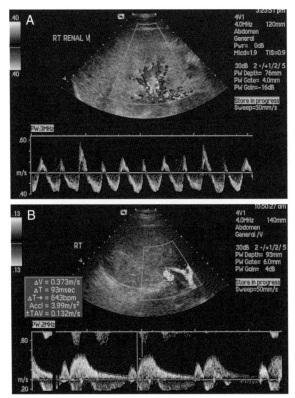

Fig. 12.12 Fluctuations to renal venous velocity. In patients with high venous pressures, changes in right atrial pressure lead to pulsatile flow waveforms. These may exhibit a combination of changes from breathing and right atrial pressure (A). If the sample volume insonates arterial and venous flow, then the individual flow waveforms may be unclear (B).

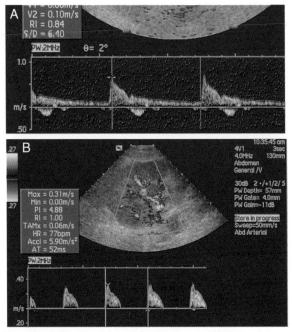

Fig. 12.13 Flow waveforms in raised renovascular resistance (RVR). As RVR increases, there is a loss of diastolic flow, evident visually in the sonogram and as measured by resistance index (A). With severely raised RVR, diastolic flow is absent (B).

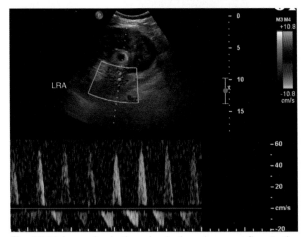

Fig. 12.14 In renal vein thrombosis there is no net flow to the kidney. Arterial waveforms show flow reversal in diastole. *LRA*, Left renal artery.

artery stenosis and higher values reflect increased stenosis severity in a similar way to the internal carotid artery so that PSVs of 400 cm/s can be regarded as approximately 90%. The renal artery to aorta PSV ratio (RAR) is described by some as helpful in normalizing the absolute velocity measurements in cases where cardiac

BOX 12.1 Indications of Referral for Investigation of Renal Artery Stenosis

- Asymmetry of kidney size (>1.5 cm length) without other explanation in elderly (>50) or young patient (<30)
- Significantly impaired renal function (elevated plasma creatinine or estimated low glomerular filtration rate) with significant arterial disease elsewhere
- Significant deterioration in renal function with angiotensin-converting enzyme (ACE) inhibitor or angiotensin receptor blocker
- Resistant hypertension, especially with evidence of arterial disease elsewhere
- Flash pulmonary edema—rare, pulmonary edema usually other cause than as a result of renal artery stenosis

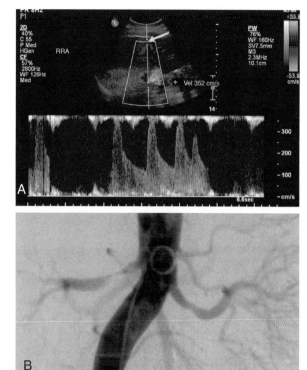

Fig. 12.16 (A) Renal artery stenosis imaged from a flank approach. Flow is toward the transducer, resulting in high Doppler frequencies. The required high pulse repetition frequency leads to an additional superficial sample volume *(arrowed)*. This increases noise in the sonogram. The renal artery moves in and out of the sample volume with breathing motion. No angle correction is made since the flow is directly toward the beam. Peak systolic velocity is 352 cm/s. (B) Angiography confirms a stenosis. *RRA,* Right renal artery.

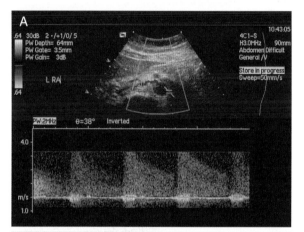

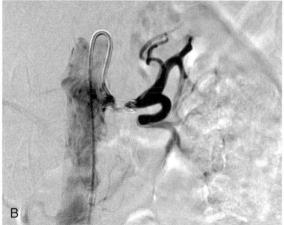

Fig. 12.15 (A) Transverse anterior approach shows high velocities exceeding 3.5 m/s in a renal artery 2 years post stenting. The high velocity leads to Doppler frequencies exceeding the pulse repetition frequency limits for the depth. The scale is restricted and there is aliasing. (B) Angiography shows a tight in-stent stenosis. *LRA,* Left renal artery.

output is low. A marked change in velocity locally has also been used as an indicator of stenosis. PSV in the stenosis is compared with that in the artery just distal to this (Souza de Oliveira et al. 2000). This aids in cases where renal artery flow is low, for example, in cases where there is a chronic reduction in RBF.

Other values for PSV have been proposed. Abu-Rahma et al. (2012) found that their optimum criteria for a RA stenosis ≥60% were 285 cm/s or RAR of 3.7. The mean PSV for RA without stenosis in the study was 173 cm/s. This is higher than our own experience and highlights possible differences of technique. We have found that velocities measured in a RA are often lower when imaged from the flank with no or little angle correction than when measured from an anterior approach with angle corrections of up to 60°. This is due to inherent errors that occur, for example, from intrinsic spectral broadening and from imperfect angle correction between the beam and the direction of flow. As is often commented, vascular laboratories or imaging departments should validate their own results.

Several studies have compared ultrasound velocities with direct measurement of the arterial pressure gradient across a stenosis at the time of angiography. This can be considered the true gold standard to define a hemo-dynamically significant stenosis, since renovascular hypertension results from a reduction in arterial pressure to the kidney downstream of a stenosis. Kawarada et al. (2006) found that a PSV of 219 cm/s had a high sensitivity and specificity for a pressure gradient of 20 mmHg and that duplex ultrasound had a better correlation with pressure gradient than angiography. Staub et al. (2007) found that the mean pressure gradient of stenoses measured at 200 cm/s was 23 mmHg and recommended this value and a RAR of ≥2.5 as indicative of severe stenosis. Drieghe et al. (2008) compared angiography and Doppler ultrasound with the ratio of pressure distal to a stenosis (Pd) and proximal to it (Pa). Using a Pd/Pa ratio of <0.9 as indicative of a significant hemo-dynamic stenosis, they concluded that a RAR of >3.5 had the best overall accuracy and that PSVs of 200 cm/s had high sensitivity but low specificity for stenoses. The variation in reported ultrasound results complicates an already contentious subject as to what is standard to us and when it is best to intervene. For ultrasound practitioners, the comparative lack of specific details of the ultrasound examinations in published papers makes it harder to judge which standard to apply.

The indirect approach uses changes in flow waveform shape from intrarenal arteries. Downstream of a severe stenosis, the waveform shows reduced pulsatility and slower acceleration and longer acceleration times, sometimes described as tardus parvus (late and weak) (Stavros & Harshfield 1994) (Fig. 12.17). Since the acceleration value is itself dependent on the velocities in the artery, care should be taken to measure these parameters consistently at a particular level in the kidney. Most authors have used measurement of flow waveform at the interlobar artery level where accelerations of <300 cm/s² and acceleration times of >70 ms are indicative of proximal stenosis. In comparison with direct measurements, indirect measurements are less sensitive but have similar specificity for stenoses >60% (House et al. 1999). This may be because distal flow waveforms are affected at higher level of stenosis and/or because the waveform is

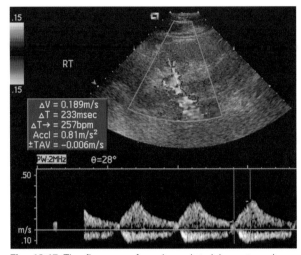

Fig. 12.17 The flow waveform in an interlobar artery downstream of a severe stenosis shows low acceleration and a long acceleration time.

> **BOX 12.2   Indications for Renal Artery Stenosis**
>
> - Peak systolic velocity (PSV) in renal artery ≥ 200 cm/s
> - Renal artery/aortic ratio PSV ≥ 3.5
> - Interlobar artery acceleration < 300 cm/s²
> - Interlobar artery acceleration time > 70 ms

---

also dependent on distal changes in vascular impedance and compliance of the aorta: all of these factors confound simple analysis.

The use of flow waveform shape to predict successful response to angioplasty and stenting has been advocated. A cutoff of RI = 0.8 in the interlobar artery vessels has been shown to be the level above which kidneys showed poor response to angioplasty. Kidneys with an RI ≤0.8 showed markedly better improvement in blood pressure and renal function (Radermacher et al. 2001), although other authors have been unable to use this level of RI to discriminate between good and poor outcome to the same degree (Garcia-Criado et al. 2005).

A summary of ultrasound indications for RAS is given in Box 12.2.

Problems When Imaging Renal Artery Stenosis

Textbook images of normal renal arteries are usually obtained from healthy, compliant, slim volunteers with good RBF and the ability to hold their breath for several seconds. Not all of these apply to all patients. Problems that occur are:

- Low RBF. Since blood velocities are used for the color flow image and spectral Doppler measurements of a stenosis, low RBF prevents accurate measurement. In patients with severely decreased RBF there may be few vessels imaged with the kidney and poor velocities in the renal artery.
- Movement. Many patients present with impaired renal and cardiac function and are unable to hold their breath for very long. In these cases, color flow should be able to show the movement of the renal artery, allowing brief snatches of the spectral Doppler to be obtained for one or two cardiac cycles at a time (see Fig. 12.16).
- Depth. Deep arteries may pose problems when imaging high velocities (see earlier). The lowest-frequency transducer possible is essential for these studies, and high PRF function should be available.
- Poor views. There are occasions when the entire course of the renal artery cannot be imaged. Use several transducer approaches and, if bowel gas obscures a view, move the patient and try again if the gas has moved. The left renal artery may appear to be in close proximity to the splenic artery in large patients and can be misleading. Ensure that the flow waveform in the renal artery matches those in the kidney and follow the renal artery and its flow waveforms from its insertion to the kidney back to the aorta to ensure continuity.

RENAL TRANSPLANTS

Renal transplants are an excellent target for Doppler ultrasound investigation. The kidney lies in the iliac fossa, is usually superficial, and does not move nearly as much as the native kidneys. In addition, the vascular anatomy, including the presence of multiple arteries, can be obtained from the operation note. Two main arterial surgical anastomoses are seen:

1 End-to-side renal artery to external iliac artery anastomosis.
2 End-to-end renal artery to internal iliac artery—seen in older transplants from living donors.

Doppler ultrasound complements B-mode ultrasound in the investigation of poor function or changes in graft function. It is most useful when investigating vascular causes of poor function, graft artery stenosis,

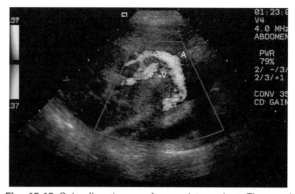

Fig. 12.18 Color flow image of a renal transplant. The renal artery *(A)* rises superficially *(red)* before turning toward the hilum where it branches *(blue)*. A section of renal vein is evident *(V)* with flow in the opposite direction. Renal transplant arteries and veins may be tortuous.

renal vein thrombosis, or arteriovenous fistula. It is helpful, but not specific, when examining flow changes as a result of rejection, drug toxicity, and acute tubular necrosis.

Scanning Kidney Transplants

Higher-frequency curvilinear arrays (2-6 MHz) are suitable to image the renal transplant and the main arteries and veins. In thin patients, low-frequency linear arrays (3–7 MHz) may be helpful if the iliac arteries are superficial. In a slim patient, the long length of the extrarenal vessels may result in a tortuous artery and vein. The position and orientation of the kidney may appear unusual (see Fig. 12.18).

The intrarenal flow arterial waveforms are measured in the upper, mid, and lower pole. In the early posttransplant period, rapid changes in the vascular resistance can occur. It is advantageous to use the pulsatility index (PI) as a measure of resistance. If there is zero flow at any point in the cardiac cycle, RI = 1. PI discriminates between a waveform with no diastolic flow and one where diastolic flow falls to zero. The range for normal-flow waveforms is wider than for a native kidney. While a normal-flow waveform usually has PIs in the range 0.8 to 1.5 (RI = 0.6–0.75), there are transplants with good long-term function with higher PIs. A change in flow waveform shape is a more important indication of changing renovascular resistance (RVR).

Arterial Stenosis

The iliac artery should be investigated to ensure there is no proximal stenosis. The normal external iliac artery waveform has high acceleration and a triphasic pattern. Damped flow in the external iliac artery is indicative of proximal disease. This can be quantified by ankle–brachial pressure index measurements and direct imaging of the upstream stenosis.

The renal artery is imaged from anastomosis to hilar level. The range of flow velocities is larger than in native kidneys, and local changes at points of tight curvature complicate the overall picture. PSV ratios of ≥2.5 or over are indicative of stenosis, as are PSVs of ≥250 cm/s (Baxter et al. 1995) (Fig. 12.19). Intrarenal flow waveforms are less helpful than for native kidneys because of the various factors that affect intrarenal flow waveforms. However, severely damped flow waveforms are indicative of upstream stenosis.

Arteriovenous Fistula

Arteriovenous fistulas are a common finding post biopsy. The appearance is of high-velocity disturbed flow at the site of the fistula, with high-velocity low-resistance flow in the artery supplying the fistula and arterial-like pulsations in the vein draining it (see Fig. 12.20). Fistulas present a risk if further biopsy is undertaken at the same site. Fistulas are occasionally associated with pseudoaneurysm and can exacerbate the effects of RAS (e.g., Fig. 12.19).

Venous Thrombosis

Renal vein thrombosis most frequently occurs in the early postoperative period. Doppler flow waveforms in the renal and intrarenal arteries show sharp systolic peaks and reversed flow in diastole with no venous flow signals.

Flow Changes in Rejection

An increase in intrarenal flow waveform resistance between visits as measured by PI or RI is a cause for concern, as it is an early sign of rejection (see Fig. 12.21). Absolute values vary considerably in the immediate posttransplantation period. High-resistance flow waveforms are also seen in cases of acute tubular necrosis, especially if there has been a comparatively long ischemic period before transplantation. The complex posttransplantation course may also include drug nephrotoxicity, which has also been associated with an increase in PI/RI. Changes in flow waveforms have been shown to lack sensitivity or specificity for rejection but are still useful as an indication of changes in RVR, which merits further investigation. Early acute tubular necrosis is often

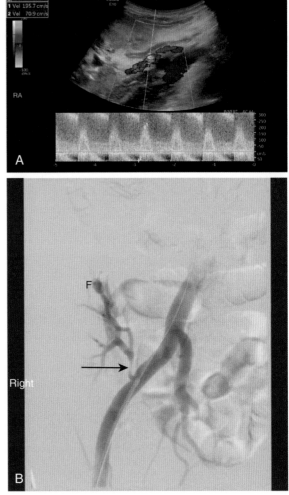

Fig. 12.19 (A) High velocities in a renal artery *(RA)*. There is aliasing, but the peak systolic velocity can be estimated by adding the value of the maximum of the scale (300 cm/s) to the aliased flow in systole (which ranges from −70.9 to +195.7). The total velocity is therefore 300 + 70.9 + 195.7 = 566.6 cm/s, approximately. (B) Angiography confirmed the stenosis *(arrowed)*. An AV-fistula *(F)* is evident as it was on ultrasound and contributes to the extremely high velocities through the stenosis.

associated with increases in edema. Changes in arterial flow waveform shape are sometimes accompanied by high intrarenal venous velocities caused by extrinsic compression on the low-pressure veins.

Chronic rejection is manifested by a steady reduction in arterial velocities throughout the kidney, which may be accompanied by a slight rise in PI. These changes are irreversible and are presaged by changes in renal function.

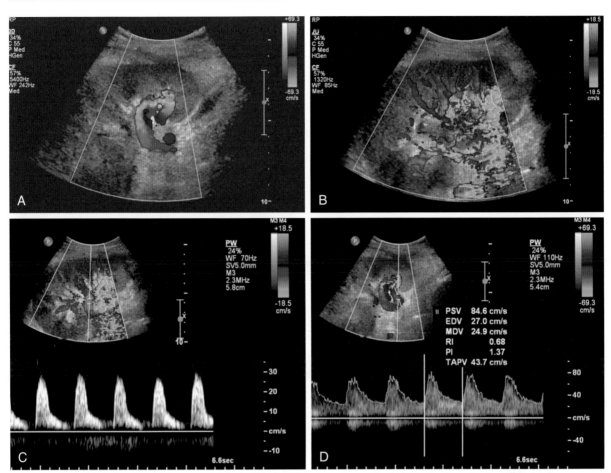

Fig. 12.20 Renal transplant arteriovenous fistula. With the color scale set high (A), the color flow imaging is of the arterial supply and venous drainage from the fistula. With the color scale reduced (B), the flow in other vessels are now detected. The flow to the fistula (D) shows high diastolic flow; in the arteries away from the fistula (C), low diastolic flow shows impaired flow.

CELIAC AXIS AND MESENTERIC ARTERIES

The CA and SMAs are readily imaged, as they rise anterior from the aorta and are usually evident as a close pair of arteries in the longitudinal view (Fig. 12.22). The CA bifurcates into the splenic and common hepatic artery a short distance (1 to 3 cm) from its origin. The left gastric artery also branches from the proximal CA but is much smaller. The origin of the inferior mesenteric artery (IMA) is distal and usually arises slightly left of the anterior midline of the aorta. There are many variants of the anatomy of the CA and SMA, the most common is the right hepatic artery arising from the SMA.

Flow waveforms and velocities in the superior and IMA change markedly after eating. Changes in the CA, which branches into the splenic, hepatic, and left gastric arteries, are less marked. Measurements should be made with the patient fasted (see Fig. 12.23).

Doppler examination of these arteries is most commonly requested in the investigation of atherosclerotic disease causing ischemia of the bowel. Elevated velocities in the proximal arteries are indicative of stenosis (Fig. 12.24). Values for SMA/CA and IMA are listed in Table 12.1 (Moneta et al. 1991; Pellerito et al. 2009). Other values for CA and SMA to distinguish between ≥50 and ≥70% stenosis have also been published (Abu-Rahma et al. 2012).

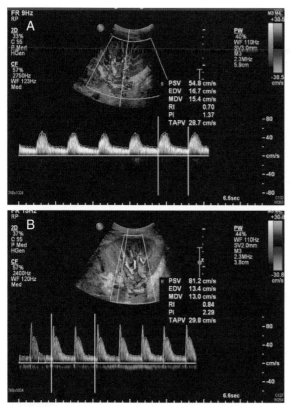

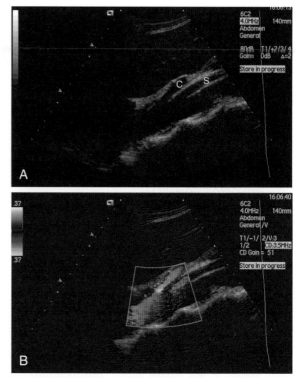

Fig. 12.21 Changes to flow waveform in acute rejection. The flow waveform at day 26 shows good diastolic flow when there was good renal function (A). Seven days later renal function had deteriorated (B) and flow waveforms exhibit greater pulsatility suggesting an increase in resistance associated with rejection.

In some patients the proximal CA may be compressed by the median arcuate ligament during expiration (see Fig. 12.25). In the example shown, the highest peak velocity exceeds the criterion for a stenosis; however, by measuring it throughout the breathing cycle, the true cause of the narrowing is evident.

VISCERAL ARTERY ANEURYSMS

Visceral artery aneurysms can be monitored by ultrasound depending on their location and the accessibility for clear ultrasound imaging. Most aneurysms are discovered incidentally during imaging by CT or ultrasound; they are usually asymptomatic. The greatest risk to the patient is from rupture. The most common site is the splenic artery, followed by the renal and hepatic arteries, but aneurysms can occur in the mesenteric arteries and CA.

Fig. 12.22 (A) B-mode and (B) color image of the celiac axis *(C)* and superior mesenteric artery *(S)* origins seen in a midsagittal plane.

Depending on the type, location, and any symptoms, intervention is usually considered when the aneurysm diameter is ≥2 cm.

The clarity of ultrasound images of an aneurysm is dependent on the location, depth, and intervening tissue. The maximum diameter of the enlarged artery is measured. If images are clear, ultrasound monitoring is effective and reliable, although the precision of caliper placement is affected by the orientation of the artery and wall structure (Figs. 12.26 and 12.27).

REPORTING

Reporting should describe major findings, including numerical values for renal artery velocities and mean intrarenal RI (or PI in renal transplants) and an interpretation of these results. Limitations of the test should be described, and it is helpful to indicate the clarity with which renal arteries were imaged and measurements were made. For renal transplants with unusual arterial or venous anatomy, a quick sketch or description can save considerable time at the next visit.

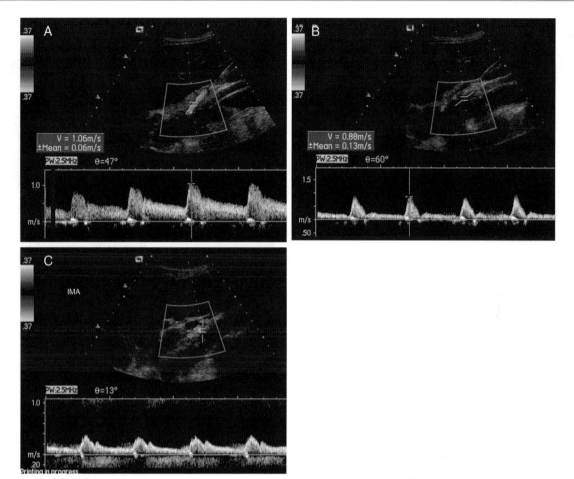

Fig. 12.23 Flow waveforms in the celiac axis (A), superior mesenteric artery (B), and inferior mesenteric artery (C) in a fasted state. *IMA*, Inferior mesenteric artery.

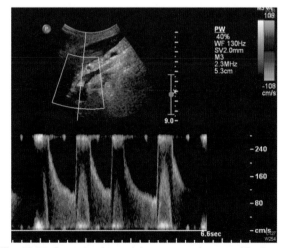

Fig. 12.24 Stenosis of a superior mesenteric artery. The beam is in line with the flow, so no angle correction is used. Despite aliasing, the velocity can be estimated as 500 cm/s.

TABLE 12.1 Indications of Stenosis of Splanchnic Arteries	
Celiac axis ≥ 70%	Peak systolic velocity ≥ 200 cm/s
Superior mesenteric artery ≥ 70%	Peak systolic velocity ≥ 270 cm/s
Superior mesenteric artery/ aorta ratios ≥ 70%	≥3.5
Inferior mesenteric artery > 50%	Peak systolic velocity > 200 cm/s

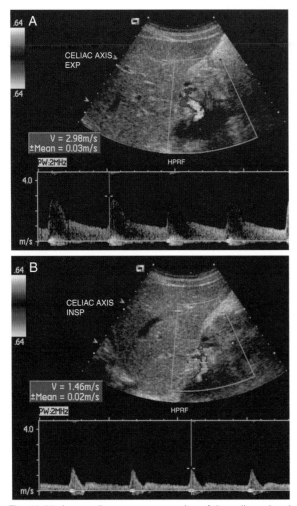

Fig. 12.25 Arcuate ligament compression of the celiac axis origin during expiration (A) causes high velocities that decrease markedly on inspiration (B).

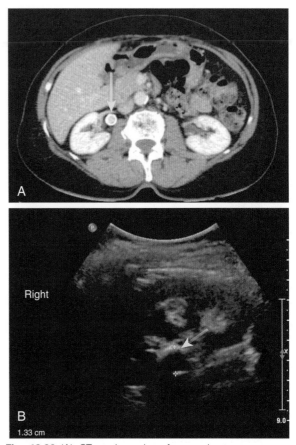

Fig. 12.26 (A) CT angiography of a renal artery aneurysm *(arrowed)*. (B) Ultrasound image of the aneurysm. In this case, calcification *(arrowed)* makes the aneurysm wall easy to detect and measure.

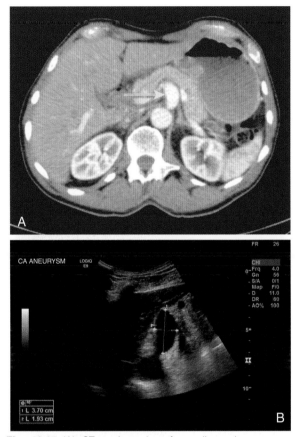

Fig. 12.27 (A) CT angiography of a celiac axis aneurysm *(arrowed)*. The orientation for ultrasound follow-up means that the diameter is measured perpendicular to the beam direction which limits precision in caliper placement (B).

13

Anatomy of the Lower-Limb Venous System and Assessment of Venous Insufficiency

INTRODUCTION

Lower-limb venous disorders are a common problem and consume a significant proportion of the resources available to health care systems. The National Venous Screening Program undertaken by the American Venous Forum in the United States (McLafferty et al. 2008) identified varicose veins and venous reflux in over 30% of participants and more advanced venous disease such as ulceration in at least 10%. Significant venous disease can cause itching, venous eczema, swelling and ultimately lead to venous ulceration, resulting in a marked loss in quality of life. Duplex scanning is the most commonly performed procedure for the detailed investigation of lower-limb venous insufficiency, including the assessment of patients with primary or recurrent varicose

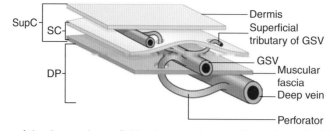

Fig. 13.1 A diagram of the deep and superficial vein compartments. The main trunk of the saphenous vein lies in the saphenous compartment *(SC)*, located within the superficial compartment *SupC* (see text). *DP*, Deep compartment; *GSV*, great saphenous vein.

veins, skin changes, postthrombotic complications, and venous ulceration. Additionally, ultrasound is used to guide endovenous ablation procedures, such as foam sclerosant injection, endovenous laser therapy (EVLT), or radiofrequency ablation (RFA), for the treatment of superficial venous insufficiency. These treatments can be performed under local anesthetic as outpatient-based procedures. In comparison with arterial duplex scanning, venous duplex investigations can be technically challenging due to the wide range of anatomical variations in the venous system. There are also wide variations in practice, technique, and interpretation. In some countries the treatment of venous insufficiency under state-run health care services is reserved for patients with skin changed and venous ulceration, with cosmetic treatments performed by private providers. Therefore, sonographers may follow different protocols and have very differing experiences in the assessment of venous insufficiency. This chapter covers the basic principles and approaches for investigating venous insufficiency but does not include detail on the assessment of very minor or cosmetic veins. It also highlights areas where there are variations in practice and interpretation. It also includes a basic description of ultrasound-guided endovenous procedures.

ANATOMY AND PHYSIOLOGY

This description is based on the consensus document covering duplex assessment of chronic venous disease of the lower limbs and anatomy published by the Union Internationale de Phlébologie (UIP; Cavezzi et al. 2006).

The lower-limb venous system is divided into the deep and superficial veins. The deep veins lie below the muscular fascia. The superficial veins lie between the muscular fascia and the dermis and drain the cutaneous circulation

(Caggiati et al. 2002; Fig. 13.1). There are numerous interconnections between the deep and superficial veins via perforating veins.

Deep Venous System

The anatomy of the deep veins is shown in Fig. 13.2. Generally, the deep veins are larger than their corresponding artery. The main deep veins of the thigh and calf are the following:

- Common femoral vein
- Deep femoral vein (also called the profunda femoris vein)
- Femoral vein (also called the superficial femoral vein)
- Popliteal vein
- Posterior tibial veins
- Peroneal veins
- Anterior tibial veins
- Gastrocnemius veins
- Soleal veins and sinuses

> **Femoral Vein Nomenclature, a Potential for Confusion**
>
> Some sonographers use the term *superficial femoral vein* to describe the vein running between the common femoral vein and popliteal vein. This is a misnomer and should be avoided, as this vein is part of the deep venous system and could be misinterpreted in subsequent reports. The Union Internationale de Phlébologie recommends the use of the term femoral vein.

The posterior tibial (PT) and peroneal veins are usually paired and are associated with their respective arteries. The paired veins join into common trunks in the upper calf before forming the below-knee popliteal vein.

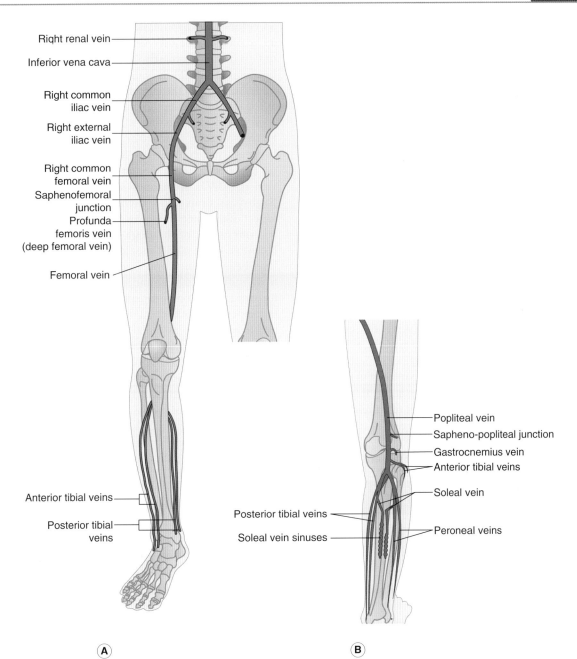

Fig. 13.2 Anatomy of the deep venous system, including the iliac veins and vena cava (A and B).

The soleal veins are deep venous sinuses and veins of the soleus muscle that drain into the proximal PT and peroneal veins. They are an important part of the calf muscle pump mechanism (see Ch. 5). The gastrocnemius veins drain the medial and lateral gastrocnemius muscles. The gastrocnemius veins normally drain into the popliteal vein through a single or multiple trunks below the level of the saphenopopliteal junction. The anterior tibial vein is paired and associated with the anterior tibial artery and drains to the popliteal vein. The above-knee popliteal vein runs through the adductor canal and becomes the femoral vein in the lower medial aspect of the thigh.

The femoral vein runs toward the groin, where it is joined by the deep femoral vein to form the common femoral vein. This confluence is distal to the level of the saphenofemoral junction (SFJ) and common femoral artery bifurcation (see Fig. 9.7). The common femoral vein lies medial to the artery, becoming the external iliac vein above the inguinal ligament (Fig. 13.2). The external iliac vein runs deep and is joined by the internal iliac vein, which drains blood from the pelvis, forming the common iliac vein. The left common iliac vein runs deep to the right common iliac artery to drain into the vena cava, which lies to the right of the aorta.

Superficial Venous System

The main superficial veins are the great saphenous vein (GSV) and small saphenous vein (SSV) (Fig. 13.3) (sometimes referred to as the long saphenous vein and short saphenous vein, respectively). The GSV and SSV are contained in a separate saphenous compartment, bounded superficially by the hyperechoic saphenous fascia and deeply by the muscular fascia (see Fig. 13.4). Branches, tributaries, and cross-communicating veins lie external to the saphenous compartment in the superficial subcutaneous regions (Caggiati et al. 2002; Fig. 13.1). The saphenous compartment often resembles the shape of an Egyptian eye when imaged.

The GSV and Saphenofemoral Junction

The Great Saphenous Vein and Bifid Trunks

- The anatomically observed image of the main trunk of the great saphenous vein and a large tributary, lying superficial to the saphenous compartment, does not constitute a true bifid or paired system. The term *bifid* is properly used when both veins are contained in the same saphenous compartment which is relatively rare.

The anatomy of the GSV is shown in Fig. 13.3A. The distal GSV is located anterior to the medial malleolus (inner ankle bone), runs up the medial aspect of the calf and thigh, and is joined by a number of superficial tributaries. It can be difficult to distinguish the GSV from tributaries below the knee, but it can be identified in transverse section lying in a triangle formed by the tibia and medial gastrocnemius muscle.

Sometimes it is hypoplastic (small) or tributaries may appear larger. The GSV drains into the common femoral vein approximately 2.5 cm below the inguinal ligament at the SFJ. It is important to have a detailed understanding of the anatomy in this area, as there are at least six other tributaries draining to the GSV at the level of the SFJ (see Fig. 13.5). These tributaries can be the source of primary or recurrent varicose veins. It is not usually possible to identify all these tributaries by ultrasound. The anterior accessory saphenous vein (AASV), sometimes called the anterolateral thigh vein, drains flow from the anterior and lateral aspect of the knee and lower thigh and runs across the anterior aspect of the thigh into the SFJ (Fig. 13.3). However, it can sometimes join the GSV at a variable level below the junction. The AASV is normally easy to identify with ultrasound, and it is contained within its own fascial compartment (Figs. 13.6 and 13.7). In the upper thigh, it runs superficial to the femoral vein: this is referred to as the alignment sign and helps to distinguish the AASV from the GSV that lies medial and posterior to the AASV (Fig. 13.7). The posterior accessory saphenous vein also runs in a facial compartment and drains flow from the posteromedial and posterior regions of the lower thigh and usually joins the main trunk of the GSV in the upper thigh. There are sometimes connections between the thigh extension (TE) of the SSV or Giacomini vein, described later in the chapter.

The SSV, Saphenopopliteal Junction, Giacomini Vein, or Thigh Extension Vein

The anatomy of the SSV is shown in Fig. 13.3B.

The distal SSV arises posterior to the outer aspect of the ankle (lateral malleolus) and runs up the posterior calf in an interfascial compartment that resembles an "Egyptian eye" (see Fig. 13.4D). In the upper calf the compartment appears as a triangular shape that is defined by the lateral and medial heads of the gastrocnemius muscle and the superficial fascia that stretches over the intermuscular groove (Cavezzi et al. 2006). It drains to the popliteal vein via the saphenopopliteal junction located superior to the insertion of the gastrocnemius vein. Typically, the saphenopopliteal junction is located 2 to 5 cm above the popliteal knee crease. However, the anatomy can be extremely variable. The saphenopopliteal junction may be located proximal to the popliteal fossa, draining to the above-knee popliteal vein or distal femoral vein (see Fig. 13.8).

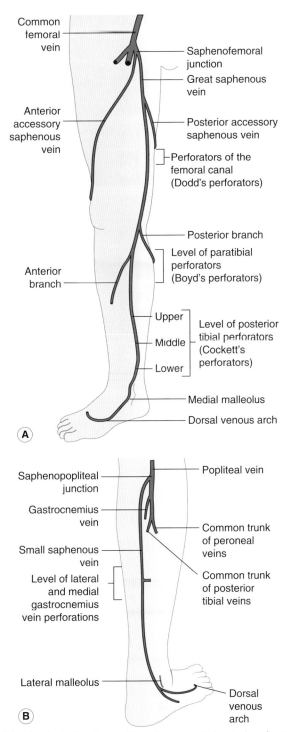

Fig. 13.3 Anatomy of the superficial veins, including the position of commonly located perforators. (A) The great saphenous vein. Posterior tibial perforators (sometimes referred to as Cockett's perforators) are located at distances of approximately 6, 13, and 18 cm above the medial malleolus. Paratibial or Boyd perforators are located in the upper calf, approximately 10 cm below the knee joint. (B) The small saphenous vein.

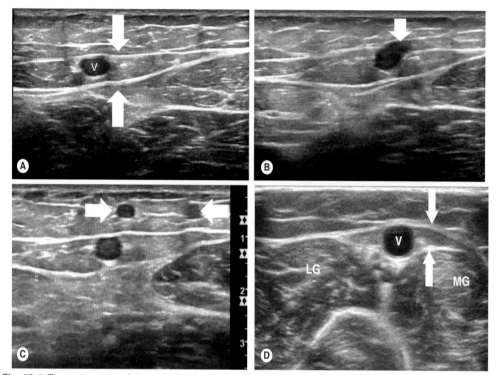

Fig. 13.4 The main trunks of the superficial veins are shown in cross-section. (A) The great saphenous vein *(V)* lies in the saphenous compartment, bounded by the deep muscular fascia *(upward arrow)* and the saphenous fascia *(downward arrow)*. (B) A tributary of the great saphenous vein (GSV) exits the saphenous compartment *(arrow)*. (C) GSV tributaries are seen in the subcutaneous region *(arrows)*. (D) The small saphenous vein *(V)* is also bounded by the deep fascia *(upward arrow)* and saphenous fascia *(downward arrow)*. The medial gastrocnemius muscle *(MG)* and lateral gastrocnemius muscle *(LG)* are shown on this image of the right leg.

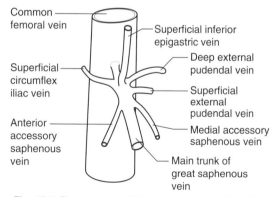

Fig. 13.5 The anatomy of the saphenofemoral junction.

The SSV can insert directly into the gastrocnemius vein with a common trunk draining to the popliteal vein, or share a common confluence at the popliteal vein (Fig. 13.8). In addition, it is common to find a TE of the SSV, described by Giacomini in 1873 running in an intrafascial

compartment or groove bounded by the semitendinous muscle, long head of biceps, and superficial fascia (Georgiev et al. 2003; Fig. 13.9).

There are a number of terminations for the TE, as shown in Fig. 13.8. The TE is often referred to as the Giacomini vein, although strictly this term should only be applied when the vein connects to the GSV. There is sometimes confusion as to whether a posterior thigh vein is the Giacomini vein or merely a superficial posteromedial tributary of the GSV. Generally, the Giacomini vein should appear to run into an intrafascial compartment in the lower thigh before joining the SSV, whereas superficial tributaries of the GSV tend to lie above the superficial fascia. Finally, there are usually intersaphenous veins in the upper calf, running between the GSV and SSV.

Perforators

There are major perforating veins in the GSV and SSV system, and these can be variable in their presence,

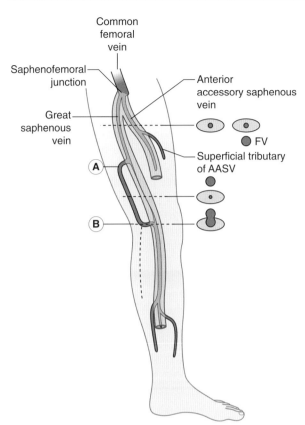

Fig. 13.6 A diagrammatic representation of the saphenous compartments containing the great saphenous vein (GSV) and anterior accessory saphenous vein *(AASV)*. In this example a large incompetent tributary inserts to an incompetent GSV in the mid-thigh *(A)*, with the GSV becoming small and competent beyond this point. The tributary communicates with the main trunk lower in the thigh *(B)*, where the GSV becomes incompetent once more. Alternatively, the large tributary could continue to run down the leg (indicated by the *short dashed lines*) and the GSV could remain small below point B. There can be many anatomical variations involving the GSV and its tributaries, especially in the knee region and mid to lower thigh. *FV, Femoral vein.*

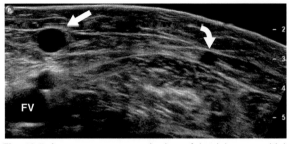

Fig. 13.7 A transverse panoramic view of the right upper thigh showing the anterior accessory saphenous vein (AASV, *straight arrow*) lying above the femoral vein *(FV)*, indicating the alignment sign. The great saphenous vein *(curved arrow)* is lying medially in its own saphenous compartment. In this example it is likely that the AASV is incompetent due to its size.

Other Superficial Veins

There is typically a lateral venous system in the leg, but the veins are often very small and difficult to detect. They may represent an embryonic system and are only relevant if there are isolated varicose veins in this area not associated with the GSV or SSV. They can become prominent in cases of Klippel–Trenaunay syndrome.

Anatomical Variations

There are numerous anatomical variations in the lower-limb venous system, and even experienced sonographers will encounter new variations from time to time. Duplicated, or bifid, vein systems mainly involve the femoral vein and popliteal vein (see Fig. 13.10). A potentially confusing anatomical variation occurs in patients who have a large deep femoral vein in the thigh running as a large trunk between the popliteal vein and the common femoral vein. In this situation, the size of the femoral vein in the thigh can be small when compared with the size of the superficial femoral artery, and this appearance may be mistaken for evidence of venous obstruction. However, good flow augmentation, with a calf squeeze, will be demonstrated in the common femoral vein just below the SFJ. Careful inspection by duplex will normally reveal the larger deep femoral vein. A low-frequency (2–4 MHz) curved array transducer may be necessary to identify this vein. A rare anomaly can occur toward the level of the SFJ, with the GSV running between the superficial femoral artery and profunda femoris artery to drain into the SFJ.

being more numerous below the knee (Fig. 13.3). They are named after their location, but historically they had eponymous names such as Dodd's and Boyd's. Large perforators are easy to identify by ultrasound. It is worth noting that some perforators do not connect directly to the main trunks of the GSV or SSV but communicate via side branches of the main trunks. There are a number of perforating veins associated with the SSV, especially from medial and lateral gastrocnemius veins and soleal veins.

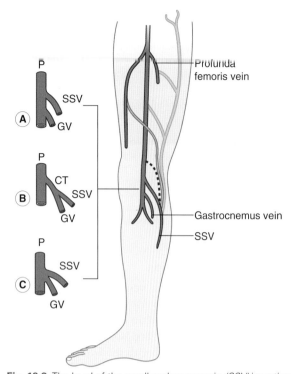

Fig. 13.8 The level of the small saphenous vein *(SSV)* insertion can be highly variable. Potential positions are shown by lettered diagrams. The SSV normally drains to the popliteal vein *(P)* in the popliteal fossa at the saphenopopliteal junction (A). It can share a common trunk *(CT)* with the gastrocnemius vein *(GV)* (B). It can share a common junction with the gastrocnemius vein (C). It sometimes has a high junction with the popliteal vein *(blue dashed line)*. The thigh extension vein, when present, runs above the level of the saphenopopliteal junction and has a variable outflow. It may drain to the femoral vein, profunda femoris vein, or branches of the internal iliac vein *(green lines)*. It may also drain to the great saphenous vein (GSV) and in this situation the vein is termed the Giacomini vein *(orange line)*. Note that it is possible to confuse the posteromedial tributary of the great saphenous vein with the Giacomini vein; see text.

Venous Valves

Veins contain bicuspid valves to prevent the reflux of blood to the extremities. There is normally a characteristic dilation of the vein at the valve site that can sometimes be seen on the ultrasound image (Fig. 13.11). Venous valves can withstand high degrees of back pressure, typically in excess of 250 to 300 mmHg. The number of valves in each venous segment varies among individuals, but there are more valves in the distal veins than in the proximal veins, as they must withstand higher hydrostatic pressures. The inferior vena cava and common iliac vein have no valves, and most of the population have no valves in the external iliac vein. Approximately two-thirds of people have a valve in the common femoral vein 4 cm proximal to the SFJ (Mühlberger et al. 2008). There is usually a valve at the proximal end of the femoral vein and an average of three to four valves along the length of the femoral and popliteal vein to the level of the knee, although the number can be inconsistent. In most people there is a valve in the below-knee popliteal vein that is sometimes referred to as the "gatekeeper," as it prevents venous reflux into the proximal calf. The deep veins in the calf contain numerous valves. The GSV and SSV contain a variable number of valves.

The configuration of the valves at the SFJ is important to consider, as there is typically a terminal valve located at the junction and a preterminal valve that is positioned in the GSV, 3 to 5 cm distal to the terminal valve (Mühlberger et al. 2009). Tributaries of the SFJ join between these two points (Fig. 13.12). This explains how it is possible for the junction to be competent but for reflux to occur across the preterminal valve into the proximal GSV due to refluxing flow from the tributaries (Caggiati et al. 2004; Fig. 13.12B). In addition, there are normally valves protecting many perforating veins so that flow is directed from the superficial venous system to the deep system. In rare cases, patients may have absent venous valves due to congenital valve aplasia (Eifert et al. 2000). This can be the cause of deep venous reflux in the young patient.

Flow Patterns in the Venous System

The flow patterns in normal deep veins are described in Chapter 5. The venous flow patterns in the superficial veins can vary, depending on patient position and external factors, such as ambient temperature. Normally there should be no, or very little, spontaneous flow in the GSV and SSV when the patient is standing or sitting. If the ambient temperature in the room is high, vasodilation may result in increased flow in the superficial veins. Evidence of high-volume spontaneous or continuous flow in the superficial veins at rest should be treated with suspicion, as this may indicate obstruction of the deep veins or could be due to infection, such as cellulitis (see Fig. 13.13).

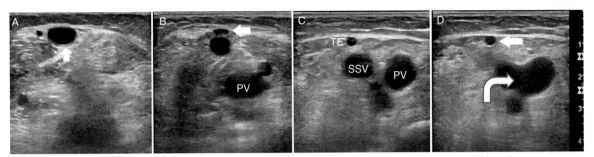

Fig. 13.9 Four transverse images showing the small saphenous vein *(SSV)*, saphenopopliteal junction, and an example of a thigh extension vein *(TE)*. (A) The SSV is seen in the upper calf *(arrow)*. In this example it is probably varicose due to its size. (B) In the lower part of the popliteal fossa, a TE divides from the SSV *(arrow)*. The popliteal vein *(PV)* is visible. (C) The SSV, PV, TE, and popliteal artery are visible in the mid-popliteal fossa. (D) In the mid-upper popliteal fossa, the saphenopopliteal junction is seen *(curved arrow)*. The TE is clearly visible *(straight arrow)* and in this example continued to course up the thigh.

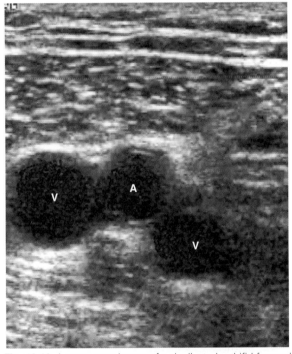

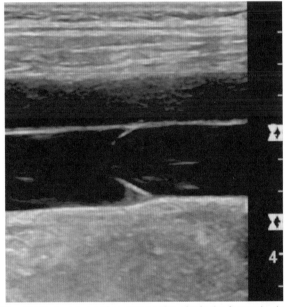

Fig. 13.11 An image of a venous valve site in the femoral vein.

Fig. 13.10 A transverse image of a duplicated or bifid femoral vein with the artery *(A)* lying between the paired veins *(V)*.

VENOUS DISORDERS AND TREATMENT

Deep-vein thrombosis (DVT) is covered in Chapter 14.

Classification of Chronic Venous Disorders

The CEAP (Clinical–Etiology–Anatomy–Pathophysiology) classification system for venous disorders was developed by an ad hoc committee of the venous forum (Eklöf et al. 2004). It has been developed to facilitate the use of consistent terminology and diagnosis within the clinical and scientific community. The clinical classes are shown in Table 13.1. For example, a patient with a painful venous ulcer due to primary venous disease that included great saphenous and popliteal vein reflux, with perforating vein reflux in the calf, would have a basic CEAP classification of $C_{6,s}, E_p, A_{spd}, P_r$. In advanced CEAP, the classification would be $C_{2,6,s}, E_p, A_{s,p,d}, P_{r2,3,18,14}$.

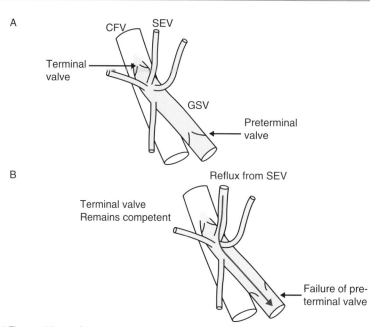

Fig. 13.12 (A) The positions of the terminal and preterminal valves are shown in this diagram of the saphenofemoral junction and proximal great saphenous vein *(GSV)*. The superficial inferior epigastric vein *(SEV)* is shown in this example, but not all tributaries of the junction have been included. (B) This example shows how it is possible for the terminal valve to be competent, but reflux is possible in the GSV due to failure of the preterminal valve with flow supplied from the SEV. *CFV,* Common femoral vein

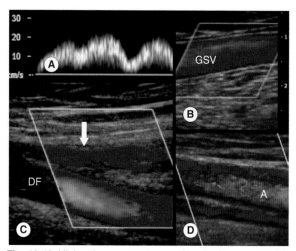

Fig. 13.13 High-volume spontaneous flow is demonstrated in the great saphenous vein *(GSV)* of a patient with popliteal and femoral vein obstruction due to chronic postthrombotic syndrome. (A) Spectral Doppler recording from the GSV shown in (B) indicating spontaneous flow. (B) A large dilated GSV. (C) The deep femoral vein *(DF)* is patent, but the femoral vein *(arrow)* is small. (D) An image of the femoral vessels in the mid-thigh demonstrating small collateral veins *(blue)* adjacent to the artery (A).

Varicose Veins

Varicose veins are common; their cause is uncertain, but there is evidence that increased age, gender, and pregnancy are risk factors (Campbell 2006; Piazza 2014; Davies 2019; NICE Guidance varicose veins 2020).

Varicose veins appear as dilated, tortuous, elongated vessels on the skin surface, especially in the calf. Abnormal superficial veins can be classified according to their size. Minor cosmetic or intradermal spider veins (telangiectasia) <1 mm in diameter are not normally visible to ultrasound without using probes with frequency greater than 20 MHz. Small dilated subdermal veins (reticular veins) 1 to 2 mm in diameter can also be difficult to image without high-frequency probes 12 to 20 MHz. Varicose veins, typically subcutaneous and measuring >3 mm in diameter, often involve the main superficial trunks, or their tributaries, or both and can be easily assessed with ultrasound. Varicose veins most commonly occur due to incompetence of the GSV or SSV, or a combination of both systems.

TABLE 13.1	CEAP (Clinical–Etiology–Anatomy–Pathophysiology) Classification		
Clinical Classification		Po	Obstruction
C0	No visible or palpable signs of venous disease	Pr,o	Reflux and obstruction
		Pn	No venous pathophysiology identifiable
C1	Telangiectasia or reticular veins	**Advanced CEAP: Same as Basic CEAP, With the Addition That Any of 18 Named Venous Segments Can Be Used as Locators for Venous Pathology**	
C2	Varicose veins		
C3	Edema		
C4a	Pigmentation or eczema	**Superficial Veins**	
C4b	Lipodermatosclerosis or atrophie blanche	1	Telangiectasia or reticular veins
C5	Healed venous ulcer	2	Great saphenous vein above knee
C6	Active venous ulcer	3	Great saphenous vein below knee
S	Symptomatic, including ache, pain, tightness, skin irritation, heaviness, and muscle cramps, and other complaints attributable to venous dysfunction	4	Small saphenous vein
		5	Nonsaphenous veins
		Deep Veins	
		6	Inferior vena cava
A	Asymptomatic	7	Common iliac vein
Etiologic Classification		8	Internal iliac vein
Ec	Congenital	9	External iliac vein
Ep	Primary	10	Pelvic: gonadal, broad ligament veins, other
Es	Secondary (postthrombotic)	11	Common femoral vein
En	No venous cause identified	12	Deep femoral vein
Anatomic Classification		13	Femoral vein
As	Superficial veins	14	Popliteal vein
Ap	Perforator veins	15	Crural: anterior tibial, posterior tibial, peroneal veins (all paired)
Ad	Deep veins		
An	No venous location identified	16	Muscular: gastrocnemial, soleal veins, other
Pathophysiologic Classification		**Perforating Veins**	
Basic CEAP		17	Thigh
Pr	Reflux	18	Calf

Modified from Eklöf et al. (2004).

It is important to identify the supply to the varicose areas and the level of incompetence in the GSV or SSV. This can be highly variable but frequently involves reflux from the saphenofemoral or saphenopopliteal junctions. In some situations, varicose veins may be independent of the GSV or SSV systems, such as those in the lateral thigh. Much debate has surrounded the development of varicose veins, but it appears that for the most part incompetence in the main trunks develops distally, in the lower leg, and progresses in an ascending direction over time (Bernardini et al. 2010). This is contrary to traditional teaching, which proposed that incompetence developed at the SFJ, leading to progressive valve failure in a descending direction. The model of progressively ascending valve failure would also explain why it is possible to observe segmental GSV reflux in the lower thigh but competence of the vein in the upper thigh and at the SFJ. Some patients with superficial varicose veins may also have coexisting deep venous insufficiency.

Skin Changes and Venous Ulcers

A serious complication of superficial or deep venous insufficiency is the development of chronic venous hypertension in the lower limb, resulting in venous ulceration (Fig. 13.14). Risk factors associated with ulceration include postthrombotic syndrome, obesity, immobility, and arthritic conditions, which cause reduced movement of the ankle joint, leading to failure of the calf muscle pump. It is important to note that some ulcers that may appear to be venous in origin are caused by other conditions, such as vasculitis, rheumatoid arthritis, or skin disorders. The underlying cause of ulceration is still unclear but is thought to involve changes in the microcirculation of the skin and subcutaneous tissues in response to local venous hypertension. The venous hypertension causes an increase in venular and capillary pressure, leading to local edema and reduced reabsorption of proteins and fluid from the interstitial tissue spaces. This is combined with damage to the capillary walls, which may cause localized tissue hypoxia. Leakage of red blood cells across the damaged capillary wall and into the interstitial tissue spaces produces the brown pigmentation associated with many ulcers. This is due to hemosiderin deposition caused by the breakdown of the red blood cells. Venous ulcers are usually reasonably shallow and vary in size, and in some cases they may be circumferential around the calf. They frequently become infected with different types of bacteria, causing odor, and can be extremely painful.

Skin changes around the ankle or lower calf are the first physical signs of venous hypertension. This is typically seen as areas of venous eczema and pigmentation, frequently associated with local skin irritation or itching. There is often development of lipodermatosclerosis, typified as hardening of the subcutaneous tissues in the lower calf and ankle, giving a hard, "woody" feel to the area. The development of an ulcer is sometimes initiated by a minor injury or abrasion that fails to heal. It is important to remember that some venous ulcers are associated with arterial disease, and patients with mixed venous and arterial ulceration pose a challenging diagnostic problem for the vascular laboratory. It is therefore routine practice to measure the ankle–brachial pressure index (ABPI) in all patients with venous ulceration to exclude a significant arterial component. However, in some situations it can be impossible to measure the ABPI due to pain, edema, or limb swelling, and a subjective assessment of the pedal artery waveforms will have to suffice. A layer of cling film or Saran wrap is ideal for wrapping around areas of ulceration to protect the ulcer and to keep the pressure cuff clean.

Historically, it was thought that venous ulceration was primarily due to deep venous insufficiency following valve failure, postthrombotic syndrome, or failure of the calf muscle pump, resulting in deep venous hypertension. However, it is clear that a significant number of patients with ulceration have superficial reflux alone,

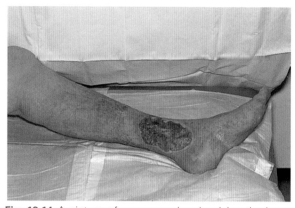

Fig. 13.14 A picture of a venous ulcer involving the lower aspect of the medial calf and ankle. Varicose veins are also seen in the great saphenous vein distribution of the mid-calf.

with the deep veins being competent. Therefore, ligation of the relevant superficial vein junction, with or without stripping of the superficial vein, results in the healing of many ulcers due to the reduction in venous hypertension. The role of perforator ligation remains controversial, but there is evidence that chronic venous insufficiency is associated with an increase in the number and diameter of medial calf perforators (Stuart et al. 2000). Presurgical marking of incompetent perforators may be performed with the aid of the duplex scanner.

Varicose ulcers caused by superficial incompetence alongside gross deep venous insufficiency are not usually treated by the ligation or stripping of superficial varicose veins, as the underlying deep venous hypertension will not be corrected. Instead, the use of compression bandaging, which reduces edema and venous hypertension, has proved to be an effective method of healing ulcers. Different grades of compression bandaging can be used depending upon the clinical situation. However, an ABPI of ≥0.8 is usually required for the application of four-layer compression dressings, in order to avoid arterial compromise in the tissues under the bandaging (NICE Guidance ABPI 2020). This can be a serious complication and can lead to limb loss in extreme cases. An ABPI > 1.3 can be due to arterial calcification giving a misleading diagnosis/result, and further specialist arterial assessment is normally required to investigate the arteries.

Treatment of Superficial Venous Disorders

A range of treatment options is available depending on the severity of the condition (NICE Guidance varicose veins 2020). Conservative treatment is with compression hosiery. Thread veins can be treated by microinjection sclerotherapy, followed by local compression to occlude the vein. They can also be treated by local laser therapy. Larger varicose veins can be treated by a variety of methods, including foam sclerotherapy, open surgery, or endovenous ablation. Some patients undergo combined procedures to achieve optimum results. In the case of open surgery for primary GSV incompetence, the SFJ and tributaries are ligated at the groin, and the main trunk stripped with a vein stripper to knee level or below. Surgery of the SSV normally involves ligation of the saphenopopliteal junction. Some surgeons strip the vein, but others leave it intact to avoid injury to the sural nerve, which is closely associated with the vein. Some surgeons also ligate large perforators, and these can be marked preoperatively with the aid of duplex scanning. Any remaining veins are then removed or avulsed using small microincisions. It is useful to observe some varicose vein surgery, as it gives a better appreciation of the anatomy seen during duplex examinations. It is possible that new techniques such as high-intensity focused ultrasound could become treatment options in the future.

What Does the Clinician Want to Know?

- Is there deep venous reflux or obstruction, or evidence of postthrombotic syndrome?
- The source of reflux
- Is there reflux in the great saphenous vein, small saphenous vein, or tributaries and at what level?
- Is there reflux across the saphenofemoral or saphenopopliteal junction or relevant perforators?
- Are there any large localized dilations (varices) present?
- Are there other sources of reflux, such as the lateral thigh system?
- Indication of veins that have been removed or stripped or are not present
- Unusual anatomy of the saphenopopliteal junction, including the presence of thigh extension or Giacomini vein
- Are the veins suitable for endovenous ablation (i.e., assessment of diameter, depth, and tortuousity) or injection treatments such as foam sclerotherapy?
- Abnormal anatomy

Practical Considerations for Duplex Scanning of Varicose Veins

The purpose of the scan is to assess the competency of the superficial and deep veins and identify the source of venous insufficiency and any associated varicose veins. At least half an hour should be allocated for a bilateral vein scan. Adopting a logical approach to the examination is useful, as this reduces the length of time required for the assessment. The patient should be asked the following questions before starting the examination:

- *Have you had any previous varicose vein treatment, either by surgery, endovenous therapy, or by injection sclerotherapy?* It is not uncommon to find that the request card has omitted previous clinical details, and the patient may have undergone some form of treatment in the past. This may be evident on the duplex scan.
- *Have you ever had a DVT or severe leg swelling?* If the patient has had a DVT, there may be chronic damage of the deep venous system, causing deep venous insufficiency or obstruction, which may be the cause of the current symptoms.

It is essential that the sonographer also visually examines the position and distribution of the varicose veins and/or ulcers or skin changes, as this can provide a clue to their supply. No preparation is required before the scan, but the legs should be accessible from the groin to the ankle. It is necessary to position the patient so that the feet are lower than the heart to generate sufficient hydrostatic pressure to assess the competency of the venous valves. If the patient is lying completely flat, there is very little pressure differential between the central venous system and the legs. Therefore, an incompetent vein may not demonstrate detectable reflux leading to false-negative result (Bonfield et al. 2012). Many units perform the examination with the patient in a standing position. When standing, partial weight should be on the examined limb with the knee slightly flexed, but most weight-bearing should be on the contralateral limb. The patient can use a hand rail, or suitable alternative, for support. Other common positions in which to assess a patient include the supine position on the examination table with the whole table tilted feet-down (reverse Trendelenburg position). Alternatively, the patient can sit on the edge of the examination table, and partial weight-bearing is achieved by placing the foot of the examined limb on a stool. It is not uncommon for patients, especially younger ones, to feel faint during the examination due to the calf compressions. When patients are standing, this can be a risk to the sonographer as the patient can fall on them. Let the patient lie down immediately if he or she feels unwell, and, if necessary, appropriate medical advice should be sought.

AUGMENTATION MANEUVERS AND VENOUS REFLUX

Before considering the practical techniques used for scanning the venous system, it is important to understand the methods most commonly employed for assessing venous valve competency (Coleridge-Smith et al. 2006). These are calf compression, to augment flow toward the heart, and the Valsalva maneuver for examining the competency of the veins in the groin. In addition, proximal compression can be used to assess flow in perforators. It is also important to understand the normal venous flow patterns observed in the legs due to respiration as discussed in Chapter 5.

Valsalva Maneuver

> **CAUTION**
>
> It is possible for enthusiastic patients performing a very strong Valsalva maneuver to generate pressures beyond the normal physiological range, leading to reflux.

The competency of the proximal deep veins and SFJ can be assessed with a Valsalva maneuver. The patient is told to inhale deeply and then to expire against a closed glottis, while at the same time bearing pressure down on the abdomen. This leads to a reduction in venous return and produces an increase in intraabdominal pressure, thus increasing the venous blood pressure in the iliac and femoral veins. It is usual to see the common femoral vein distending during a Valsalva maneuver. Provided that the venous valves are competent, there should be no reflux across the SFJ or proximal superficial femoral vein during Valsalva testing (see Fig. 13.15). There should be a temporary cessation of the normal respiratory phasic flow pattern in the femoral and common femoral veins. If the SFJ is incompetent, the increase in abdominal pressure will produce significant reflux across the junction (Fig. 13.16). The Valsalva maneuver is not used for the assessment of more distal veins.

Calf Compression

To assess the competency of the valves, the flow in the veins toward the heart should be temporarily increased or augmented. The easiest way to produce flow augmentation is to place a hand around the back of the calf and give a firm squeeze that is then briskly released. It is important to squeeze the bulk of the muscle rather than a small portion or next to bone (Fig. 13.17). In our experience flow augmentation should be sufficiently strong to produce a transient peak flow velocity of >30 cm/s in the main superficial vein trunks so that valve closure should be rapid on the squeeze release. However, this velocity can be difficult to achieve in very small veins. Variation in the strength and duration of augmentation, the speed of squeeze release, the size of the vein, and degree of valve failure will influence any reflux pattern observed (see Fig. 13.18A). Multiple calf squeezes over a short time will empty the calf reservoir of blood, resulting in decreasing flow augmentation (Fig. 13.18B). If an inadequate calf squeeze is performed, flow augmentation may be poor or not seen at all. It can also be difficult to maintain the probe position while augmenting flow, as both hands are required (one for holding the probe and the other squeezing the calf). In challenging situations, an assistant can help to squeeze the calf. The problem is demonstrated in Fig. 13.19. Good coordination and technique are required. Some sonographers prefer to use transverse imaging for the assessment of reflux, as it is easier to maintain an image of the vein even if there is some leg or probe movement during augmentation maneuvers (see Fig. 13.20). If assessing for reflux in the transverse plane, it is important to create an angle between the probe and the vein to detect flow (Fig. 13.20B).

To overcome the problems involved with flow augmentation described earlier, some units prefer to use a rapid cuff inflator with cuffs around the calf or thigh. The system inflates the cuff to a preset pressure before rapid deflation to provide reproducible compression. The disadvantage of this method is that it can be time-consuming and cumbersome. Manual compression of vein clusters is useful if the varicose veins are in less common positions,

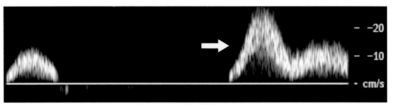

Fig. 13.15 The Valsalva maneuver demonstrates competency of the proximal femoral vein. There is a cessation of normal phasic flow during the Valsalva maneuver followed by a surge of flow during expiration *(arrow)*.

such as the lateral aspect of the calf or thigh. It is also possible to augment flow by asking the patient to dorsiflex and relax the foot a couple of times.

Augmenting flow to assess perforators competence can be inconsistent and frustrating, as discussed later in the chapter.

GRADING OF SUPERFICIAL AND DEEP VENOUS REFLUX

Inconsistent Reflux

Ultrasound evaluation of the degree of venous reflux and even the detection of its presence or absence can be poorly reproducible. Many factors change venous tone and hence venous reflux. Limb muscle tone also influences venous flow and reflux. A consistent degree of weight-bearing seems to introduce some reproducibility:

- Reflux is more likely to be recorded later in the day due to hydrostatic effects on the venous system and loss of venous tone. If assessing patients with small varicosities, it can be better to do it at this time.
- If the examination room is very cold, the periphery may be vasoconstricted, resulting in reduced filling of the veins, which in some cases may lead to reflux being missed or classed as normal.
- If the patient is anxious, the leg muscles may be tense; it may be difficult to produce an adequate calf squeeze to augment flow. Make sure the patient relaxes the calf muscle.
- If the patent is sitting with the mid-thigh on the edge of the examination table, this can have the effect of compressing or "cutting into" the thigh muscles, making imaging and assessment of the femoral vein difficult, and can also distort the position of the great saphenous vein.
- A degree of weight-bearing can be achieved with the legs dependent by placing the foot of the examined leg on a stool.
- Weight-bearing can have a variable effect on venous reflux; for example, there are cases when a calf perforator in an edematous leg will show continuous reflux on dependency, but this reflux cannot be reproduced with partial or full weight-bearing.
- Variation in the squeeze, duration, and release time (rapid or slow) can affect the reflux pattern.
- Multiple calf squeezes over a short time will empty the calf reservoir of blood, as there will be insufficient time for refilling, resulting in decreasing flow augmentation and reflux.
- Poor or inconsistent augmentation techniques may fail to demonstrate reflux.

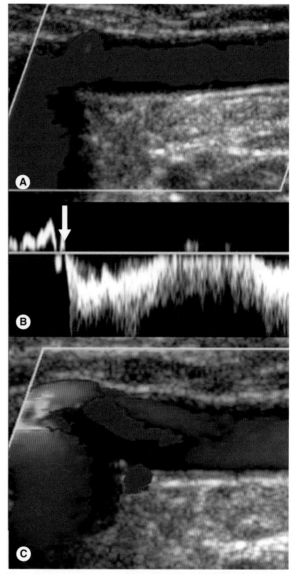

Fig. 13.16 Incompetence of the saphenofemoral junction is demonstrated by color flow imaging and spectral Doppler during a Valsalva maneuver. (A) During inspiration, flow is toward the heart *(flow coded blue)*. (B) The *arrow* indicates the start of the Valsalva maneuver, with marked reflux demonstrated. (C) Color flow imaging also demonstrates the reflux *(flow coded red)*. Note that the saphenofemoral junction and great saphenous vein are distended during the maneuver.

Considerable debate surrounds the grading of venous reflux, especially as different patterns of reflux can be observed in the venous system. The following protocol is suggested as a starting point.

With the relevant segment of vein imaged in longitudinal section, the color box is steered to obtain the

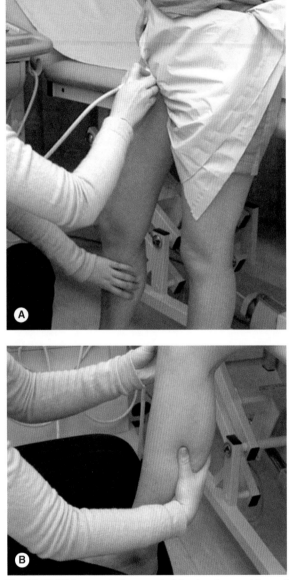

Fig. 13.17 (A) Incorrect placement of the hand around the calf will result in poor augmentation. (B) The bulk of the calf muscle should be firmly squeezed, as shown in this example.

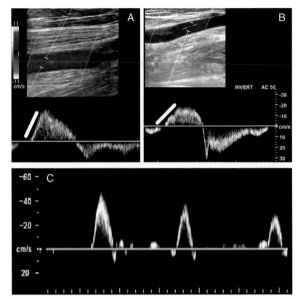

Fig. 13.18 Variation in flow augmentation. (A and B) Doppler recordings taken from two patients demonstrate a brisk calf squeeze and augmentation in the left image as shown by the slope of the white line. On the right side the calf squeeze was more prolonged. Despite this, there is significant reflux recorded in the right image. (C) Three calf squeezes in quick succession result in progressively decreasing flow augmentation in a competent great saphenous vein due to emptying of the venous reservoir with insufficient time for refilling from the arterioles.

best angle of insonation to the vein. A calf squeeze is performed and the augmentation of flow demonstrated with color flow imaging. It is often possible to tell from the color flow display if the vein is normal or incompetent. A competent vein will display a burst of flow toward the heart during a calf squeeze, followed by an abrupt cessation of flow during squeeze release, although a very brief period of retrograde flow may be seen as the valves close. Significant venous reflux will be demonstrated

by a sustained period of retrograde flow following calf release (Figs. 13.21 and 13.22). However, the grading of venous reflux based on color flow imaging alone can sometimes be misleading. This is because the color flow image may give little impression of the flow volume or may not detect low-volume reflux at all. Spectral Doppler is used to grade the degree and duration of venous reflux (Fig. 13.23). The spectral Doppler sample volume should be large enough to cover the vein lumen, and ideally the angle of insonation should be equal to or less than 60° to obtain a good spectral Doppler trace (Fig. 13.18A).

Table 13.2 categorizes the degrees of venous reflux. The same criteria are used for grading venous reflux by calf compression or the Valsalva maneuver. Although the classification of venous reflux can sometimes be subjective and poorly reproducible, many scientific publications have used a reflux duration of >0.5 seconds to indicate abnormal valve function (Evans et al. 1998; Ruckley et al. 2002). However, some departments use a reflux duration of >1 second or different cutoff times for the superficial

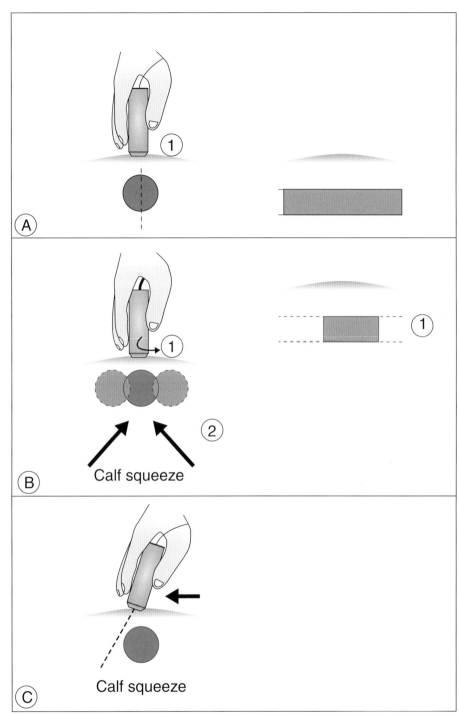

Fig. 13.19 Movement of the probe or skin and tissue below the probe during manual augmentation can result in the loss of the vein image and spectral Doppler trace. (A) The probe is positioned to provide a longitudinal image of the vein. (B) As the calf is squeezed, the probe may be inadvertently twisted *(1)*, so that only a short section of the vein is visible. It is also possible that during the squeeze the vein and tissue may move or "role" out of the image plane *(2)*. (C) The probe can be accidentally tilted during augmentation as both hands are working simultaneously.

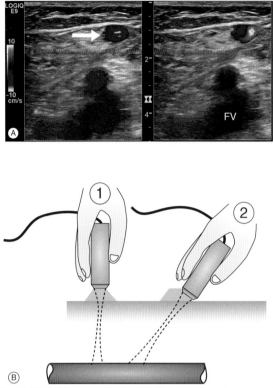

Fig. 13.20 (A) A transverse image of the great saphenous vein *(arrow)* demonstrating reflux following calf augmentation (right image). The femoral vessels are shown in these images, and there is no reflux in the femoral vein *(FV)* in the right image. (B) It is important to create an angle between the transducer and vein in transverse section to adequately demonstrate flow. In position *1*, the probe is 90° to the vein. In position *2*, the probe is tilted to provide a better Doppler angle.

and deep veins (Labropoulos et al. 2003). In some cases, the reflux may be so severe that retrograde flow persists for more than 4 seconds. Finally, it may be possible to misinterpret a competent segment of a large vein as incompetent due to helical motion of flow during augmentation. This is especially true for the popliteal vein just above the knee, as the vein is large at this level, having been joined by several veins across and just below the knee.

Some patterns of reflux can be difficult to interpret, and attempts have been made to measure the volume of reflux using ultrasound volume flow measurements. In practice this is too time-consuming to be used routinely, but subjective assessment of the reflux volume can be useful. Trickle or low-velocity reflux can occur due to partially incompetent valves (Fig. 13.24). This can be observed in many veins but is common in the popliteal

vein below the knee. Leaking valves can demonstrate a high-velocity jet between the leaflets, which can be eccentric to the vein lumen (Fig. 13.24A). It has been speculated that incipient deep venous reflux may occur due to gross superficial varicose veins causing overload of the deep venous system. This may cause some degree of dilation of the deep veins in the lower leg, which impairs normal valve function (Adam et al. 2003).

Another problem of interpretation can occur when a vein is very large or dilated, as the duration of reflux may be relatively short. However, the volume of reflux can be high due to the large diameter of the vein. In this situation, significant reflux may be suspected if the shape of the spectral Doppler reflux pattern is the same as the augmentation pattern (see Fig. 13.25). It may be difficult to augment flow in the veins of patients with gross venous stasis, and very little reflux will occur following distal release. However, the B-mode image often displays aggregation of the blood in the dilated vein as a speckle pattern (Fig. 13.26). Only a small amount of movement in the speckle pattern will be seen during augmentation. The deep venous sinuses in the calf may be dilated and congested with blood, and this appearance can be mistaken for a DVT (see Ch. 14). DVT can be ruled out by compression of the veins. In some cases, it may be necessary to complement the duplex scan with other diagnostic tests, such as ambulatory venous pressures or plethysmography.

SCANNING PROTOCOL FOR THE LOWER-LIMB VENOUS SYSTEM

ADVICE

- It is often quicker to image the varicose veins distally and follow them back to their supply.
- Don't be overwhelmed if the clinical presentation looks complex. Break the assessment down into logical stages and answer the key questions: Is there reflux, and where is the source?
- Don't become fixated on assessing small varicosities at the expense of missing more significant pathology.
- Make sure you adopt a good posture and technique to avoid repetitive strain injury and work-related upper-limb disorders. Venous insufficiency scanning is particularly high risk while trying to image veins and augment flow at the same time, as it can result in twisting of the torso.

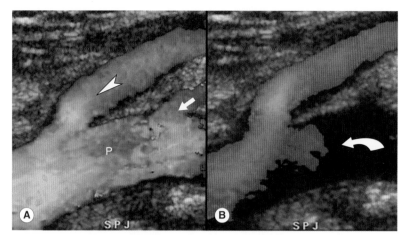

Fig. 13.21 (A) In this color flow image of the saphenopopliteal junction, flow in the small saphenous vein *(arrow head)* and popliteal vein *(P)* is toward the heart *(coded blue)* during distal augmentation. The *straight arrow* shows the insertion of the gastrocnemius vein. (B) Following squeeze release there is significant retrograde flow *(coded red)* in the small saphenous vein and popliteal vein above the junction, due to saphenopopliteal junction incompetence. However, no retrograde flow is demonstrated in the popliteal vein below the level of the saphenopopliteal junction, indicating popliteal vein competency at this level *(curved arrow)*.

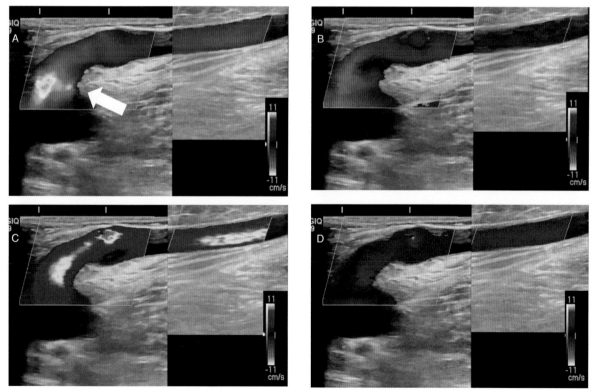

Fig. 13.22 Incompetence of the saphenofemoral junction and great saphenous vein is demonstrated with color flow imaging. Images *A to D* show flow across the junction *(arrow)* and proximal GSV during distal augmentation and release. In image *A*, flow *(coded red)* is toward the heart just before squeeze release. In image *B*, there is early transition to retrograde flow with areas of flow coded blue. In image *C*, there is significant retrograde flow *(coded blue)*. In image *D* the velocity of reflux is decreasing, demonstrated by the *darker blue color hue*.

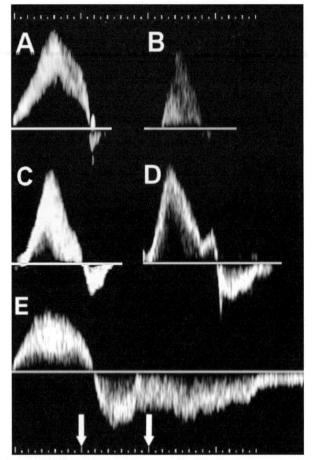

Fig. 13.23 Spectral Doppler is used to assess venous reflux. The scale between the arrows is 1 second. (A) Augmentation of flow in the great saphenous vein following calf compression shows a short duration of normal retrograde flow below the baseline on squeeze release, indicating competent valves. (B) Poor spectral traces can be obtained due to transducer movement during calf augmentation, and the measurement should be repeated (see Fig. 13.19). (C) Borderline reflux is demonstrated (approximately 0.5 seconds). (D) Moderate venous reflux of 0.8 seconds duration. (E) Severe venous reflux >1 second duration.

TABLE 13.2	**Grading of Venous Reflux**
Grade	**Reflux Duration**
Normal valve function	Rapid valve closure. Reflux duration <0.5 s
Moderate reflux	Reflux duration of 0.5–<1 s, mild-to-moderate retrograde flow
Significant reflux	Reflux duration of ≥1 s, large volume of retrograde flow

A venous preset should be selected on the duplex scanner, which should typically set the pulse repetition frequency at 1 KHz, or set the color scale to approximately 10 cm/s. The color wall filter should also be set at a low level. A high-frequency transducer is normally used for scanning superficial varicose veins, although a mid-frequency transducer may be needed for large legs. A mid-frequency transducer is usually required for imaging the deep veins and junctions. A combination of B-mode, color flow imaging, and spectral Doppler is used throughout the examination. The assessment of venous reflux is best and more consistently performed with the transducer in a longitudinal plane to the vein, but initial identification of reflux is often better performed in transverse with transducer angulation. Also, the assessment of perforator competency may be easier in the transverse section. It is necessary to perform an examination of the femoral and popliteal veins during any vein assessment to assess their

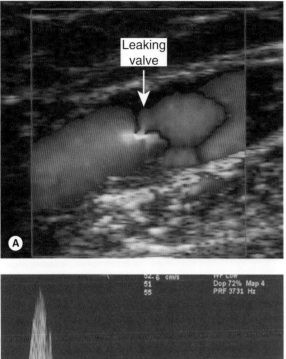

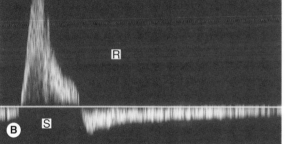

Fig. 13.24 (A) Partial incompetence of a venous valve is demonstrated by an area of retrograde flow *(arrow)* between the two valve cusps. (B) Spectral Doppler demonstrates trickle or low-velocity reflux *(R)* in the popliteal vein following distal augmentation *(S)*.

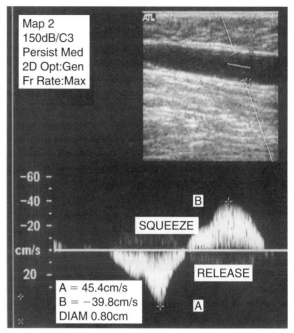

Fig. 13.25 There can be problems in quantifying venous reflux. In this example the great saphenous vein was very large (8 mm diameter), but the duration of reflux (0.9 seconds) is shorter than that shown in Fig. 13.23E. However, the volume of reflux is similar to that demonstrated during augmentation. In this example, the volume of blood flow during reflux is likely very significant due to the size of the vein. It should be noted that volume flow calculations are not routinely used in venous examinations.

patency and competency, as the superficial veins can act as collateral pathways if the deep veins are damaged or obstructed due to postthrombotic syndrome, and surgery of the superficial veins would be contraindicated and potentially damaging. During the examination it is important to remember key characteristics. Veins should be compressible and have thin smooth walls. Evidence of spontaneous phasic flow with respiration is normally seen in proximal deep veins and sometimes the GSV.

Assessment of the GSV and Deep Veins of the Thigh and Knee

1. The SFJ is located by first identifying the common femoral vein in transverse section just below the level

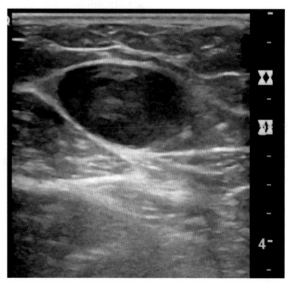

Fig. 13.26 Venous stasis is demonstrated as an echogenic speckle pattern in this B-mode image of a varix (dilated area) of the great saphenous vein.

of the inguinal ligament. The anatomy in this region is demonstrated in Fig. 9.7. The common femoral vein lies medial to the common femoral artery and is normally larger than the artery. The SFJ will be seen on the anteriomedial side of the common femoral vein (Fig. 13.27). It is usual to see other tributaries

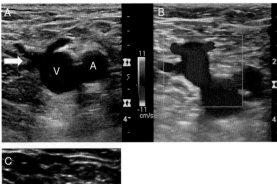

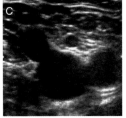

Fig. 13.27 The saphenofemoral junction. (A) A transverse B-mode image of the left common femoral vein demonstrating the position of the saphenofemoral junction *(arrow)* and some of its tributaries, common femoral vein *(V)*, and common femoral artery *(A)*. (B) A color flow image of the saphenofemoral junction demonstrating flow in tributaries. (C) This view is sometimes called "Mickey Mouse," for obvious reasons. This junction is reasonably large and would need investigation for incompetence.

joining the SFJ. Remember that these tributaries may be the main supply to the varicose veins, especially the AASV (Fig. 13.28).

2. The transducer should then be rotated so that the common femoral vein and SFJ can be seen in longitudinal section (Fig. 13.29). The competency of the common femoral vein, SFJ, and proximal GSV can be assessed using distal compression and the Valsalva maneuver. The origin of the femoral vein, which lies below the level of the SFJ, should also be assessed for competency. Large visible branches dividing from the SFJ, especially the AASV, can also be checked for competency. Check for spontaneous flow and respiratory phasicity of the common femoral vein. Absence could indicate a proximal obstruction or occlusion.

3. The GSV is examined in transverse section along the medial thigh to the knee. In transverse section, it is often possible to see the GSV running directly into varicose areas. Large perforators and tributaries are relatively easy to identify. Large thigh perforators should be assessed for competency. The GSV is then followed in longitudinal section from the SFJ to the knee and assessed for competency at frequent intervals. This is because the SFJ and proximal GSV may be competent, but there may be segmental reflux in the upper, mid-, or lower thigh, beyond incompetent valve sites, perforators, or branches. It is even possible for the main trunk of the GSV to be competent, with isolated incompetence of side tributaries that supply superficial varicose areas in the thigh or calf. Another common

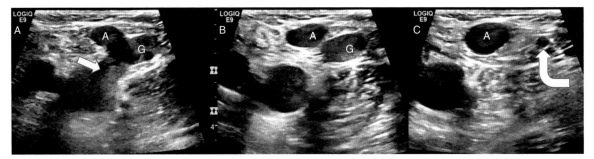

Fig. 13.28 Three transverse views at the level of the right saphenofemoral junction (SFJ). (A) The SFJ *(arrow)* is seen along with the confluence of the great saphenous vein *(G)* and anterior accessory saphenous vein *(A)*. (B) Just distal the SFJ, the anterior accessory saphenous vein (AASV) and great saphenous vein (GSV) both appear dilated and varicose. (C) A short distance distal to point in image (B), the AASV appears dilated and varicose but the GSV is now small *(curved arrow)* and was found to be competent due to normal function of the preterminal valve. The AASV supplied the varicose areas in the leg.

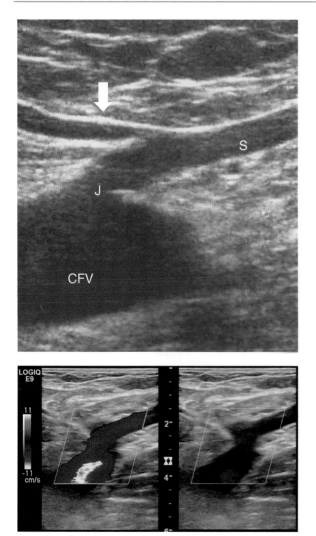

Fig. 13.29 (A) A longitudinal image of the distal common femoral vein *(CFV)*, saphenofemoral junction *(J)*, and proximal great saphenous vein *(S)*. A superior tributary is seen draining to the great saphenous vein, just proximal to the junction *(arrow)*. It is often not possible to image the femoral vein distal to the saphenofemoral junction in the same plane. (B) Competency of the great saphenous vein is demonstrated with color flow imaging. In the left image, flow augmentation *(coded blue)* is demonstrated but no reflux is evident in the right image following augmentation.

finding is incompetence of the proximal GSV to the level of an incompetent superficial thigh tributary that exits the saphenous compartment. Beyond the incompetent tributary, the GSV can be competent, very small, hypoplastic, or absent (see Fig. 13.6). It is also not infrequent to find a superficial tributary

reentering the saphenous compartment lower down in the leg and for the GSV to become incompetent again beyond this point. The size of the GSV is often seen to increase where the tributary joins. The GSV or a large tributary can also be incompetent proximally, flowing into a competent perforator in the mid-thigh, becoming competent below the perforator. There can be numerous variations to the patterns described earlier, especially in the thigh and knee region.

4. The femoral vein and proximal popliteal vein above the knee should be assessed for patency and competency. They are imaged from a medial thigh position in transverse and longitudinal section. The femoral and popliteal veins lie deep to their respective arteries when imaged from this position.

5. The GSV is then followed in transverse section across the knee along the medial aspect of the calf to the ankle. Assessment of the superficial foot veins, comprising the dorsal arch and medial and lateral marginal veins, is not normally necessary. These veins are the anatomic origins of the GSV and SSV. It is common to see large tributaries dividing from the main trunk of the GSV in the calf. Posteromedial varicose tributaries of the GSV in the upper calf sometimes interconnect to the SSV system in the posterior calf, causing SSV incompetence below this level (Fig. 13.30). The GSV and its major tributaries are then assessed in a longitudinal section using distal compression to augment flow. However, the varicose veins may be so obvious in the calf that little time needs to be spent on assessing the GSV at this level if it is the supply to the varicose areas. The GSV can also supply varicose areas on the lateral aspect of the calf, via incompetent tributaries that run over the front of the shin. There is considerable debate about the need to examine all calf perforators by duplex, and whether this is undertaken may depend upon local protocols. In many cases perforators connect to side branches of the GSV and not to the main trunk.

6. The popliteal vein above and below the knee is examined from the popliteal fossa and assessed for patency and competency. The popliteal vein lies superficial to the popliteal artery when imaged from the popliteal fossa. Some clinicians request an assessment of the gastrocnemius veins. The investigation then continues with an assessment of the SSV.

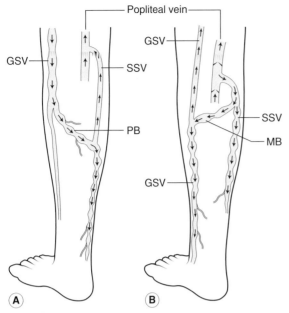

Fig. 13.30 (A) Posterior varicose branches *(PB)* of the great saphenous vein may interconnect to the small saphenous vein *(SSV)* distribution in the posterior calf, causing SSV incompetence below the point of communication. (B) Medial varicose branches *(MB)* of the SSV can interconnect to the great saphenous vein *(GSV)* in the calf, leading to segmental GSV incompetence. ↑, Competent veins; ↓, incompetent veins.

Assessment of the SSV

Preoperative Marking of the Position of the Saphenopopliteal Junction

The position of the saphenopopliteal junction can be marked preoperatively with the aid of duplex scanning, because of its highly variable position. Some surgeons ask for a mark to be made on the skin corresponding to the position of the junction. However, others prefer a mark over the small saphenous vein just distal to the junction, or at a point where it becomes superficial so that the vein can be identified and followed back to the junction. Alternatively, a cross can be placed over the junction with a line drawn indicating the path of the small saphenous vein to the point where it becomes superficial (Fig. 13.31). Try to avoid any transverse tilt of the transducer when marking, as the mark can be made at the wrong position (Fig. 13.32). It is important for the surgeon and sonographer to agree on a system of marking to avoid any misunderstandings.

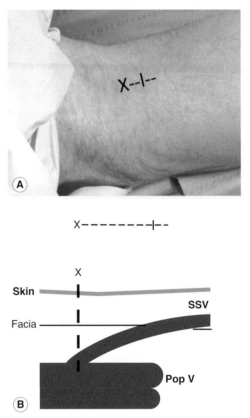

Fig. 13.31 (A) An example of a system for marking the position of the saphenopopliteal junction. Point X indicates the level of the junction. The *dashed line* shows the direction of the small saphenous vein *(SSV)* and *I* represents the point where the SSV becomes superficial (see text). (B) A diagrammatic representation showing the positions described in (A).

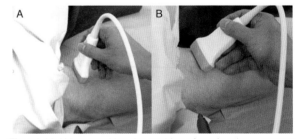

Fig. 13.32 When marking the position of a vein prior to surgery in transverse section, it is important to keep the probe perpendicular to the point that requires ligation as shown in image (A). Transverse tilting of the transducer (B) will result in imaging and subsequent marking of the vein below (as would occur in this example), or above the point that requires ligation.

1. The SSV is initially easier to locate just below the popliteal fossa in transverse section, where it will be seen lying within the superficial saphenous compartment (Fig. 13.33). It is sometimes very small and easy to miss. The SSV is followed proximally into the popliteal fossa in transverse section, where it will be seen to perforate the muscular fascia and run deep to join the popliteal vein at the saphenopopliteal junction. The proximal SSV can curve medially or laterally toward the saphenopopliteal junction (Figs. 13.9 and 13.33C). The actual junction can be located on the anterior, medial, lateral, or, occasionally, posterior aspect of the popliteal vein when viewed from the popliteal fossa. In some situations, the junction and proximal SSV can be extremely tortuous, with the vein doubling back on itself in a S-shape

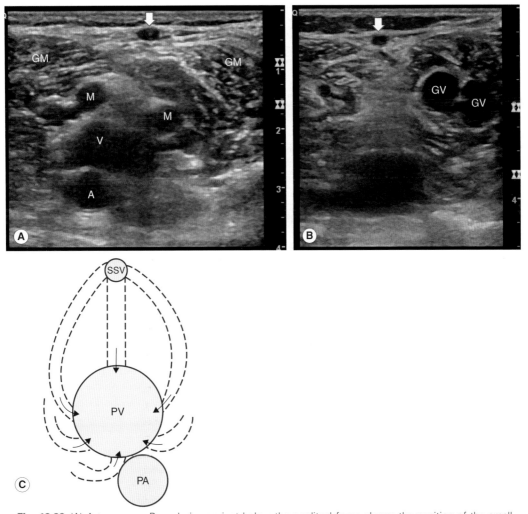

Fig. 13.33 (A) A transverse B-mode image just below the popliteal fossa shows the position of the small saphenous vein (arrow) lying in the superficial, saphenous compartment, with the gastrocnemius muscles (GM) visible. The popliteal vein (V) and muscular veins (M) are seen below the fascia. The popliteal vein lies superficial to the popliteal artery (A) when imaged from this position. (B) A transverse B-mode image just below the popliteal fossa shows the position of the small saphenous vein (arrow) and dilated gastrocnemius veins (GV). It can be possible to confuse gastrocnemius veins with the SSV, particularly if they are superficial within the muscle. (C) A diagram showing potential positions of the saphenopopliteal junction. PA, Popliteal artery; PV, popliteal vein; SSV, small saphenous vein.

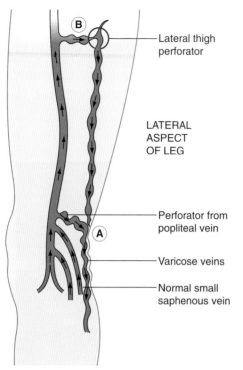

Lateral thigh perforator

LATERAL ASPECT OF LEG

Perforator from popliteal vein

Varicose veins

Normal small saphenous vein

Fig. 13.34 The saphenopopliteal junction and small saphenous vein may be competent, but an incompetent perforator dividing from the popliteal vein can supply varicosities in the popliteal fossa and calf, as shown in this diagram (A). Varicose areas on the lateral thigh and calf can also be supplied via upper lateral thigh perforators (B). It is often difficult to trace the perforator to its connection to the deep vein.

longitudinally, while following a tortuous path in either the medial or lateral direction. This leads to a very confusing image in which it is even possible to see different sections of the proximal SSV in the same scan plane. Slow, careful movement of the probe should be used to track the vein back to the popliteal vein. It is also possible to mistake tributaries of the gastrocnemius vein for the SSV if they run superficially within the gastrocnemius muscle. Care should be used when identifying the anatomy in this area, and it is important to be able to identify the saphenous compartment for correct identification of the SSV. Finally, a large perforator from the popliteal vein, separate from the SSV, can sometimes be found in the popliteal fossa, supplying superficial varicose areas (Fig. 13.34). It is more common for this perforator to be located on the lateral aspect of the popliteal fossa or lower thigh. The varicose veins supplied

by the perforator can be completely independent of the SSV, which may be normal throughout its length.

2. The saphenopopliteal junction and proximal SSV are then imaged in longitudinal section (Fig. 13.35). In some cases, the junction is tortuous, and rotation of the probe is required to allow the junction to be visualized. The saphenopopliteal junction and proximal SSV should then be assessed for reflux with a strong calf squeeze. If not already performed previously, the competency of the above- and below-knee popliteal vein should be assessed.

3. As described previously, there is considerable anatomical variation in the position and configuration of the saphenopopliteal junction (Figs. 13.8 and 13.35). In some cases, it may be impossible to identify, owing to the height of the junction in the posterior thigh. The TE, if present, can be the source of SSV incompetence. In this situation, it is possible to follow the TE, which will be seen to run as a continuation of the SSV, in transverse section up the posterior thigh to its origin, which may be from a number of sources, as shown in Fig. 13.8. The Giacomini vein tends to run in a layer of fascia as it courses toward the GSV, which can aid its identification. It is possible to misidentify very superficial posterior thigh branches of the GSV as the Giacomini vein.

4. In transverse section, the SSV is followed distally from the popliteal fossa along the posterior aspect of the calf, to the posterolateral aspect of the ankle. The SSV is then assessed for reflux along its length in longitudinal section. If the vein is small (for instance, less than 2 mm in diameter), it can be difficult to demonstrate flow during augmentation and little time needs to be spent on the assessment of the SSV. Large perforators can be assessed for competency. Varicose tributaries from the GSV can interconnect to the SSV system. Conversely, medial varicose tributaries of the SSV may also interconnect to the GSV system (Fig. 13.30B). The SSV can also supply varicose areas on the lateral and anterior aspects of the calf via branches. Varicose tributaries of the lateral thigh system can also join the SSV at a variable level, with the SSV being competent proximal to this point.

Assessment of Perforators

Perforators are easiest to identify in transverse section, but some rotation of the probe may be required

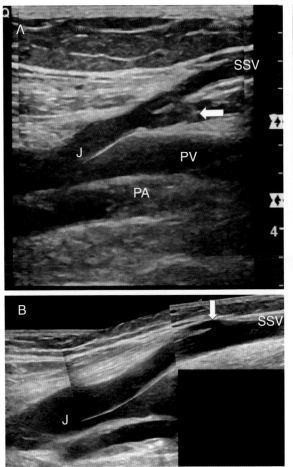

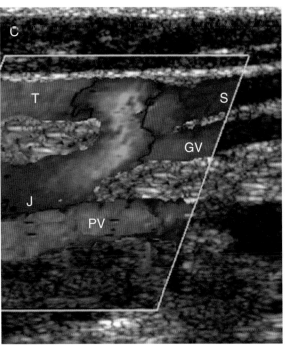

Fig. 13.35 (A) A composite longitudinal image of the popliteal fossa demonstrating the saphenopopliteal junction *(J)* and proximal small saphenous vein *(SSV)*. In this example there is a gastrocnemious vein *(arrow)* draining to the SSV forming a common trunk. The popliteal vein *(PV)* and popliteal artery *(PA)* are shown in this image. It is not always possible to see the junction in this plane or this clearly, especially if it lies to the medial or lateral side of the popliteal vein. (B) A composite longitudinal image of the popliteal fossa demonstrating the saphenopopliteal junction *(J)* and proximal SSV. In this image it is possible to see a short section of the confluence between the thigh extension vein and SSV *(arrow)*. (C) An anatomical variation involving the proximal SSV. In this image the SSV *(S)* continues to run up the posterior thigh as the thigh extension *(T)*. A gastrocnemius vein *(GV)* also drains to the SSV just proximal to the saphenopopliteal junction *(J)* forming a common trunk. The PV is demonstrated in this image. Flow coded red is toward the head, and the image demonstrates reflux across the junction going up the thigh extension.

to image an adequate length for assessment. Color flow imaging and spectral Doppler are used to identify reflux and grade reflux, but color flow imaging can give a misleading impression of the duration and degree of reflux, as the direction of the perforator is often parallel with the beam leading to aliasing. Spectral Doppler will generally provide better diagnostic information. Perforator assessment can prove challenging, and it is worth trying distal and proximal compression,

especially over any localized varicose areas. It may take several attempts to assess perforator competency, and the results may be inconsistent. Generally, if the perforator is very small (<2 mm diameter) and is not associated with any varicose areas, it is unlikely to be clinically significant. Perforators >3 mm in diameter and above are far more likely to be incompetent and clinically significant, especially large mid-thigh perforators in cases of recurrent varicose veins.

Concluding the Scan

Some varicose veins may lie in more unusual distributions, such as the anterior aspect of the calf or lateral aspect of the thigh. In these situations, it is important to follow the varicose areas proximally in transverse section to identify the supply. The supply is frequently from varicose branches of the GSV or SSV, depending on the location of the varicose areas. One such example is incompetence of the AASV from the SFJ. This vein often supplies varicose areas on the anterior aspect of the thigh and lateral calf and these varicose areas can also join the SSV in the upper or mid-calf. The main proximal trunk of the GSV can be competent or incompetent in this situation. Varicose veins running along the lateral aspect of the thigh and calf can be related to isolated perforators located on the lateral or posterolateral aspect of the upper thigh and buttock (Fig. 13.34). Varicose veins in the lower thigh and calf can be supplied by the TE. In this unusual situation, blood flows in a loop, across an incompetent saphenopopliteal junction and up the TE vein, which then feeds the superficial varicosities running down the leg. This paradoxical situation is like a siphon effect, but flow will eventually make its way down into the calf via the incompetent veins, in the correct gravitational direction (Georgiev et al. 2003; Fig. 13.36). The main trunk of the SSV can be competent or incompetent in this situation. In some patients, it may be impossible to clearly define the source of the varicose veins, especially if they are very small, are diffusely distributed, and generally run into very small superficial tributaries.

Vulval Varicosities and Pelvic Incompetence

Vulval varicosities can develop during pregnancy and most regress after delivery. However, persistent vulval varicosities are due to incompetence of the pelvic veins, including the ovarian or internal iliac veins. Vulval varicosities can supply varicose veins in the leg and this source is sometimes overlooked or missed by clinicians. These veins may either render the GSV incompetent or remain isolated from it. The sonographer should always be suspicious of veins that are running toward the inner aspect of the groin, especially if they run behind the adductor longus tendon, which is normally easy to feel. The detailed investigation of ovarian veins requires transvaginal ultrasound scanning, and the description is

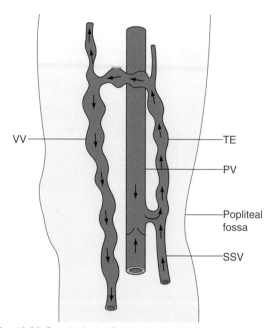

Fig. 13.36 Paradoxical reflux can occur in the thigh extension *(TE)* vein of the small saphenous vein *(SSV)* due to incompetence of the saphenopopliteal junction leading to a siphon effect, causing blood to flow up the TE which feeds into the varicose veins *(VV)*. *PV*, Popliteal vein.

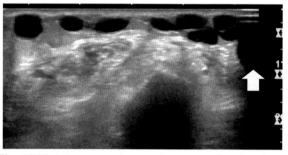

Fig. 13.37 A transverse image of tortuous dilated varicose veins. The right-hand side of the probe has lost contact with the skin due to the contour of the leg *(arrow)*.

outside the scope of this book. Ovarian and pelvic vein reflux can be treated effectively by coil embolization.

B-Mode Appearance of Veins, Varicose Veins, and Perforators

Varicose veins are easy to identify on the B-mode image. They appear as single- or multiple-dilated tortuous vessels that vary randomly in diameter as the probe is swept across the varicose area (Fig. 13.37). They are superficial and can be located in the thigh as well as the calf. The

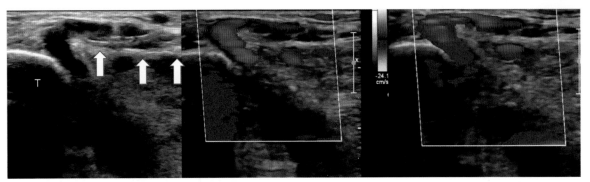

Fig. 13.38 An incompetent paratibial perforator is demonstrated with B-mode and color flow imaging. There is a clear break in the fascia as the perforator runs between the deep and superficial compartments adjacent to the tibia *(T)*. The *arrows* mark the facia. It may be difficult to display the entire path of a perforator clearly in a single image. The color flow images demonstrate flow augmentation *(coded red)* and subsequent reflux *(coded blue)*.

main trunk supplying varicose areas, such as the GSV in the thigh, may be dilated but often has a reasonably even caliber and is frequently not visible on the skin surface. Generally, if the GSV or SSV is greater than 5 mm in diameter, they are likely to be incompetent. Occasionally a large localized dilation can be seen in the main trunk, called a varix (Fig. 13.26). The easiest way of locating perforators is to run the transducer steadily along the trunk of the superficial vein in transverse section. A break in the fascia will be seen on the B-mode image as the perforator runs between the subcutaneous and subfascial areas (Fig. 13.38).

INVESTIGATION OF RECURRENT VARICOSE VEINS

Some patients develop recurrent varicose veins over a variable time period following surgery. Recurrent varicose veins are veins that have become varicose after the original treatment and can be due to inadequate preoperative assessment, inappropriate or incomplete surgery, and development of new sites of venous reflux as a consequence of disease progression or neovascularization (Kostas et al. 2004; Fig. 13.39). The scanning technique for the investigation of recurrent varicose veins is very similar to that used for the investigation of primary varicose veins. However, it is important to keep an open mind as to the source of the recurrent veins, as their supply can be unpredictable. It is often easier to begin the examination at the level of the varicose areas in transverse section and work proximally to the point of supply. The use of color flow imaging during calf augmentation can allow smaller varicose veins to be followed proximally if the B-mode imaging is poor. Some of the main causes of recurrent varicose veins are summarized below.

Possible Causes of GSV Recurrences
Incomplete Ligation of the Saphenofemoral Junction
Normally the junction should be ligated and any tributaries divided (Fig. 13.40A). However, due to misidentification or inadequate dissection, it is possible to ligate only a tributary during surgery, rather than the main junction. The level of the SFJ should be examined in transverse section, where it is easy to identify a large patent junction. Sometimes the scan demonstrates that the main trunk of the GSV has been ligated just distal to the SFJ but a tributary has been left intact. This tributary then supplies the varicose veins or intact GSV trunk, if the GSV has not been stripped. This is often the case when the AASV is found to be intact at the level of the SFJ. It frequently supplies varicose areas in the anterior and medial aspects of the thigh, which in turn run into the calf (Fig. 13.39A). Occasionally, there may be a very small recurrent junction that can be difficult to identify without the aid of color flow imaging (Fig. 13.40B).

Incompetent Tributaries
In some cases, the SFJ has been ligated, but small tributaries from the inner aspect of the groin or from the lower abdominal wall supply varicose areas in the GSV

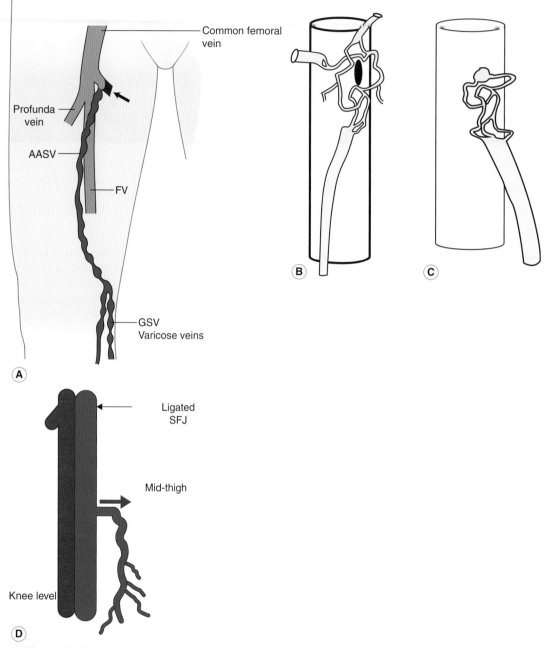

Fig. 13.39 Recurrent varicose veins have many causes. (A) The anterior accessory saphenous vein *(AASV)* has been left intact following incomplete ligation of the junction *(arrow)*. The AASV now supplies the varicose areas shown in the diagram. (B) The saphenofemoral junction has been ligated, but small tributaries in the groin supply a varicose trunk (this could be the great saphenous vein if it has not been stripped). (C) Neovascularization has occurred between the saphenofemoral junction and small veins supplying a varicose trunk. (D) Incompetent mid-thigh perforators are a common cause of reoccurrence. *FV,* Femoral vein; *GSV,* great saphenous vein; *SFJ,* saphenofemoral junction.

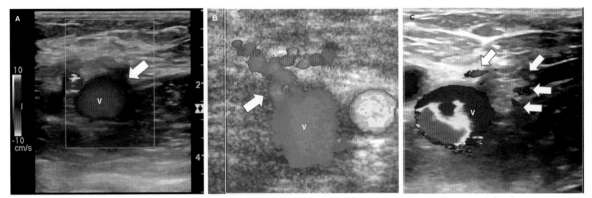

Fig. 13.40 Three examples of ultrasound findings at the level of the saphenofemoral junction following surgery. The femoral vein *(V)* is seen in all three images. (A) The saphenofemoral junction *(arrow)* has been completely ligated by surgery. (B) A small recurrent junction *(arrow)* is seen to supply a diffuse network of small veins. (C) The saphenofemoral junction has been ligated but small veins or tributaries are seen adjacent to the vein *(arrows)*.

distribution or the main GSV trunk, if it has not been stripped. These tributaries are often supplied from pudendal, perineal, or superficial epigastric veins. Typically, the scan will demonstrate varicose veins, or an intact trunk if this has not been stripped in the upper thigh, breaking up into small tributaries before disappearing toward the inner aspect of the groin. These tributaries are usually seen as a fine, diffuse web of veins on the color flow image. Sometimes these tributaries may run close to the femoral vein, but no direct connection will be identified (Figs. 13.39B and 13.40C). It is also possible for recurrent varicose veins to be supplied from veins running from the lower abdominal wall.

Neovascularization

It is generally accepted that neovascularization or regrowth can occur between the femoral vein and superficial varicose veins at the groin following ligation of the SFJ (Brake et al. 2013; Fig. 13.39C). These small veins then supply the GSV, if it had not been stripped, or proximal recurrent varicose veins. Duplex scanning will reveal a diffuse web of small tortuous veins in the groin, with a small connection to the femoral vein that may be impossible to follow without the aid of color flow imaging.

Thigh or Calf Perforators

Recurrent varicose veins can be supplied by thigh or calf perforators (Fig. 13.39D). Large thigh perforators are relatively easy to identify by following the varicose trunk up the medial thigh in transverse section, where it will be seen to connect directly, or via side branches, to the perforator. Perforators to the deep veins can have very tortuous courses. If a mid-thigh perforator is the main supply to the varicose areas, there may be only small or no varicose veins seen above the level of the perforator. Duplex scanning can be used to mark the location of perforators preoperatively.

Incomplete Stripping of the GSV Trunk in the Thigh

Sometimes the SFJ has been ligated, but the vein stripper has been passed down a tributary of the GSV, leaving the majority of the main trunk intact. The image will demonstrate the presence of an incompetent GSV trunk that breaks into small tributaries toward the groin with a variable supply, as described in some of the examples earlier.

Incompetence of the SSV

Varicose veins in the GSV distribution of the calf can occur due to incompetence of the SSV. In this situation, posteromedial varicose branches of the SSV interconnect to the GSV distribution (Fig. 13.30B).

Nonidentifiable Source

In some instance small diffuse tortuous varicose veins may be present superficially in the GSV distribution and no obvious major source can be located. These veins can be avulsed or treated with sclerotherapy.

Possible Causes of SSV Recurrences
Incomplete Ligation of the Saphenopopliteal Junction

Recurrence can occur if there has been incomplete ligation or misidentification of the saphenopopliteal junction during surgery. With the transducer in transverse section, the SSV can be followed proximally, where it will be possible to see the saphenopopliteal junction clearly.

Incompetent Thigh Extension Vein or Giacomini Vein

In some circumstances a large incompetent TE vein may run directly into the SSV, or varicose areas, at the popliteal fossa. Starting in a transverse section just below the popliteal fossa, the SSV is identified and followed proximally. The saphenopopliteal junction should not be seen if it has been correctly ligated. However, the SSV continues to course up the posterior thigh as the TE. The TE vein can have a variable supply, as described previously.

Incompetent Perforators

These perforators may arise from variable positions and can be found above the popliteal fossa, at the popliteal fossa, or arising from the gastrocnemius and soleal veins. Perforators arising in the region of the popliteal fossa can follow very tortuous routes. Perforators supplying varicose areas in the SSV distribution are easiest to identify in transverse section.

GSV Incompetence

Varicose veins in the SSV distribution can occur due to GSV incompetence. Incompetent posterior veins in the GSV distribution, which are not prominent on the skin surface, may run into the SSV system in the upper posterior calf, where the veins become more prominent. The surgeon performing the original surgery may have assumed that these varicose veins were related to saphenopopliteal junction incompetence and ligated the junction, but in fact the SSV was competent above the point of communication between the GSV and the SSV. Therefore, ligation of the saphenopopliteal junction will not have controlled the varicose veins (Fig. 13.30A).

Diffuse Varicosities in the Popliteal Fossa

Diffuse varicosities distinct from the saphenopopliteal junction or SSV may resupply the SSV. In this situation, although the saphenopopliteal junction has been ligated, the SSV trunk is supplied by numerous small superficial tributaries that are difficult to follow to any major source.

ASSESSMENT OF PATIENTS WITH SKIN CHANGES AND VENOUS ULCERATION

Many patients with venous ulcers have never had varicose vein surgery, whereas others may have had several previous operations. However, the basic technique for assessing patients with venous ulceration is the same technique for the assessment of varicose veins. Many patients are elderly and are unable to stand during the examination, but the leg should be in a dependent position to assess for reflux. This is best achieved by hanging the leg over the side of the examination table with the feet resting on a stool. It is necessary to remove any pressure or compression dressings, as these may reduce venous reflux, leading to false results. Patients with venous ulceration are more likely to have deep venous incompetence or obstruction than patients with simple varicose veins. Therefore, it is important to assess the deep veins carefully. It is often easier to start the scan by examining the popliteal vein from the popliteal fossa, as many surgeons will not perform superficial surgery if there is gross reflux in the popliteal vein below the knee, and a less detailed scan of the superficial vein system may be required.

There are a number of problems associated with the assessment of patients with venous ulcers. It can be difficult to image the deep veins in obese patients with large legs. In this situation, it may be worth trying a low-frequency curved array transducer to image the deep veins. Sometimes the calf is too ulcerated or sore to perform calf compression for the assessment of reflux. In such cases, try squeezing the upper portion of the calf, where there may be less ulceration or skin change. If in doubt, warn the patient that the test could be uncomfortable, as many patients are willing to cooperate but may be distressed if no prior warning of discomfort is given. In rare cases, some analgesia may be required. It can be difficult to assess the competency of veins in patients with continuous high-volume flow (hyperemic flow) in the superficial and deep veins due to infection. The high-volume flow toward the heart can lead to a reduction in reflux duration (Fig. 13.41). In these circumstances it is very

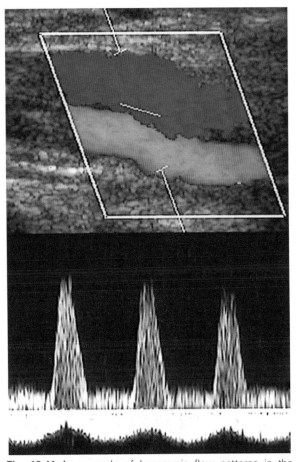

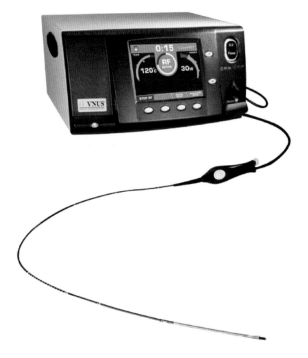

Fig. 13.42 A VNUS ClosureFAST radiofrequency catheter and VNUS RFG. (Courtesy of VNUS Medical Technologies.)

Fig. 13.41 An example of hyperemic flow patterns in the superficial femoral artery and femoral vein due to infection in the lower leg. The arterial signal, above the baseline, demonstrates high-volume flow throughout the cardiac cycle. There is continuous high-volume flow in the vein, shown below the baseline.

difficult to examine the function of the veins, but it may be an indication that the leg is infected. Appropriate action, such as antibiotic therapy and leg elevation, may need to be taken to reduce the infection or cellulitis. The leg can be reassessed when the hyperemia subsides. In contrast, it can be difficult to generate flow or reflux in some immobile patients with edema.

There are also a group of patients who have skin pigmentation, eczema, and other signs associated with venous insufficiency, but the scan demonstrates normal deep and superficial veins. Some of these patients have dermatological conditions.

ENDOVENOUS ABLATION OF VARICOSE VEINS

EVLT and RFA of varicose veins are minimally invasive catheter-based techniques that can avoid the need for open surgery and vein stripping (see Fig. 13.42). Both systems use heat to destroy the vein, but different methods are used to generate the heat. The treatment procedure is similar for EVLT and RFA, with the tip of the catheter positioned just below the relevant junction, usually the SFJ or saphenopopliteal junction. The injection of diluted local anesthetic solution (tumescent anesthesia), to surround the length of the vein, protects perivenous tissue from heat damage by acting as a heat sink once heating is activated. The tumescence also reduces the vein diameter by compression, removing blood and ensuring better contact between the vein wall and catheter and more efficient transfer of energy or heat. The catheter is then withdrawn at a predetermined rate to destroy the vein. Specialized stylet-type catheters are also available to treat perforators.

Technology

Introduction

Medical devices and accessories are undergoing constant development and refinement, and for this reason we are not providing detailed specification of catheters or accessories, as this is beyond the remit of this book. For comprehensive information concerning equipment, accessories, and device-specific protocols (catheter pullback speeds, etc.), the reader should contact the appropriate manufacturer.

Endovenous Laser Therapy

Laser (light amplification by stimulated emission of radiation) creates high-energy bundled light that is monochromatic (all one wavelength) and releases direct thermal energy that heats both the blood and adjacent vein wall, causing destruction of the cells in the vein wall (van den Bos et al. 2008). The tip reaches temperatures in the region of 800°C. The use of tumescence to compress the vein increases the contact surface area. The term *fluence* refers to the total amount of energy applied per unit area and is measured in J/cm^2. The laser energy delivered to the vein depends, among other factors, on the output setting of the device and the pullback speed of the catheter. The quicker the pullback speed, the less energy is delivered to the surface area of the vein. The energy produced by the laser is sufficient to vaporize the blood, creating bubbles that can be seen on the ultrasound image (see Fig. 13.46).

Radiofrequency Ablation

A radiofrequency generator delivers high-frequency alternating electromagnetic energy (radiofrequency) to the treatment element, which at the time of writing is 7 cm in length, but shorter lengths are available for treatment of the SSV. The radio waves do not conduct the heat, but it is the resistance to these waves in the surrounding tissue, causing excitement of the molecules in the tissue, that causes resistive heating. The injection of tumescence anesthesia to collapse the vein ensures good contact between the vein wall and treatment element. The element target temperature is typically 120°C, and a thermocouple allows for accurate monitoring and automatic maintenance of this temperature. The heat induces venous spasm and collagen shrinkage, damaging the vein wall, leading to occlusion. The catheter is withdrawn in segmental stages at specific time intervals (normally 20 seconds intervals) dependent on the vein being treated (Dietzek 2007).

Ultrasound Scanners

Almost all modern ultrasound scanners used for imaging peripheral venous disease should be suitable for guiding endovenous procedures. This also includes most portable scanners, providing they have a large enough screen. Typically, flat linear array transducers with a frequency in the range of 5 to 12 MHz are suitable for guidance, providing good images of wires and catheters. High-frequency probes can provide excellent resolution of the main superficial venous trunks but may provide suboptimal images of the SFJ or saphenopopliteal junction in larger patients and in certain cases could lead to problems in the precise positioning of the catheter tip relative to a junction. Catheters are often easier to visualize with compound imaging switched off as the beam steering employed in compound imaging can make the catheters and fibers less prominent (see Fig. 2.33). To ensure sterility of the procedure, the transducer is placed in a sterile probe cover containing ultrasound gel with a sterile sleeve covering the transducer cable.

The Procedure

This is a general description of the procedure, but the reader should be aware that advances in treatment and technology may occur. A pretreatment scan should have been performed to ensure the veins are suitable for endovenous treatment. In most cases, the main trunk of the GSV or SSV is treated but it is possible to treat other veins providing they fulfill treatment criteria (see Table 13.3). The following description is for EVLT treatment of the GSV.

The patient should be in a supine position on the treatment table. Prior to vein puncture, the GSV should be scanned to identify the optimum site for catheter access. For the GSV, this is around or just below knee level where the vein is usually superficial and nerve injury is less likely to occur. It is also useful to image the SFJ to ensure that good images of the junction can be obtained. This also allows the operator to optimize the gray-scale image controls for guiding the procedure. As the procedure is commenced, the operating table is tilted in a foot-down position to distend the vein for easier identification and puncture of the vein. For patients undergoing a local anesthetic procedure, some local anesthetic can be injected into the skin at

TABLE 13.3 Suggested Criteria for Endovenous Thermal Ablation of Varicose Veins
The main inclusion and exclusion criteria can include the following, although these may change with technological development:
Inclusion Criteria
• Primary or recurrent truncal varicosities without significant tortuousity • Veins >2 mm in diameter but preferably >3 mm • Treatable length of at least 10–12 cm
Exclusion Criteria
• Very small veins <2 mm diameter • Tortuous veins • Grossly dilated veins (local clinician definition) • Veins containing acute thrombophlebitis • Chronic scarring due to previous thrombophlebitis preventing passage of wire and catheter • Patients with acute deep-vein thrombosis

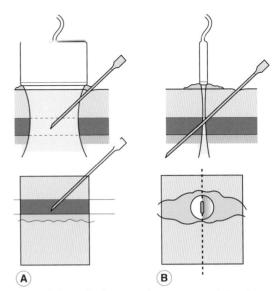

(A)   (B)

Fig. 13.43 Schematic diagrams of venous cannulation that can be performed in the longitudinal (A) and transverse imaging planes (B). The disadvantage of the transverse plane is that the needle tip may be out of plane and lie deeper than suspected from the image, as shown by the *dashed parts* of the line.

the region of the puncture site. The vein is then cannulated under ultrasound guidance. This can be performed using transverse or longitudinal imaging of the vein, as shown in Fig. 13.43, and depends on personal preference. The advantage of longitudinal imaging is that the tip and shaft of the cannula can be seen within the image once the cannula is in alignment with the vein. Using transverse imaging, it is possible that the cannula may be inserted too deep, with the tip lying below the vein, but the ultrasound image may show an oblique image of a short section of the shaft close to the vein, giving the false impression that this represents the tip (Fig. 13.43). However, the transverse plane is sometimes easier to use if the vein is lying in a very superficial position.

When the needle tip makes contact with the vein, it will cause an indentation of the vein wall, and at this point slightly more pressure is applied to the needle to pierce the wall.

Once the vein has been cannulated, a guide wire is then passed into the vein. The wire is advanced so that it runs across the SFJ (Fig. 13.44A). The passage of the guide wire is followed by ultrasound. It is not uncommon for the wire to loop or snag, especially in dilated or tortuous areas of the vein. Local external compression or "stretching" of the vein with fingers will usually solve this problem and facilitate passage of the guide wire. The introducing cannula is then removed and a flexible

sheath passed over the guide wire and advanced across or to the level of the SFJ. The sheath has markings every centimeter to enable accurate pullback speed when the laser is activated. Some sheaths have a pre-dilator with a sharp tip to increase rigidity and improve venous access. Manufacturers have also produced sheath tips that are loaded with tungsten or ceramic material to make imaging easier.

The guide wire and pre-dilator are then removed. The sheath should be in a position so that it is approximately 2 to 4 cm distal to the junction as seen on a longitudinal ultrasound image (Fig. 13.44B). The laser fiber is then inserted into the sheath. The laser fiber has a locking device so that it can be inserted to the correct length and will be seen to project 2 cm beyond the sheath (Fig. 13.44C). It is essential to confirm that the laser tip extends beyond the end of the sheath, otherwise the end of the sheath will be transected once the laser is activated and will remain in the patient. The laser tip also has a red guide light that should be visible through the skin in nonobese patients.

The next important stage is to position the laser tip so that it lies 2 cm from the SFJ, as seen on longitudinal imaging, by gently withdrawing or advancing the sheath. It is advantageous to do this before the injection

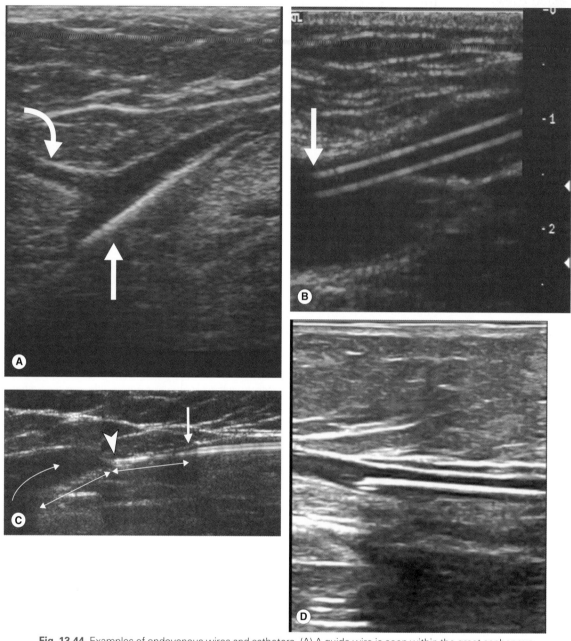

Fig. 13.44 Examples of endovenous wires and catheters. (A) A guide wire is seen within the great saphenous vein (GSV) and across the saphenofemoral junction (SFJ: *straight arrow*). Note the superficial epigastric vein *(curved arrow)*. The laser or radiofrequency catheter tip should be placed distal to this tributary (see text). (B) The sheath tip is clearly seen *(arrow)*. (C) A laser catheter has been positioned below the SFJ. The tip *(arrowhead)* can be seen protruding 2 cm beyond the sheath. The small step indicating the end of the sheath is visible *(straight arrow)*. The *curved arrow* runs through the center of the GSV from the SFJ toward the laser tip. The double-headed lines indicate 2-cm distance. (D) The heating element of a VNUS catheter.

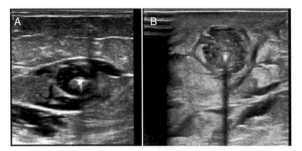

Fig. 13.45 (A) A transverse image of great saphenous vein following injection of tumescence creating a "halo" of fluid around the vein. There is a bright echo produced by the catheter in the vein. (B) The tumescence will sometimes diffuse into surrounding tissue, particularly if some fluid has been injected outside the saphenous compartment or if the vein is not located in an obvious compartment. An acoustic shadow is seen in the image deep to the catheter within the vein. This can help to identify the position of the vein if imaging of the vein is poor after tumescence has been injected and is clearer if spatial compounding is turned off.

of tumescence, as imaging of the junction can be more difficult once the tumescence has infiltrated the tissues in this area. Some clinicians place the tip slightly closer to the junction or just distal to the junction of the superficial epigastric vein, which is normally the first tributary of the SFJ (see Fig. 13.44A). Theoretically this preserves flow at the junction and prevents thrombus extending from the GSV across the junction.

The operating table is now placed into a head-down (Trendelenburg) position to empty the vein of blood, providing better contact between the laser tip and vein wall and allowing more efficient transfer of heat to damage the vein wall. The next phase of the procedure involves the injection of tumescence, normally saline containing local anesthetic, in the perivenous space along the length of the vein, with the aim of producing a "1-cm halo" around the vein when viewed on a transverse image (Fig. 13.45). This can be done manually via a syringe system or by using an infusion pump controlled by a foot pedal. The infusion pump method provides more control and flexibility. The tumescence has four main functions. First, it provides cooling and offers some perivascular tissue protection against heating or burns. Second, it provides pain relief. Third, the vein tends to collapse, removing blood and improving surface contact between the laser and vein wall. Finally, injection of

the tumescence will "sink" the position of superficial veins relative to the skin surface, to ensure that there is at least 1 cm between the vein and the skin surface to avoid skin burns. Superficial veins that often sit above the saphenous compartment may require a substantial amount of tumescence to achieve this.

The GSV usually lies in the saphenous compartment, which has a layer of fascia superficial to the vein, and it is important to penetrate this layer of fascia with the needle tip so that the anesthetic fluid enters the saphenous compartment. Starting distally, the needle tip is advanced so that the tip is adjacent to the vein, and then the solution is injected so that there is obvious splaying of the perivenous tissues, indicating that the vein is surrounded by a cuff of fluid. The tumescence will tend to diffuse more with veins that lie superficial to the saphenous compartment. With a good tumescence technique, it is possible to image the fluid tracking along the perivenous space well above the puncture site as the fluid is being injected to avoid too many injections. Once the vein is surrounded by tumescence, the position of the laser tip can be rechecked to ensure it has not become accidentally displaced.

Finally, the laser is activated and the catheter withdrawn at an appropriate speed to destroy the vein. As the fiber is withdrawn, some clinicians will apply some pressure with the scanning probe to ensure good contact between the vein walls and the fiber. The energy supplied to the laser tip also heats the surrounding blood, and this can be clearly seen as echogenic areas. It is very common to see streaming of echogenic reflections moving proximally toward the common femoral vein. This probably represents steam bubbles and may appear disconcerting when first seen (Fig. 13.46). The length of the vein is treated down to a few centimeters above the puncture site, and finally the sheath and laser are withdrawn. Ultrasound can then be used to ensure the patency of the common femoral vein. Finally, compression bandaging is applied to the leg, normally for a number of days.

The main complications of the procedure are shown in Table 13.4. The most serious procedural complication involves misidentification of anatomy leading to the placement of the tip in the wrong position or even a deep vein. In addition, the treatment tip must always extend beyond the sheath tip.

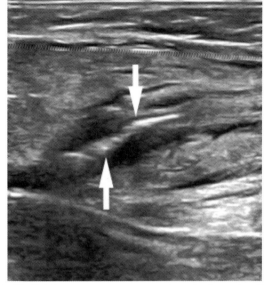

Fig. 13.46 It is common to see streaming of echogenic reflections *(upward pointing arrow)* moving proximally from the laser tip or heating element *(downward pointing arrow)* once it is activated *(arrow)*. This probably represents gas bubbles as the blood is vaporized.

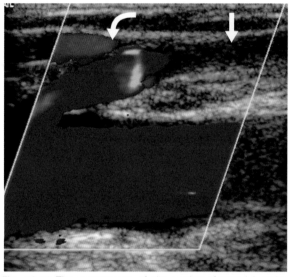

Fig. 13.47 The appearance of the saphenofemoral junction after successful endovenous treatment. The great saphenous vein is occluded *(arrow)*. The saphenofemoral junction remains patent due to flow entering from a preserved superficial epigastric tributary *(curved arrow)*.

TABLE 13.4 **Complications Associated With Endovenous Ablation**	
Procedural	**Comment**
Inability to cannulate vein	May be due to spasm or inexperience. If spasm occurs, the vein may need to be punctured above the original puncture site
Vein spasm	Can make passage of the sheath difficult
Incorrect placement of catheter tip	Rare and can be avoided by following protocols
Post-procedure	
Excessive pain	Usually resolves with analgesia
Skin burns	Rare
Recanalization of vein	
Deep-vein thrombosis	
Thrombophlebitis	

The treatment of the SSV is the same as the procedure described earlier, but the anatomy is far more variable and care should be used in the positioning of the tip of the catheter. There is some evidence that DVT is more likely to be associated with the treatment of an SSV that drains directly to the saphenopopliteal junction with no other tributaries, unlike the SFJ where flow in the superficial inferior epigastric vein or other tributaries can maintain patency of the SFJ (see Fig. 13.47). It has also been suggested that greater volumes of tumescence may be required during ablation of the SSV to prevent any thermal injury to the sural nerve, which is in close proximity to the vein. It is also possible to treat incompetence of the Giacomini vein with endovenous techniques.

Shorter fibers or stylets can be used for treating incompetent perforators.

Radiofrequency Treatment

The ultrasound guidance follows a similar pattern to that described for EVLT but a shorter introducer sheath is used. Different element lengths are available for treating the SSV.

Follow-up

Data on the effectiveness of endovenous ablation suggest good outcomes with low recanalization rates and high patient satisfaction. A randomized trial comparing EVLT with surgery has indicated comparable results but an earlier return to normal activity following EVLT (Darwood et al. 2008). Ultrasound is the ideal modality for follow-up to assess outcomes and complications

FOAM SCLEROTHERAPY AND OTHER TECHNIQUES

These techniques use ultrasound guidance, and it is essential that the operator understands how to operate an ultrasound scanner and how to identify cannulas and catheters on the ultrasound image.

For foam sclerotherapy the foam is formed by mixing liquid sclerosant with air using two syringes linked by a three-way tap. Foam sclerotherapy can be used to treat varicose veins and the main trunks of the GSV and SSV. Ultrasound can be used to guide the cannulation of the vein. The injection of foam displaces the blood and causes damage to the endothelium of the vein wall and subsequent fibrosis and occlusion. Ultrasound can be used to guide the cannulation and injection of the foam into the appropriate superficial veins. Some clinicians elevate the leg before injecting the foam to empty blood from the vein or use an injection of saline solution. The progress of the foam can be monitored with ultrasound during the injection, as it is easy to observe the echogenic reflections due to the air. The foam can be milked along the vein with the aid of the transducer. Ultrasound compression of the saphenofemoral or saphenopopliteal junction is often used to prevent the foam entering the deep system. In practice, it is not infrequent to see some foam that has entered the deep venous system via perforators, but this will be rapidly diluted.

Emerging treatments include mechanochemical endovenous ablation (MOCA). The device uses a technique that combines mechanical endothelial damage using a rotating wire with the infusion of a liquid sclerosant. Glue treatments have also been developed to occlude veins.

OTHER DISORDERS OF THE VENOUS SYSTEM

Superficial Thrombophlebitis

Superficial thrombophlebitis is an inflammatory process that involves the superficial veins, which is discussed in detail in Chapter 14. The superficial vein may become partially or fully thrombosed. Typically, the area around the phlebitis is reddened, tender, and hot, and the superficial vein may be swollen and hard. Phlebitis is normally treated with analgesia and antiinflammatory drugs, but superficial vein stripping or saphenofemoral or saphenopopliteal junction ligation may be required. If thrombus is extensive or close to the SFJ, it is treated as DVT (see Ch. 14).

Klippel–Trenaunay Syndrome

Klippel–Trenaunay syndrome (KTS) is a congenital condition and consists of a range of abnormalities that can involve the skin capillaries, often causing nevi (birthmarks or portwine stains), bone and soft-tissue hypertrophy (excessive limb growth), and venous varicosities. Each case of KTS is unique, and often only one limb is affected, but other areas of the body may also be involved. Abnormalities of the venous system range in severity (https://ghr.nlm.nih.gov/condition/klippel-trenaunay-syndrome#genes). Visible varicose veins vary from very minor to severe and can be widely distributed throughout the leg. Varicosities are commonly seen on the lateral aspect of the thigh and calf. In some cases of KTS, the deep veins may be abnormal. Abnormalities can include absence of parts of the deep venous system, unusually small deep veins, or large, dilated deep veins with nonfunctioning valves. It is therefore very important to scan the deep venous system in all patients with KTS to detect any deep venous abnormalities before treating any large superficial varicosities by surgery.

Venous Hemangioma

Venous malformations can occur anywhere in the body and consist of an abnormal network of veins. Venous hemangiomas vary in size and can be very extensive. They can occur in the superficial tissues, muscles, or organs. They can cause pain and swelling and may be disfiguring when they are superficial. Duplex scanning can be useful for imaging venous malformations to exclude evidence of arteriovenous fistulas, but it can be difficult to define the full extent of the lesion, especially if it is deep or involves joints. Large venous spaces are sometimes seen within the lesion, which will compress with transducer pressure. When imaging very superficial lesions, it is important not to apply too much pressure with the transducer, as this may occlude the veins. Other imaging techniques, such as magnetic resonance imaging, are often used to investigate the extent of the malformation, especially if it is diffusely distributed in muscles.

REPORTING

Duplex assessment of varicose veins is a dynamic technique, and it can be difficult to demonstrate this quality on hard copy, although recordings of reflux patterns, as seen on the spectral Doppler display, may be useful. It is therefore easier to provide a functional map of the venous system, as shown in Fig. 13.48. The superficial veins can be drawn on to the diagram, and black arrows pointing toward the heart indicate normal competent veins. Red arrows pointing toward the feet indicate venous reflux. The size of veins and other features such as anatomical variants can be included, along with comments regarding suitability for endovenous treatments. The diagram can be accompanied by a brief report outlining any limitations of the scan. This type of report is easy for the surgeon to interpret in a busy outpatient clinic rather than having to read a page or two of text and is also useful to show to the patient, as it provides a clear explanation of the problem.

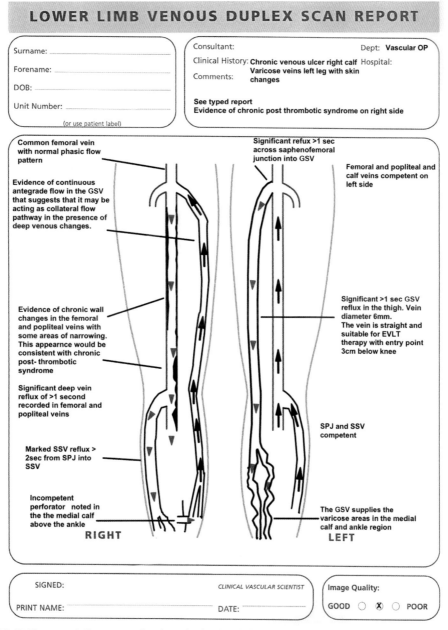

LOWER LIMB VENOUS DUPLEX SCAN REPORT

Surname: _____

Forename: _____

DOB: _____

Unit Number: _____

(or use patient label)

Consultant: _____   Dept: **Vascular OP**

Clinical History: **Chronic venous ulcer right calf** Hospital:

Comments: **Varicose veins left leg with skin changes**

See typed report
Evidence of chronic post thrombotic syndrome on right side

Common femoral vein with normal phasic flow pattern

Evidence of continuous antegrade flow in the GSV that suggests that it may be acting as collateral flow pathway in the presence of deep venous changes.

Evidence of chronic wall changes in the femoral and popliteal veins with some areas of narrowing. This appearnce would be consistent with chronic post- thrombotic syndrome

Significant deep vein reflux of >1 second recorded in femoral and popliteal veins

Marked SSV reflux > 2sec from SPJ into SSV

Incompetent perforator noted in the the medial calf above the ankle

RIGHT

Significant reflux >1 sec across saphenofemoral junction into GSV

Femoral and popliteal and calf veins competent on left side

Significant >1 sec GSV reflux in the thigh. Vein diameter 6mm. The vein is straight and suitable for EVLT therapy with entry point 3cm below knee

SPJ and SSV competent

The GSV supplies the varicose areas in the medial calf and ankle region

LEFT

SIGNED: _____   *CLINICAL VASCULAR SCIENTIST*

PRINT NAME: _____   DATE: _____

Image Quality:

GOOD ○ ⊗ ○ POOR

Fig. 13.48 The use of diagrams makes it easier for the clinician to interpret the findings of a venous duplex examination (see text). *GSV,* Great saphenous vein; *SSV,* small saphenous vein.

14

Duplex Assessment of Deep Venous Thrombosis and Upper-Limb Venous Disorders

OUTLINE

INTRODUCTION

Deep venous thrombosis (DVT) is a common disorder that can lead to fatal pulmonary embolism (PE). The condition of venous thromboembolism (VTE) is defined when patients present with DVT, PE, or both. Duplex scanning is the method of choice for the imaging of DVT in lower and upper limbs, with alternative imaging techniques reserved for technically incomplete or difficult duplex examinations or detailed examination of iliac veins. Duplex scanning can be used for repeat investigations to monitor for propagation of thrombus. In addition, duplex scanning can be useful for assessing the long-term damage to veins and valve function from chronic postthrombotic syndrome (Haenen et al. 2002). This can lead to the development of lower-limb venous hypertension due to venous insufficiency or obstruction and can result in chronic symptoms including leg ulceration. This chapter provides a description of duplex scanning techniques for the diagnosis of DVT in the lower and upper limbs and considers other pathologic conditions that may mimic the symptoms of venous thrombosis. We have avoided reference to specific drugs used for prophylaxis and treatment of VTE as these may change over time. The reader should also be aware that guidelines and recommendations undergo continual revision and examples included in this chapter may be superseded.

EPIDEMIOLOGY AND PATHOLOGY OF DVT

DVT usually affects the lower-limb veins, but it can also occur in the upper limbs, especially in conjunction with catheter access or malignancy. The published data on the epidemiology of DVT and PE demonstrate some variability, and reported rates of DVT and VTE appear to be partly dependent upon methods of data collection (diagnosis, discharge, and autopsy records) and the patient population studied. In the United States it is estimated that 1 to 2 per 1000 people could be affected each year. However, the incidence differs by age, race, and gender. For instance, in the young it may be 1 per 100,000 increasing to about 1 per 100 people aged >80 years (Beckman et al. 2010). The condition has significant morbidity and mortality impacts with 10% to 30% of all patients with VTE dying within 30 days, although most deaths are due to PE. It can also be the cause of sudden death in up to 25% people who suffer a PE (Centers for Disease Control and Prevention 2020). At least a third of patients with DVT develop postthrombotic syndrome that can lead to swelling, skin changes, pain, and venous ulceration. The early detection and treatment of DVT can therefore reduce the subsequent risk of mortality or long-term morbidity.

Virchow (1846) described the association between thrombosis in the legs and emboli in the lung. The factors predisposing to thrombosis are described by his famous triad of coagulability of the blood, damage to the vein wall or endothelium, and venous stasis. Venous thrombi are believed to originate in valve cusp pockets (Fig. 14.1) or in the deep venous muscular sinuses, such as the soleal and gastrocnemius veins. DVT most commonly occurs in the calf veins and can propagate to the proximal veins. In the lower limb the popliteal vein is usually described as a proximal vein. It is not necessary for all the calf veins to be affected for proximal propagation to occur. The reported incidence of calf vein propagation is variable and not clearly defined. It is believed that approximately 5% to 20% of calf vein thrombi propagate to the deep veins across and above the knee (Khaw 2002; Labropoulos et al. 2002; Utter et al. 2016). This is thought to be associated with an increased risk of PE. Isolated thrombosis of the proximal veins, such as the femoral or iliac veins, is less common and can be due to trauma, surgery, pregnancy, compression, or malignancy. Proximal and distal propagation of thrombus can occur in this situation. The main risk factors associated with the development of venous thrombosis are shown in Table 14.1. Patients undergoing periods of bed rest or immobility are at greater risk of

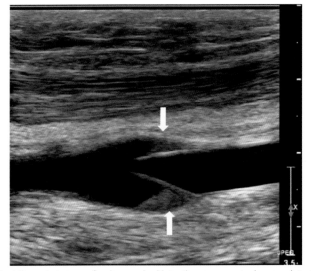

Fig. 14.1 A longitudinal B-mode image of a deep vein. Note the venous stasis associated with the valve sites (arrows).

TABLE 14.1	**Risk Factors for the Development of Deep Venous Thrombosis**	
Genetic	**Changes Through Life**	**Temporary or Nonpermanent**
Family history	Advancing age	Oral contraceptives
Protein C and S deficiency	Previous DVT	Pregnancy
Other coagulation disorders	Stroke reducing mobility	Hospitalization for treatment
Sickle-cell disease	Obesity	Surgery
	Heart failure	Trauma
	Cancers	Immobilization
		Long distance or air travel
		Infection/septicemia

DVT, Deep venous thrombosis.

developing thrombosis due to venous stasis. Hospitalized patients with medical illnesses have a similar risk of VTE as those undergoing major general surgery (Anderson & Spencer 2003).

There is evidence to suggest that long-haul air travel is associated with an increased risk; this risk may be low but increases with the duration of the journey. As with VTE generally, the risk of DVT will increase if there are a combination of factors. In the early stages of a DVT, it is possible for a large proportion of the clot to be nonadherent to the vein wall. This is termed a *free-floating thrombus*. In this situation there is a risk of detachment, leading to PE. As thrombus becomes older (7–10 days), it becomes more organized and adherent to the vein wall.

Signs, Symptoms, and Treatment of VTE

The symptoms of PE include the following:
- Acute dyspnea (sudden breathlessness)
- Pleuritic chest pain
- Hemoptysis (coughing up blood)
- Right-sided heart failure or cardiovascular collapse.

The clinical diagnosis of DVT is unreliable and inaccurate in up to 50% of cases (Cranley et al. 1976; Beyer & Schellong 2005). However, typical symptoms include the development of acute calf pain associated with localized tenderness, heat, and swelling. The superficial veins may also be dilated. If the thrombosis involves the proximal veins, there may be significant swelling of the calf. Unfortunately, other conditions, such as cellulitis and edema, can mimic the symptoms of DVT. In some cases of DVT the patient may be asymptomatic, especially if the thrombus is small or distal. In extensive cases of DVT the outflow of the limb is so severely reduced that the arterial inflow may become obstructed, leading to venous gangrene. This condition is called *phlegmasia cerulea dolens*. It is relatively rare but can be confused with ischemia. The foot may appear blackened and the limb swollen and blue, even when elevated.

PE occurs when a segment of thrombus breaks loose, travels through the right side of the heart, and lodges in branches of the pulmonary artery, leading to a perfusion defect in the arterial bed of the lungs. Computed tomographic pulmonary angiography (CTPA) is used for imaging and diagnosing PE. The high risk of VTE among both medical and surgical hospital inpatients has resulted in guidelines from various national and professional bodies such as the National Institute for Health and Care Excellence (NICE 2019) as to the best preventive measures. The prophylaxis of DVT includes the use of mechanical prevention in the form of graduated compression stockings and pneumatic compression devices that increase venous return and therefore reduce the risk of venous stasis. Patients at higher risk may be given antiplatelet or anticoagulation prophylaxis. In the presence of DVT, the aim of treatment is to prevent thrombus extension and pulmonary embolus and in the longer term to reduce the likelihood of recurrent DVT and postthrombotic syndrome. Treatment is usually with anticoagulation drugs, which can be prescribed for short-term or long-term use to prevent recurrence. Occasionally, devices called vena cava filters are positioned in the vena cava to capture thrombi when there is a high risk of embolization to the lungs. These can be temporary or permanent devices. Interventional treatments to dissolve or remove the thrombus can include mechanical or pharmomechanical thrombectomy, plus or minus stenting to maintain patency.

The investigation and treatment of isolated calf vein thrombosis remain a contentious issue (Kearon 2003; Utter et al, 2016). It is beyond the scope of this book to consider the debate in any detail, but sonographers should be aware of the controversies surrounding this area; most DVTs start in the calf and most resolve, but proximal progression does occur. Issues related to scanning of calf veins are the extra time to extend the scan from the distal popliteal vein to calf veins, the ability to visualize calf veins adequately, and accuracy of detecting DVT in the calf.

Investigations for Diagnosing DVT

The assessment for people presenting with signs or symptoms of DVT should begin with a medical history and physical investigation. If a DVT is suspected, a two-level DVT Wells score (Wells 2007) is used to predict if a DVT is likely or unlikely (see Fig. 14.2). The test assigns a score to clinical features and ongoing or previous conditions, such as a previously documented DVT. Currently a score of 2 or higher indicates a DVT is likely. The next

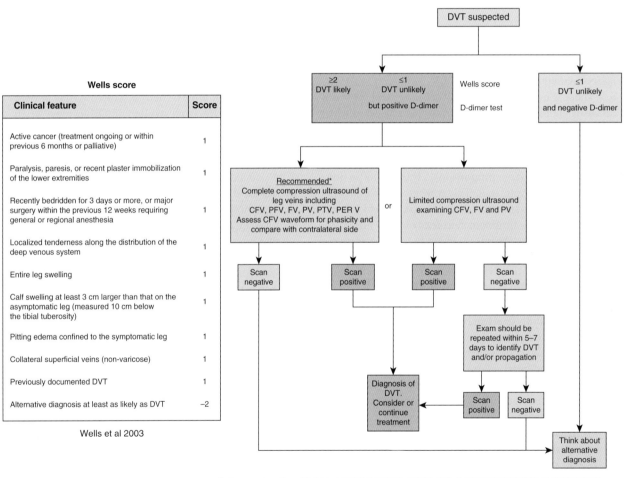

Wells score

Clinical feature	Score
Active cancer (treatment ongoing or within previous 6 months or palliative)	1
Paralysis, paresis, or recent plaster immobilization of the lower extremities	1
Recently bedridden for 3 days or more, or major surgery within the previous 12 weeks requiring general or regional anesthesia	1
Localized tenderness along the distribution of the deep venous system	1
Entire leg swelling	1
Calf swelling at least 3 cm larger than that on the asymptomatic leg (measured 10 cm below the tibial tuberosity)	1
Pitting edema confined to the symptomatic leg	1
Collateral superficial veins (non-varicose)	1
Previously documented DVT	1
Alternative diagnosis at least as likely as DVT	−2

Wells et al 2003

*In the presence of persistent or worsening symptoms, or if the study is technically incomplete or compromised, consider a repeat scan in 5–7 days

* This flow chart does not include initial anticoagulant and therapeutic drug management as this will vary between health care systems and countries

Fig. 14.2 An example of a visual summary of the diagnosis for venous thromboembolism including the two-level deep venous thrombosis Wells score. This summary has been developed using data from UK and USA sources (NICE 2020 and Needleman et al 2018).

stage of the assessment is dependent on specific local or national healthcare system guidance. Fig. 14.2 demonstrates an example pathway This shows that following a two-level DVT Wells score test, especially when there is no rapid access to an ultrasound scan, a D-dimer blood test can be performed to aid in initial management. This is a biochemical assay to measure D-dimer levels in the blood. D-dimers are products that are formed by the interaction of fibrin, contained in thrombus, and plasmin. Increased levels of D-dimer are associated with the presence of DVT. Unfortunately, increased levels of D-dimer are also found in other conditions, such as malignancy, infection, and trauma. Therefore, the D-dimer test has a high sensitivity but low specificity for the presence of DVT. Ultrasound scanning is used to exclude or confirm a DVT. In the NICE pathway a proximal ultrasound examination is indicated, which includes the popliteal and femoral veins but not the calf veins. However, there is considerable variation in ultrasound protocols used in different departments and healthcare systems. Two- and three-point compression ultrasound has been used in emergency departments (Zuker-Herman et al. 2018). However, reported sensitivity and specificity are variable with reports of errors and inadequate visualization (Zitek et al. 2016). Fig. 14.3 shows these different protocols, but we would recommend a minimum of a complete femoral and popliteal vein examination. The following protocols have been described in publications:

- A full evaluation of the leg veins including the calf veins to the ankle
- A full evaluation of the common femoral vein, femoral vein, and popliteal vein to below knee
- A limited compression test involving two- or three-point compression. Two-point includes the common femoral vein and popliteal vein. Three-point compression includes the proximal femoral vein (tends to be used in emergency departments)
- Investigation of the nonsymptomatic leg to exclude asymptomatic DVT.

Multidisciplinary recommendations from the Society of Radiologists in Ultrasound consensus conference (Needleman et al. 2018) suggested that limited imaging protocols are not recommended as these protocols often require a second scan 5 to 7 days later.

CT scanning and magnetic resonance venous imaging are generally reserved for imaging the iliac veins and vena cava or when ultrasound imaging is inadequate or

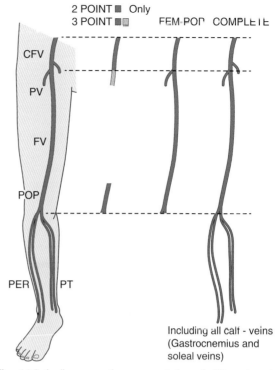

Fig. 14.3 A diagrammatic representation of different protocols used for compression ultrasound in the detection of deep venous thrombosis (see text for description). *CFV,* Common femoral vein; *FV,* femoral vein; *PER,* peronral vein; *POP,* popliteal vein; *PT,* posterior tibial vein; *PV,* profundal vein.

impossible. The assessment of superficial thrombophlebitis is discussed later in this chapter.

PRACTICAL CONSIDERATIONS FOR DUPLEX ASSESSMENT OF DVT

OBJECTIVES OF THE SCAN

- Exclude or confirm the presence of a deep venous thrombosis
- Identify the location of the thrombus, which veins are involved, and its proximal extent, as this will influence subsequent treatment
- Determine the age of thrombus (can be subjective and prone to error, especially acute on chronic thrombus)
- Monitor change or extension of thrombus
- Diagnose postthrombotic limb mimicking DVT
- Identify other conditions that may mimic deep venous thrombosis, such as cellulitis

ADVICE

It is important not to overextend the knee when examining the popliteal vein, as this can lead to partial collapse of the vein and also make compression with the probe more difficult due to tightening of the skin and subcutaneous tissues caused by the extension.

The main diagnostic criterion used to exclude DVT is complete collapse of the vein under transverse plane transducer pressure. Color flow imaging and spectral Doppler can also be used during the assessment. Color flow imaging may aid vein identification and improve diagnostic confidence. Between 20 and 30 minutes should be allocated for a full scan of one leg from the groin to the distal veins. Limited scans will require less time.

The legs should be accessible, and the patient made as comfortable as possible. In rare situations, the patient may require some sedation or analgesia before the examination if the limb is extremely painful. The limb should be visually examined and the patient asked to point to any areas of discomfort or tenderness, especially in the calf, as this can often be located over the site of the thrombosis. This region should be carefully examined by duplex scanning. In our experience, pain is usually most pronounced in calf vein DVTs and cases of superficial vein thrombosis (thrombophelbitis). Superficial vein thrombosis is discussed later in this chapter.

The examination room should be at a comfortable ambient temperature to prevent vasoconstriction (>20°C). Ideally, the patient should be examined with the legs tilted downward from the head, as this will help to fill the veins to enable visualization (reverse Trendelenburg position, or partially sitting up). The leg can be externally rotated (frog leg) to aid access, but it is important that it is relaxed without any muscle tension, as this will make compression more difficult and can be uncomfortable for the patient. Alternatively, the patient can be examined in a standing position, with the leg to be examined minimally weight-bearing and the patient holding a hand-rail or equivalent for support, but for elderly patients this can be difficult and often impossible. The calf veins and popliteal fossa are easier to scan with the legs hanging over the side of the examination table and the feet resting on a stool, or by rolling the patient onto their side with feet tilted down off the examination table. Wherever possible, immobile or sick patients should be tilted into a reverse Trendelenburg position, although there may be situations in which the patient cannot be moved, such as in the intensive care unit.

It is important to tell the patient that probe compression will be used before commencing the examination, as occasionally there can be some discomfort. Patients are more likely to tolerate this if they are advised that some compression is being used. Many cases of patients experiencing discomfort are due to poor patient positioning or tension in the leg. Spending a few minutes ensuring the patient is relaxed and comfortable can prevent problems during the examination.

DEEP-VEIN EXAMINATION FOR ACUTE DVT

It is important to have a good understanding of venous anatomy (see Ch. 13). The deep veins lie deep to the fascia separating the superficial and deep venous compartments and between the muscle facia and have an accompanying artery of the same name. Below the knee they are normally paired and are often referred as *vena comitantes*. Intramuscular veins such as the gastrocnemius and soleal veins lie within the muscle. A mid-frequency, linear array transducer should be used for examining the femoral, popliteal, and calf veins, although in large legs a lower-frequency curvilinear transducer is useful in the femoropopliteal segment. The iliac veins are examined using a low-frequency curvilinear transducer. The scanner should be configured for a venous examination. Where color flow imaging and spectral Doppler are required, the color pulse repetition frequency should be low, typically 1000 Hz, or color scale set to roughly 10 m/s, to detect low-velocity flow. The color wall filter should also be set at a low level, and the spectral Doppler sample volume should be increased in size to cover the vessel so that flow is sampled across the lumen.

Transverse ultrasound compression with B-mode only is the main method of confirming vein patency (Fig. 14.4). If direct transducer pressure is applied over a vein, it should completely collapse, as the blood pressure in the deep veins is low, unlike the pressure in the adjacent artery, and the anterior and posterior walls will appear to meet (Figs. 14.5, 14.6, and 14.7). The adjacent artery should demonstrate little or no distortion. In contrast, if there is thrombus in the vein, it will not collapse (see Fig. 14.13). It should be noted that fresh thrombus, which is soft, can partially deform. Compression should be applied at frequent intervals along the length of a vein, every 3 to 4 cm, to confirm patency

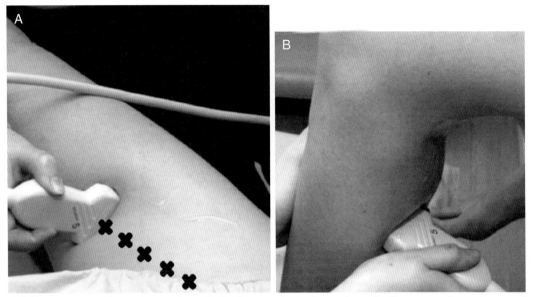

Fig. 14.4 (A) Transverse transducer pressure is applied at frequent intervals, as shown by the crosses, to compress and collapse the vein to confirm vein patency. (B) Placing a hand on the opposite side of the thigh or calf, as shown in this example, can help to bring the veins closer to the transducer to aid compression.

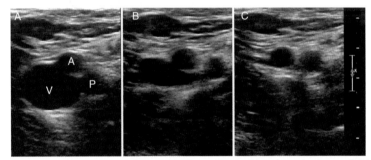

Fig. 14.5 (A) A transverse image of the left common femoral vein *(V)* and proximal superficial femoral artery *(A)* and proximal profunda artery *(P)*. (B) As pressure is progressively increased the vein begins to collapse. (C) With further transducer pressure the vein is fully collapsed indicating patency.

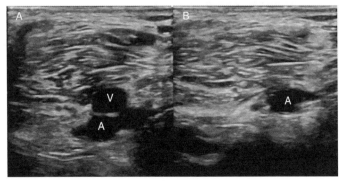

Fig. 14.6 (A) A transverse image from the popliteal fossa demonstrating the popliteal artery *(A)* and popliteal vein *(V)*. (B) The popliteal vein collapses with transducer pressure confirming patency.

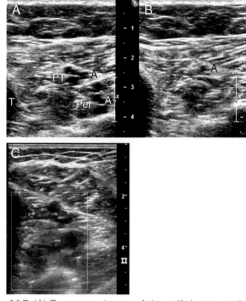

Fig. 14.7 (A) Transverse image of the calf demonstrating the posterior tibial *(PT)* veins and arteries and peroneal *(Per)* veins and arteries. The respective arteries *(A)* are shown between the paired veins. The border of the tibia is visible *(T)*. (B) There is complete collapse of the veins with transducer compression but, in this image, the PT artery *(A)* is still visible. Note that it can sometimes be difficult to differentiate the image of the veins from the surrounding tissue. (C) If the veins are difficult to locate, color flow imaging can be used to identify the tibial arteries (shown in *red*) as the veins should be adjacent to their respective arteries.

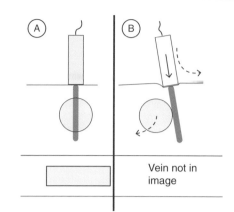

Fig. 14.8 This diagram shows that assessment of vein patency in longitudinal section by compression should generally be avoided. (A) A longitudinal image of a vein is obtained without compression. (B) As transducer pressure is applied it is possible for inadvertent tilting of the probe to occur or the position of the vein to move with compression *(dashed arrows)*. This would give the false impression of the vein lumen collapsing within the image.

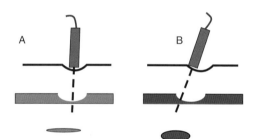

Fig. 14.9 When applying transverse pressure with the transducer it is best to apply this perpendicular to the skin as shown in (A). If excessive tilting of the probe is applied as shown in (B), the image may show a section of the vein proximal or distal to the point of maximum probe compression, giving the impression of partial collapse and nonoccluding thrombus.

(see Fig. 14.4). Partial collapse of the vein suggests the presence of nonoccluding thrombus. In this situation, the adjacent artery may be seen to deform as the probe pressure is increased to confirm partial obstruction in the vein. Transducer compression should be applied in the transverse imaging plane rather than the longitudinal plane. This is because it is easy to slip to one side of the vein, as pressure is applied in the longitudinal plane and may mimic compression of the vein when observed on the B-mode image (Fig. 14.8). It is also important not to tilt the probe in transverse plane as compression is applied, as the B-mode image of the vein will not lie directly under the point where the probe pressure is being applied and could result in an impression of partial collapse (see Fig. 14.9). For some patients with high BMI or very swollen legs, the veins in the adductor canal or calf may lie too deep for effective probe compression. Color flow imaging is useful for demonstrating patency in this

situation. To display flow when using color flow imaging in the transverse plane, some tilting of the transducer is often necessary to obtain an adequate Doppler angle to the vein (see Fig. 13.20).

The following guidelines can be used in any sequence, dependent on the veins that require assessment. It is sometimes easier to locate a specific vein by looking for the adjacent artery, especially in the calf with color flow imaging. The reader should also refer to Chapter 9 for more details on the probe positions for imaging the calf vessels and the main vessels in the thigh and pelvis:

1. Starting at the level of the groin, the common femoral vein is imaged in transverse section and will be seen to lie medial to the common femoral artery (see Fig. 9.7). The common femoral vein should be compressed to demonstrate patency and is followed distally beyond the saphenofemoral junction, to the junction of the femoral vein and deep femoral vein. The proximal segment of the deep femoral vein should also be assessed for patency if possible, with compression. With the transducer turned into the longitudinal plane, the flow pattern in the common femoral vein should be assessed with color flow imaging and spectral Doppler. Flow should appear spontaneous and phasic at this level if there is no outflow obstruction (see Fig. 14.18). Absence of phasicity or very minimal changes, or no response to a breath holding or Valsalva maneuver, could indicate a proximal problem requiring investigation of the iliac veins as discussed later in the chapter. It is useful to compare the velocity changes with those from the contralateral common femoral vein; a discrepancy in pattern should alert the sonographer to the possibility of proximal obstruction if there is little flow change when compared with that from the opposite side. A calf squeeze can provide evidence of good flow augmentation in the proximal femoral vein, which is a useful indirect indicator of probable femoral and popliteal vein patency. Alternatively, strong foot flexion will also normally augment flow.

2. The femoral vein is then followed in transverse section along the medial aspect of the thigh to the knee, using compression to confirm patency at frequent intervals. The vein normally lies deep to the superficial femoral artery. In the adductor canal the vein may be difficult to compress. It is sometimes helpful to place a hand behind the back of the lower thigh and push the flesh toward the transducer, which will bring the vein and artery more superficial to the transducer. Color flow imaging can also be used to confirm patency in this segment, but areas of nonoccluding thrombus could be missed. Remember that duplication of the femoral vein is relatively common, which will be seen when imaging in transverse plane (reported as 20%–30%), and both trunks should be examined (see Fig. 14.10).

3. The popliteal vein is examined by scanning the popliteal fossa in a transverse plane. Starting in the middle of the popliteal fossa, the vein is followed proximally

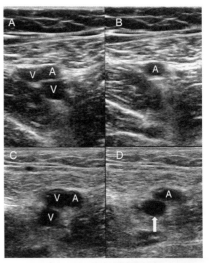

Fig. 14.10 (A) A bifid femoral vein *(V)* is demonstrated in this image. The superficial femoral artery *(A)* is seen adjacent to the veins. (B) Transducer compression confirms collapse of both vein trunks. (C) A further example of a bifid femoral vein *(V)*. (D) With compression, one of the trunks has not collapsed *(arrow)*, indicating thrombus in this trunk. The thrombus is anechoic and therefore likely to represent an acute deep venous thrombosis.

as far as possible to overlap the area scanned from the medial lower thigh. The popliteal vein will be seen lying above the popliteal artery when imaged from the popliteal fossa (Fig. 14.6). The below-knee popliteal vein and gastrocnemius tributaries are then examined in the transverse plane. The popliteal vein can also be duplicated. Sometimes it can be difficult to apply adequate pressure in the proximal popliteal fossa due to the presence of tendons and ligaments. Ask the patient to relax the leg as much as possible to overcome this problem.

4. The calf veins are often easier to identify distally. They are then followed proximally to the top of the calf. The posterior tibial and peroneal veins can be imaged in a transverse plane from the medial aspect of the calf (Fig. 14.7A). From this imaging plane the peroneal veins will lie deep to the posterior tibial veins. It can sometimes be difficult to compress the peroneal veins from this position. Color flow imaging in the longitudinal plane may be useful for demonstrating patency (Fig. 14.11), although confirmation with compression is preferable. The peroneal veins can frequently be examined from the posterolateral aspect of the calf (see Fig. 9.11). The common trunks of the posterior tibial and peroneal veins can

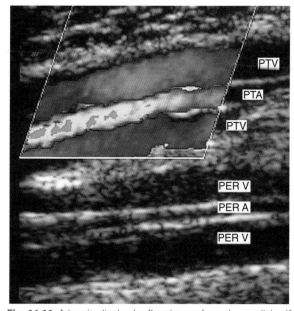

Fig. 14.11 A longitudinal color flow image from the medial calf demonstrates patency of the posterior tibial veins *(PTV)*, which are seen lying on either side of the posterior tibial artery *(PTA)*. Color filling is seen to the vein walls. The peroneal veins *(PER V)* and artery *(PER A)* are seen lying deep to the posterior tibial vessels. The peroneal vessels may not always be seen in the same scan plane.

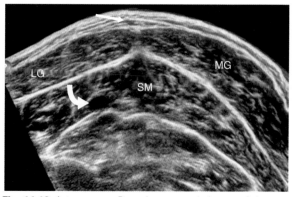

Fig. 14.12 A transverse B-mode panoramic image of the posterior aspect of the right mid-upper calf to demonstrate the position of the soleus muscle *(SM)*. A soleal vein *(curved arrow)* is seen within the muscle. The lateral and medial gastrocnemius muscles *(LG* and *MG,* respectively) lie above the SM, separated by a band of echogenic muscular fascia. The small saphenous vein is also visible in the saphenous compartment lying above the muscular fascia *(arrow).*

also be difficult to image, and medial and posterolateral transducer positions may be needed to examine this region at the top of the calf.

5. Examination of the anterior tibial veins is often not performed, as isolated thrombosis of these veins is rare. However, assessment of the anterior tibial veins is usually easier with color flow imaging, in the longitudinal plane, as the veins are small and frequently difficult to identify with B-mode imaging.

6. The examination of the calf is completed with an assessment of the soleal veins and sinuses located in the soleus muscle, which lies deep to the gastrocnemius muscle. They drain to the posterior tibial and peroneal veins. These veins are imaged from the posterior calf (Fig. 14.12). In practice, they can be difficult to identify unless dilated with thrombus.

7. If there is a clinical indication, such as in pregnancy or abdominal carcinoma, then the iliac veins are examined. In addition, May-Thurner syndrome is relatively rare condition in which patients develop iliofemoral DVT due to an anatomical variant in which the right common iliac artery overlies and compresses the left common iliac vein against the lumbar spine, that can cause a stenosis and venous stasis distal to the point of compression leading to DVT. This can sometimes be imaged directly with ultrasound. The patient should be examined supine, but as the iliac veins lie behind the bowel, an oblique or lateral approach with the patient in the lateral decubitus position can prove advantageous. The iliac veins lie slightly deeper and medial to the iliac arteries. Compression of these veins is not possible, and patency should be confirmed using color flow imaging; however, nonocclusive thrombus can be difficult to rule out. In addition, spectral Doppler can be used to examine flow patterns with flow augmentation maneuvers. The main limitation of examining this area is incomplete visualization due to overlying bowel gas.

8. In some cases, the vena cava may need to be examined. This vessel usually lies to the right of the aorta when imaged in transverse section but in rare instances can lie to the left, crossing to the right proximally. Color flow imaging can be used in the transverse plane to look for filling defects, but some transverse tilt may have to be applied to the transducer to produce a reasonable Doppler angle. Flow should also be assessed in longitudinal section with color flow and spectral Doppler ultrasound. Examination of this area should

be undertaken by a sonographer with considerable experience. Other imaging modalities are generally preferable.

SCAN APPEARANCES FOR THE ASSESSMENT OF ACUTE DVT

B-Mode Images

Normal Appearance

The vein should appear clear, contain no echoes, and be easily compressible with transducer pressure. In practice, there are often speckle and reverberation artifacts in the image, but the experienced sonographer should have little difficulty in identifying these. Smaller veins can be difficult to distinguish from tissue planes. It is sometimes possible to image static or slowly moving blood as a speckle pattern within the lumen, owing to aggregation of blood cells, but the vein should collapse under transducer pressure (see Figs. 14.5 and 14.6). In addition, if the vein is patent, the speckle pattern will clear or appear to move with a calf squeeze or by getting the patient to flex the foot a few times (see Fig. 2.13) The deep calf veins can sometimes be difficult to identify without the help of color flow imaging. The common femoral vein should normally distend with a Valsalva maneuver if there is patent venous outflow through the iliac veins.

Abnormal Appearance

In the presence of thrombus, the vein will not compress (Figs. 14.13 and 14.14). In the early stages of thrombosis, the clot often has a degree of echogenicity due to the aggregation of red blood cells in the thrombus. Within 1 to 2 days, the clot becomes more anechoic, owing to changes occurring in the thrombus, and it can be difficult to define on the B-mode image (Fig. 14.10 and Fig. 14.14D and E). However, in practice, with advanced transducer technology, it is often possible to see subtle echoes. If the vein is totally occluded in the acute phase, it may appear distended. The thrombus can be free-floating, with large areas being nonadherent to the vein wall. It is usually possible to identify the upper limit of the thrombosis, and the thrombus tip often demonstrates slightly increased echogenicity (Fig. 14.15). The tip is much easier to identify if it extends to the popliteal or femoral veins. Smaller areas of nonocclusive thrombus may not cause the vein to distend, but they can be demonstrated by incomplete collapse of the vein during compression. Older thrombus, beyond 2 weeks in age, becomes more echogenic. The varying ultrasonic appearances of acute and chronic thrombus are illustrated schematically in Fig. 14.16, but there are limitations in aging thrombus with ultrasound (Yusof et al. 2019)

Color Flow Images

Normal Appearance

Spontaneous phasic flow is usually seen in the larger proximal veins. There should be complete color filling of the lumen in both longitudinal and transverse planes during a calf squeeze. Color aliasing is sometimes observed if the distal augmentation causes a significant transient increase in venous flow. If it is difficult to squeeze the calf, owing to size or tenderness, it can be possible to augment flow by asking the patient to flex the ankle backward and forward, activating the calf muscle pump. The posterior tibial veins and peroneal veins are usually paired, which should be clearly demonstrated on the color flow image (see Fig. 14.11). However, anatomical variations can occur with single or triple vein systems. Color flow imaging of the gastrocnemius and soleal veins can be difficult, as blood flow velocities following augmentation can be low, especially if a degree of venous stasis is present.

Abnormal Appearance

There is an absence of color filling in occluded veins, even with distal augmentation. Collateral veins may also be seen in the region of the occluded vein. The color flow pattern around free-floating thrombus is very

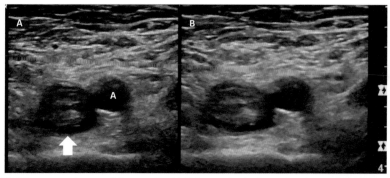

Fig. 14.13 (A) A transverse image of the proximal left femoral vein *(arrow)* and superficial femoral artery *(A)*. The femoral vein appears distended and contains echoes. (B) The femoral vein does not collapse during firm transducer pressure, confirming deep venous thrombosis.

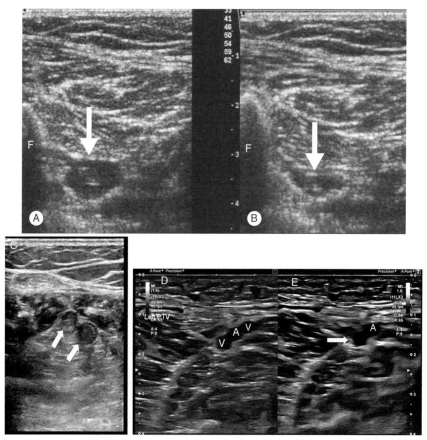

Fig. 14.14 (A) A transverse B-mode image of a peroneal vein thrombosis *(arrow)*. The image is taken from the posterolateral aspect of the calf and the veins are lying adjacent to the fibula *(F)*. (B) There is only partial collapse of the vein with transducer pressure *(arrow)* indicating a deep venous thrombosis. (C) Transverse image of soleal vein thrombus *(arrows)* with marked distension of the veins that did not compress. (D) The posterior tibial veins *(V)* and artery *(A)* are seen in this image. (E) There is noncollapse of one of the vein trunks during compression *(arrow)* indicating thrombosis. The thrombus is anechoic. The artery *(A)* is still visible.

characteristic, with flow seen between the thrombus and vein wall (Fig. 14.17). This can be demonstrated in both longitudinal and transverse sections. Color flow imaging can be useful for demonstrating the position of the proximal thrombus tip, as full color filling of the lumen will be seen just proximal to the tip. Smaller areas of non-occluding thrombus will be demonstrated as flow voids within the lumen. However, some care should be used in interpreting partially occluding thrombosis based on color flow imaging alone, and probe compression should

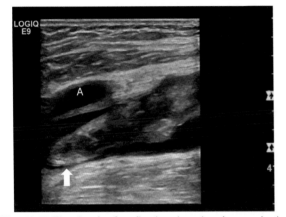

Fig. 14.15 The tip of a free-floating thrombus is seen in the femoral vein. The thrombus demonstrates heterogenous echoes *(arrow)*. The superficial femoral artery *(A)* is seen in the image.

be used for confirmation if possible. Color flow imaging can be helpful in the groin where reverse flow into tributaries can indicate proximal obstruction in the iliac veins with flow returning through collateral pathways.

Spectral Doppler
Normal Appearance
Spectral Doppler is the least-used modality in the assessment of venous thrombosis and should not be used as the only method of investigation. However, patent veins should demonstrate normal venous flow patterns. In our experience, it should be possible to augment flow velocity in the main trunks by at least 100% with a squeeze distal to the point of measurement. For example, there should be augmentation of flow in the femoral vein with a distal calf squeeze (see Ch. 13); however, this will not exclude small areas of nonoccluding thrombus. The Doppler spectral sonogram at the level of the common femoral vein should exhibit a spontaneous phasic flow pattern, which temporarily ceases when the patient takes a deep inspiration or performs a Valsalva maneuver. The degree of flow pulsatility is dependent on posture, venous pressure, breathing, and right heart pressure changes. Phasic flow suggests that there is no outflow obstruction through the iliac veins to the vena cava. However, the presence of small amounts of nonoccluding thrombus cannot be excluded based on spectral Doppler alone. Comparison with the contralateral

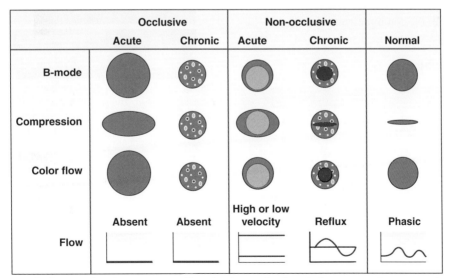

Fig. 14.16 A diagram showing transverse B-mode views of veins, their response to compression, and appearance on color flow imaging in the absence or presence of occlusive and nonocclusive deep venous thrombosis. The respective Doppler flow patterns are demonstrated at the bottom of the diagram.

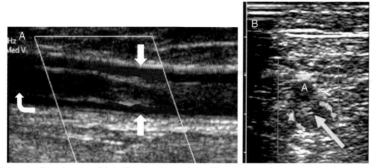

Fig. 14.17 (A) A color flow image of free-floating thrombus. Flow is seen between the thrombus and vein wall *(arrows)*. The proximal end of the thrombus toward the tip *(curved arrow)* is anechoic, which would indicate an acute thrombus. (B) A transverse image showing a crescent of flow around a floating thrombus in the femoral vein *(arrow)*. The artery *(A)* is seen adjacent to the vein.

side can help to confirm if flow changes are consistent or indicative of a unilateral proximal obstruction.

Abnormal Appearance

There is an absence of a spectral Doppler signal when the vein is completely occluded. When the vein contains a significant amount of partially occluding or free-floating thrombus, there is normally a reduced flow pattern that demonstrates little or no augmentation following distal compression. However, there are potential pitfalls when using this criterion, as there may be good collateral circulation between the point of distal calf compression and the position of the probe. An occlusive thrombosis in the iliac vein system usually results in a low-volume continuous flow pattern in the common femoral vein, with little or no response to a Valsalva maneuver (see Fig. 14.18).

Diagnostic Problems

> **OBSERVATION**
>
> It is possible to misidentify veins in the deep venous system and even confuse them with superficial veins. This occurs most commonly in the popliteal fossa and upper calf. The gastrocnemius vein can be mistaken for the popliteal vein or for the small saphenous vein. It is important to be able to identify the fascial layer that separates the superficial and deep venous systems to avoid this type of error (see Figs. 13.4 and 13.33).

The investigation of DVT can be difficult, and it is important to use a logical protocol when performing the examination. There can be considerable variation in the anatomy of the venous system, as outlined in Chapter 13. Duplication of the femoral vein and popliteal vein is

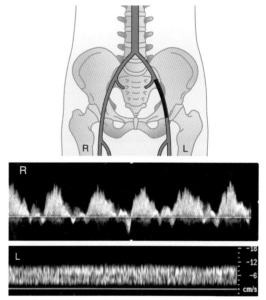

Fig. 14.18 The diagram demonstrates an occlusion of the left external iliac vein. The common femoral vein waveform distal to the obstruction demonstrates continuous low-velocity flow with a loss of phasicity, in contrast to the normal waveform shown on the right side.

not uncommon. A historical study by Gordon et al. (1996) reported duplication of the femoral vein in 25% of healthy volunteers. This could lead to potential diagnostic errors if one-half of the system is occluded and the other is patent, as it is possible to miss the occluded system during the examination (Fig. 14.10). Scrutiny of the transverse sectional image should demonstrate any bifid vein systems. The sonographer should also be highly suspicious of veins that appear small in caliber or located in abnormal positions with respect to their corresponding arteries, or contain fibrous webs, as this might indicate anatomical variation or evidence of post-thrombotic changes (Fig. 14.19). Another potentially difficult situation occurs when there is a large deep-lying thigh vein running between the popliteal vein and the deep femoral vein, as the femoral vein may be unusually small. Both the femoral vein and the deeper vein should be carefully examined for defects.

Investigation of patients with a history of intravenous drugs misuse presenting with leg swelling, or pain, can be challenging. If venous access becomes more difficult due to damaged arm veins, the femoral vein in the groin can become an alternative. Repeated injection or the substance itself can damage the vein, leading to thrombosis. In addition, infection and edema can be present. Appropriate infection control measures should be taken. Imaging can be difficult and the images may be poor quality. In some cases, this is compounded by a scarred "trumpet" or funnel-shaped depression in the groin caused by repeated injection and infection. This may cause shadowing due to air caused by poor transducer-skin contact. It may be impossible to clearly identify the major veins due to fibrosis and scarring of the veins and surrounding tissue. Color flow imaging and the use of a low-frequency curvilinear array transducer can help. In some cases obstruction and damage can be limited to the femoral vein at the groin but more extreme damage can involve the majority of veins in the thigh, knee, and even calf. Injections can also be mistakenly made into the femoral artery resulting in symptoms mimicking a DVT in the lower leg, with associated microembolization in the foot and calf.

Investigation of the iliac veins can be extremely difficult, especially in situations in which the vein may be under compression by structures in the pelvis, or by tumors, as this can be misinterpreted as a partially occluding thrombus. Compression of the iliac vein can also occur during pregnancy and is observed more frequently on the left side. This may lead to unilateral limb swelling and a reduction in the normal venous flow pattern in the femoral vein. The examination can be helped by rolling the patient on their side, to reduce compression of the vein and to confirm normal venous flow return.

IMAGING OF VENOUS STENTS

The treatment of acute and chronic venous obstruction is undergoing technological advances. The focus of treatment using stents is usually directed at iliac vein thrombosis. Catheter-directed thrombolysis can be used for thrombus dissolution and the underlying lesions or obstruction then

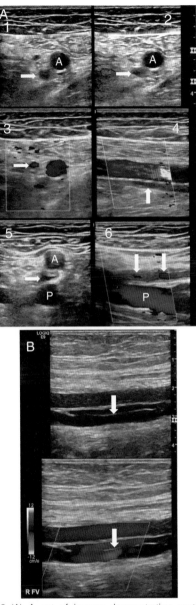

Fig. 14.19 (A) A set of images demonstrating postthrombotic changes and damage in the femoral vein. *(1)* The femoral vein *(arrow)* has a small caliber compared to the superficial femoral artery *(A)*. *(2)* With compression there is some distortion of the vein but no collapse *(arrow)*. *(3)* Color flow imaging demonstrates a small area of flow in the vein *(blue)*. There is flow in a possible collateral vein *(arrow)*. *(4)* A longitudinal image demonstrates a "cord" appearance to the vein *(arrow)*. *(5)* The femoral vein is imaged in transverse section just distal to the confluence with the profunda vein *(P)* and is seen to contain echogenic echoes *(arrow)*, suggesting chronic postthrombotic changes. *(6)* Color flow imaging shows only small regions of flow *(arrows)* in the chronically damaged femoral vein with wall thickening and scarring. The profunda vein appears widely patent. (B) A long web is seen in the lumen of the femoral vein *(arrow)* in the B-mode and color image due to postthrombotic syndrome.

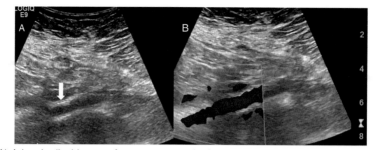

Fig. 14.20 (A) A longitudinal image of a venous stent is demonstrated in the external iliac vein. The lattice structure of the stent can be seen *(arrow)*. (B) Color flow imaging demonstrates the stent is widely patent.

treated by venous stenting. Ultrasound is a useful modality for assessing or surveying flow through venous stents due to the real time flow information provided (see Fig. 14.20). It is possible to identify in-stent stenosis with color and spectral Doppler. In addition, changes in venous flow patterns such as loss of phascity or low velocity may provide an indication of problems during surveillance scans.

ACCURACY OF DUPLEX SCANNING FOR THE DETECTION OF DVT

Many studies have been performed to compare the accuracy of duplex scanning with venography. Generally, ultrasound has good sensitivity and specificity (>90%) for the detection of femoropopliteal DVT but is less accurate for the detection of calf vein thrombus. There are a number of publications related to the accuracy of ultrasound in the diagnosis of DVT with some variation in the reported results. This may reflect factors such as patient population, operator experience, or equipment quality. The fact that ultrasound is the main modality used for imaging DVT indicates that it is widely accepted as an accurate diagnostic technique. Ultrasound image quality has improved greatly since early studies of the effectiveness for ultrasound investigation for DVT in the 1990s, and developments in scanner and probe technology are likely to improve the accuracy further. To implement a high-quality service, it is essential that staff are professionally trained and scanning protocols clearly defined.

NATURAL HISTORY OF DVT

The natural history of a DVT is variable and is dependent on the position and extent of the thrombi

(O'Shaughnessy & Fitzgerald 2001; Kearon 2003; Needleman et al. 2018). In addition, the patient's age and physical condition will have a significant bearing on the outcome. The thrombus can:

- Spontaneously lyse
- Propagate or embolize
- Recanalize over time
- Permanently occlude the vein.

Complete lysis of smaller thrombi can occur over a relatively short period of time due to fibrinolytic activity. Full recanalization of the vein will be seen, and the lumen will appear normal on the ultrasound image. Valve function can be preserved in these circumstances. If there is a large thrombus load, the process of recanalization can take several weeks. The thrombus becomes more echogenic over time as it becomes organized. The vein frequently diminishes in size due to retraction of the thrombus. As the process of recanalization begins, the developing venous flow channel within the vein lumen may be tortuous due to irregularity of lysis in the thrombus. It is even possible to see multiple flow channels within the vessel. In cases of partial recanalization, old residual thrombus can be seen along the vein wall, producing a scarred appearance. It is sometimes possible to see fibrosed valve cusps, which appear immobile and echogenic on the B-mode image. Deep venous insufficiency is frequently the long-term outcome of slow or partial recanalization.

If the vein remains permanently occluded, fibrosis causes the thrombus to become echogenic. The thrombus retracts over time, leading to shrinkage of the vein. It may even appear as a small cord adjacent to its corresponding artery, and in some cases the vein is difficult to differentiate from surrounding tissue (Fig. 14.19). Color flow imaging frequently demonstrates the development of collateral veins in the region of the occlusion. In the case of chronic common femoral and iliac vein occlusion, visible distended superficial veins, which act as collateral pathways, are often seen across the pelvis and lower abdominal wall. The great saphenous vein can act as a collateral pathway in the presence of a femoral or popliteal vein occlusion. High-volume continuous flow recorded in the great saphenous vein should always be treated with suspicion (see Fig. 13.13).

There is considerable debate about the accuracy of duplex scanning for determining the age of thrombus. A range of terms are used, such as acute, subacute, indeterminate, and chronic (Needleman et al. 2018; Yusof et al. 2019). It is generally accepted that it is possible to differentiate the acute phase, within the first week or two, from the chronic phases of venous thrombosis. Veins with chronic postthrombotic changes normally contain echogenic material or webs and bands. There can be calcification and fibrosis present and irregularity of the vein wall. If the vein is patent or partially patent, venous reflux is normally detected and filing defects may be seen due to old thrombus or webs and bands (Fig. 14.19). However, there is much less certainty about differentiating subacute and chronic thrombus. This is because the process of formation may not have been synchronous, and there are also irregularities in the process of lysis and fibrosis within the thrombus, producing a heterogeneous appearance.

Recurrent Thrombosis

Recurrent thrombotic events are common after acute DVT (Orbell et al. 2008). There are considerable diagnostic problems in attempting to detect fresh thrombus in a vein that has been damaged by a prior DVT. If the patient has had a previous scan or venogram, it is possible to check the extent of the thrombosis on the last report and compare it with the current scan. However, old reports may not be available, or the patient may not have had any previous investigations. In these situations, the vein should be examined carefully with B-mode and color flow imaging to look for areas of fresh thrombus. These will appear as anechoic areas on the B-mode image, and color flow imaging will demonstrate filling defects. In practice, this can be an extremely difficult examination to undertake. If there is a high degree of suspicion, a repeat scan can be performed a couple of days later to look for changes in the appearance of the vein or possible extension of thrombus.

SUPERFICIAL VEIN THROMBOSIS (THROMBOPHLEBITIS)

Superficial vein thrombosis, often termed *superficial thrombophlebitis*, occurs due to thrombus formation in a superficial vein with associated inflammation of the surrounding tissue. This normally affects the great saphenous vein or small saphenous veins, or tributaries of these systems. In many cases this is in association with varicose veins (Fig. 14.21). It can be felt as a hard cord in the superficial tissues. In the acute phase it is associated with erythema, localized heat, pain, and tenderness. Superficial thrombosis is generally not a serious condition compared with DVT, although be aware that DVT or PE can also develop in association with superficial vein thrombosis. However, there is a reported increased risk of DVT (Cosmi 2015; NICE 2020) in the following circumstances, when:

- The superficial vein thrombosis of the long saphenous vein is within 3 cm of the saphenofemoral junction (Fig. 14.21). This is considered to be an equivalent risk to a DVT (Cosmi 2015).
- The superficial thrombus is 5 cm or greater in length.
- The person has reduced mobility.
- The superficial thrombus is not associated with varicose veins.

If the thrombus tip extends across the saphenofemoral or saphenopopliteal junction or projects well into the deep vein, this should be clearly reported to the referring clinician, as treatment will normally be required. Care should be exercised when using compression to examine any thrombus in this position, to avoid disrupting the thrombus tip.

Imaging of superficial vein thrombus is relatively easy. Transverse imaging should be used, and it is easiest to begin in an area where there is tenderness, swelling, or hardness. It is advisable to check the saphenofemoral junction and saphenopopiteal junction even if the thrombus does not appear to affect these areas. Most cases are treated with pain relief and nonsteroidal anti-inflammatory drugs, but in the circumstances outlined earlier, anticoagulation can be required. Thrombophlebitis can cause permanent damage to superficial veins that can result in:

- Permanent occlusion
- Partial recanalization with reflux
- Full recanalization with reflux.

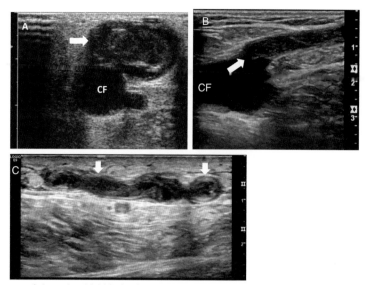

Fig. 14.21 Images of thrombophlebitis in the great saphenous vein (GSV). (A) A transverse image of distended great saphenous vein *(arrow)* at the saphenofemoral junction (SFJ). The common femoral *(CF)* vein is visible. (B) A longitudinal image of a GSV showing the proximal extent of the phlebitis *(arrow)* adjacent to the SFJ. (C) Thrombophlebitis is seen in a tortuous section of the GSV *(arrows)*.

Chronic damage is visible as fibrotic or echogenic material in the vein, webs, or irregularity and scarring of the vein wall. If a patient is being examined for a venous insufficiency scan, and evidence of previous thrombophlebitis is identified, it is important to be aware that the patient may have experienced a previous DVT or may have increased risk for DVT.

One potential complication in the diagnosis of superficial thrombophlebitis can occur if a patient presents having had recent endovenous treatment for varicose veins by laser or radiofrequency ablation. The appearance of postendovenous treatment can be similar to thrombophlebitis. If the sonographer is unaware the patient has undergone recent treatment, they may mistake this appearance for phlebitis. It is of course possible that the patient may have had a DVT posttreatment, so the patient should be investigated carefully.

OTHER PATHOLOGIC CONDITIONS THAT CAN MIMIC DVT

Hematoma

Hematomas are accumulations of blood within the tissues that can clot to form a solid swelling. They can be caused by external trauma or other mechanisms such as muscle tears, can be extremely painful, and can lead to limb swelling, especially in the calf. Blood in the hematoma may also track extensively along the fascial planes. The sonographic appearance of a hematoma is of a reasonably well-defined hypoechoic area in the soft tissues or muscles (see Fig. 14.22). Hematomas can be very variable in size and shape. It is sometimes impossible to image the veins in the immediate vicinity, owing to the size of the hematoma or the pain the patient experiences. The hematoma may also partially or completely compress the deep veins in the local vicinity.

Lymphedema

Lymphedema is observed as chronic limb swelling due to reduced efficiency or failure of the lymphatic drainage system. This may be due to a primary abnormality of the lymphatic system or to secondary causes that lead to damage of the lymph nodes and drainage system in the groin and pelvis. These include damage following surgery, trauma, malignancy, and radiotherapy in the groin region. Lymphedema is usually most prominent in the calf but can extend throughout the leg, and two-thirds of cases are unilateral. Other sites can be affected by lymphedema, including the arms. The B-mode appearance of lymphedema demonstrates the subcutaneous layer to be thickened, and a fine B-mode speckle is observed in this region, making the image appear grainy (see Fig. 14.23).

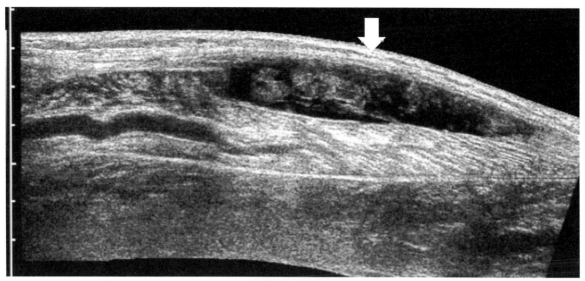

Fig. 14.22 An extensive area of hematoma *(arrow)* is seen in this panoramic view of thigh muscle.

The ultrasound image of lymphedema is usually different from that caused by simple fluid edema. Ultrasound can be used to confirm the patency of the deep veins, but unfortunately the presence of lymphedema degrades the ultrasound image, making many deep-vein scans technically challenging.

Cellulitis

Cellulitis is caused by infection of the subcutaneous tissues and skin; it produces diffuse swelling in the lower limb, often associated with pain, tenderness, and redness. There is usually evidence of edema in the region of swelling. A duplex examination can confirm patency of the deep veins. In addition, there may be hyperemic flow in the veins and arteries of the limb due to the infection (see Fig. 13.41).

Edema

Patients can develop edema in the calf due to infection, leg ulceration, local trauma, or as a result of significant venous insufficiency. This is characterized as fluid or edema in the superficial tissues. The ultrasound appearance of edema demonstrates tissue splaying by numerous interstitial channels (Fig. 14.24). Patients with congestive heart failure often develop edema in the legs due to the increased pressure in the venous system and the right side of the heart. Another characteristic of congestive heart failure is the pulsatile flow pattern that is often observed in the proximal deep veins, which can be

mistaken for arterial flow (Fig. 14.25). Careful attention to the color display will confirm the direction of flow.

Baker's Cysts

A Baker's cyst is a distension of the semimembranosus-gastrocnemius bursa and normally originates on the medial side of the knee. This bursa usually communicates with the knee joint. Bursae are pouches containing synovial fluid that prevents friction between a bone joint or tendon. Baker's cysts occur due to a number of knee disorders, such as arthritis and repetitive trauma due to exercise. Baker's cysts can rupture, causing severe pain and symptoms similar to those of acute vein thrombosis. Large Baker's cysts can compress the popliteal vein or deep veins of the popliteal fossa, causing a DVT. It is always necessary to identify and confirm the patency of the deep veins in the popliteal fossa, even when a Baker's cyst has been diagnosed, as the Baker's cyst may be an incidental finding. Baker's cysts can also be clinically misdiagnosed as popliteal aneurysms.

Baker's cysts are easiest to define in a transverse scan plane from the popliteal fossa. They are normally anechoic due to the fluid in the cyst, but some may contain debris and osteocartilaginous fragments, which are echogenic. Many Baker's cysts have a typical oval or crescent shape, with a characteristic neck (Fig. 14.26). If the cyst is excessively large, it may distort the anatomy in the popliteal fossa. It is difficult to define a ruptured Baker's cyst with ultrasound. However,

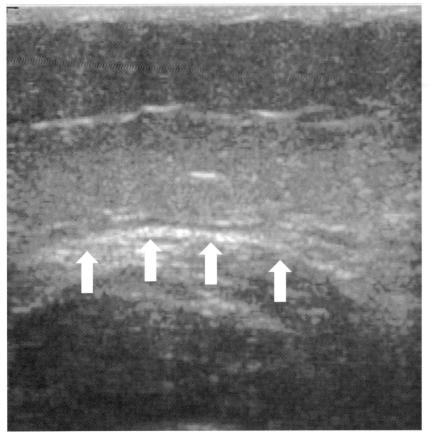

Fig. 14.23 Lymphedema produces a grainy appearance in the subcutaneous tissues, as demonstrated on this transverse B-mode image. The superficial tissue is relatively thick. The muscular fascia is demonstrated by the *arrows*. Note the degraded image quality, typical of this disorder.

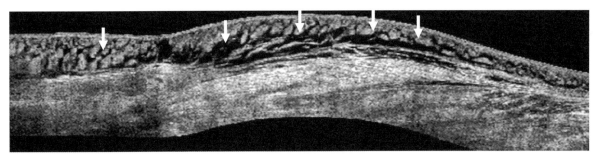

Fig. 14.24 In this panoramic image of the calf, fluid edema is demonstrated in the subcutaneous tissues as numerous anechoic channels *(arrows)* splaying the tissue.

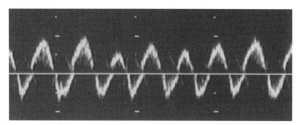

Fig. 14.25 The venous flow signals recorded from the common femoral vein of a patient with congestive cardiac failure demonstrate a pulsatile flow pattern.

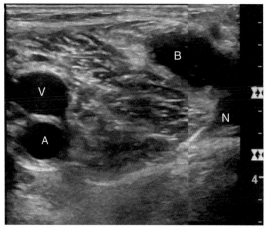

Fig. 14.26 A Baker's cyst *(B)* is demonstrated in this transverse image of the popliteal fossa. Some subtle echoes are seen in the main body of the cyst. The popliteal artery *(A)* and vein *(V)* are also seen. The neck of the cyst *(N)* is seen.

ruptured Baker's cysts may be seen to track down into the upper calf

Enlarged Lymph Nodes

Enlargement of lymph nodes can occur due to pathologic conditions including infection and malignancy. The inflow of lymphocytes and other substances into the node exceeds the outflow, leading to enlargement of the node. The main sites for enlargement visualized during venous duplex examinations are the groin and axilla, and the nodes can become so large that they compress the adjacent vein. Enlarged nodes may be tender, and localized redness and heat (erythema) may be present. They can also be clinically misdiagnosed as femoral artery aneurysms if the pulsation of the artery is amplified to the skin surface by the enlarged node.

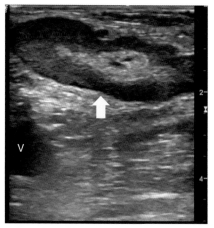

Fig. 14.27 An enlarged lymph node *(arrow)* is demonstrated in this transverse image at groin level. The common femoral vein *(V)* is seen below the node.

Enlarged lymph nodes are imaged as oval or spherical masses that are found in groups (Fig. 14.27). They are mainly hypoechoic in appearance but may contain stronger echoes within the center of the node and can be mistaken for a thrombosed vein. Color flow Doppler usually demonstrates blood flow in larger nodes, especially if infection is present.

The following conditions may also mimic DVT:
- Abscesses
- Muscle tears
- Hyperperfusion syndrome following arterial bypass surgery or angioplasty for lower-limb ischemia
- Immobility resulting in leg swelling
- Prolonged leg dependency resulting in edema
- Arteriovenous fistulas
- Heart failure resulting in leg edema.

Be aware that a DVT could be present even if these conditions are diagnosed or encountered.

UPPER-LIMB VEINS

Anatomy of the Deep Upper-Limb Veins

The upper-limb veins can also be divided into the deep and superficial veins (Fig. 14.28), and there are a number of anatomical variations. Usually, paired veins are associated with the radial and ulnar arteries. They normally join at the elbow to form the brachial vein but can run separately to form the brachial vein higher in the upper arm. The brachial vein is usually paired and associated with the brachial artery. At the top of the arm, the brachial vein becomes the axillary vein, which is usually a single trunk. The axillary vein becomes the subclavian vein as it crosses the border of the first rib. The subclavian vein enters the thoracic outlet but runs separately from the artery in front of the anterior scalene muscle. The internal jugular vein, from the neck, joins the proximal subclavian vein, which then drains via the brachiocephalic vein to the superior vena cava. The left brachiocephalic vein is longer than the right brachiocephalic vein. It is generally difficult to image the brachiocephalic veins clearly with ultrasound.

Anatomy of the Superficial Upper-Limb Veins

The cephalic vein and the basilic vein are the two major superficial veins in the arms (Fig. 14.28). The cephalic vein drains the dorsal surface of the hand and runs up the lateral (radial) aspect of the forearm to the antecubital fossa at the elbow and then continues in a subcutaneous path along the lateral aspect of the biceps muscle. Toward the shoulder, it runs in the deltopectoral groove between the deltoid and pectoralis muscles and then pierces the clavipectoral fascia to join the axillary vein in the infraclavicular region. The basilic vein drains blood from the palm and ventral aspects of the hand and runs along the medial (ulnar) side of the forearm to the medial aspect of the antecubital fossa. The basilic vein then penetrates the fascia in the lower aspect of the upper arm to join the brachial vein. However, its insertion can be variable, and sometimes the basilic vein may run directly into the distal axillary vein.

Thrombosis of the Upper Limbs

The incidence of upper-limb deep-vein thrombosis (ULDVT) has increased with the widespread use of central venous catheters; the number of investigations requested has increased commensurately. The subclavian and axillary veins are the commonest sites for thrombosis and can lead to upper-limb swelling with distension of superficial veins. The causes of upper-limb thrombosis are similar to those that lead to lower-limb DVT. In addition, catheters can damage the axillary and subclavian veins and can restrict flow causing venous stasis. Venous thoracic outlet syndrome can also cause thrombosis of the subclavian vein. Effort-induced thrombosis of the subclavian vein, referred to as Paget–Schroetter syndrome, is associated with strenuous upper-body

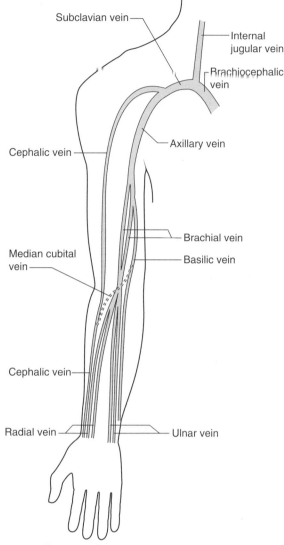

Fig. 14.28 The venous anatomy of the arm.

exercise or repetitive movements and is mainly seen in younger patients.

Upper-limb superficial vein thrombosis (ULSVT), most commonly in the cephalic, median cubital and basilic veins, is associated with needling, catheters, and damage from lines. The patient may suffer from local swelling and pain. Ultrasound is used to confirm the extent of the thrombus and the involvement of the deep veins.

The appearance of thrombosis in the upper extremities is similar to that seen in the lower extremities. A combination of compression, color flow imaging, and spectral Doppler is required to confirm patency, as it is sometimes difficult to apply satisfactory probe compression, particularly in the supraclavicular fossa. However, duplex scanning provides good results when compared to contrast venography in areas where compression can be applied, but caution should be used when attempting to diagnose DVT on the basis of Doppler flow patterns (Baarslag et al. 2002). Upper-limb swelling can also be caused by lymphedema, following mastectomy with removal of lymph nodes in the axilla and the effects of radiotherapy. When combined with clinical score and D-dimer tests, ultrasound has been shown to be effective in the diagnosis of ULDVT (Kleinjan et al. 2014).

TECHNIQUE FOR ASSESSING THE BRACHIAL, AXILLARY, AND SUBCLAVIAN VEINS

Imaging of the subclavian vein, proximal axillary vein, internal jugular vein, and brachiocephalic veins is easiest with the patient lying supine so that the veins are distended. Conversely, the distal axillary vein, brachial veins and distal veins, and the basilic and cephalic veins are scanned with the patient sitting. The scan normally takes 15 to 30 minutes for each arm. Remember, it can be useful to compare the scan appearance from both sides in cases of suspected unilateral thrombosis. It should also be noted that the color flow image of the proximal subclavian vein can look rather confusing and cluttered because of the proximity of other vessels and the often pulsatile appearance superimposed on the venous flow pattern, due to atrial contractions (see Fig. 16.8). Imaging of the subclavian vein is also discussed in Chapter 16:

1. The arm should be abducted and placed on a comfortable support. It is easier to start the examination distally in the brachial vein, which will be seen lying adjacent to the brachial artery in the upper arm.
2. The brachial vein is imaged in transverse section and should be compressible with relatively light transducer pressure. Like lower-limb DVT, the appearance of a distended vein containing echoes is suspicious for thrombus and DVT (Fig. 14.29), and where possible, compression should be used for confirmation. Color and spectral Doppler recordings should demonstrate flow augmentation in the brachial vein

with a manual squeeze of the forearm. The basilic vein is seen medial to the brachial vein at lower to mid humerus level and should be compressible. Basilic vein thrombus associated with lines should be followed to confirm the proximal extent.

3. The axillary vein can be imaged using a combination of transaxillary and infraclavicular transducer positions (see Fig. 16.3 and Chs. 10 and 16). The vein will be seen lying adjacent to the artery, but color flow imaging can aid identification, particularly if B-mode imaging is poor. A combination of compression and color flow imaging may be needed to confirm patency in this region. The cephalic vein may act as a collateral pathway to the subclavian vein in the presence of a distal axillary vein thrombosis.
4. The distal end of the subclavian vein is initially imaged from the infraclavicular fossa in transverse section, where it will be seen lying inferior to the subclavian artery. The mid-subclavian vein is imaged from the supraclavicular fossa. A large acoustic shadow will be seen as the subclavian vein runs under the clavicle. Compression of the subclavian vein is extremely difficult, owing to the contour of the neck and the presence of the clavicle, and color flow imaging in transverse and longitudinal planes is used to confirm patency. Irregular echoes or changes in size of the vein should be investigated carefully (Fig. 14.30). In addition, spectral Doppler should demonstrate spontaneous phasic flow with respiration if there is no outflow obstruction. It is also usual to observe a pulsatile flow pattern superimposed on the phasic flow pattern due to atrial contractions of the heart (see Ch. 5). It should be noted that it is extremely easy to miss a proximal thrombosis in the subclavian vein, owing to poor visualization of this area, especially if it is a partially occluding thrombus. It is possible to image indwelling catheters, such as Hickman lines, in the subclavian vein. Always state any limitations or doubts about the scan in this region, as other imaging tests may be required.
5. Two breathing maneuvers can be used for assessing flow in the subclavian vein. The first is a Valsalva maneuver, in which there should be cessation of flow or flow reversal during Valsalva. This is followed by an enhancement in flow toward the heart during expiration. The second involves multiple sniffing through the nose. During continued sniffing the subclavian

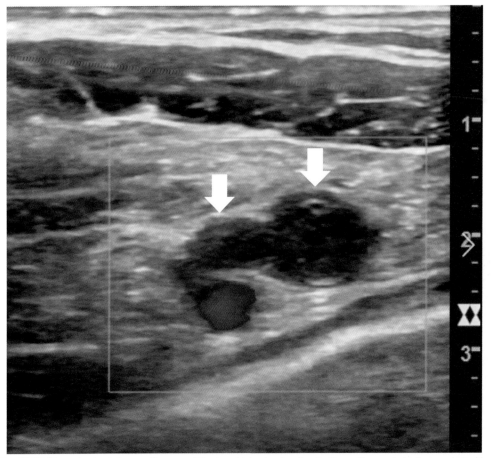

Fig. 14.29 Thrombosis at the confluence of the brachial veins leading to the axillary vein is demonstrated by thrombus echoes within the veins *(arrows)*, with distension and an absence of color flow filling with augmentation. Thrombosis was confirmed, as the veins did not collapse with compression. The artery is coded *red*.

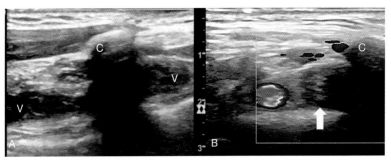

Fig. 14.30 Thrombosis of the subclavian vein at the level of the clavicle. (A) The longitudinal image demonstrates significant echoes within the vein *(V)* and, in this case, irregular diameter of the vein. (B) Transverse color flow imaging demonstrates flow in the subclavian artery but no flow in the vein and evidence of thrombus *(arrow)*. The clavicle *(C)* is causing an acoustic shadow.

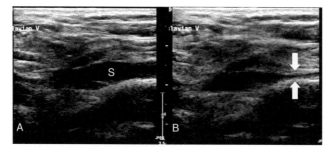

Fig. 14.31 An indirect method of assessing subclavian vein patency involves a series of short sniffs through the nose. (A) A longitudinal image of a patent subclavian vein *(S)* during normal breathing. (B) With two to three short sniffs through the nose, the vein is seen to collapse *(between arrows)* and collapsed completely after a couple of further sniffs.

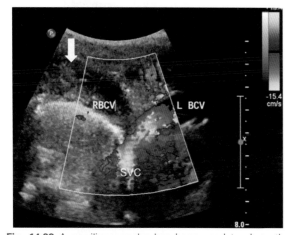

Fig. 14.32 A curvilinear probe has been used to show the confluence of the right *(RBCV)* and left *(LBCV)* brachiocephalic veins. The RBCV is occluded with thrombus *(arrow)*, but there is unimpeded flow from the LBCV to the superior vena cava *(SVC)*.

vein will be seen to contract (see Fig. 14.31). Neither of these maneuvers can exclude DVT, as there may be nonoccluding thrombus present. However, if an abnormal flow pattern or response is recorded, it may indicate a potential abnormality.

6. Thrombosis may involve the internal jugular vein in the neck, and a scan of the jugular vein is recommended for all upper-limb DVT investigations. The jugular vein can be imaged in cross-section from the mid-neck and followed to its confluence with the subclavian vein.

7. It is usually difficult to image the brachiocephalic veins fully (see Fig. 16.4), but a thrombosis may

be indirectly suggested if there is an abnormality in the subclavian and axillary vein flow patterns. Curvilinear arrays are useful in providing adequate penetration and a wider view from the limited supraclavicular acoustic window (Fig. 14.32).

If patients have indwelling venous catheters, lines, or wires for treatment, and there is clinical suspicion of thrombosis, the veins proximal to the insertion point should be carefully examined, along with the general assessment for upper-limb DVT. The appearance of a central line catheter associated with thrombosis is shown in Fig. 14.33. Dependent on the catheter size and composition, there can be multiple reflections observed in the B-mode image. The appearance of thrombus can be subtle and easily missed or obscured by the catheter.

Other Upper-Limb Venous Disorders

Phlebitis of the superficial veins can occur due to repeated catheter access or intravenous drug abuse. Arteriovenous malformations are sometimes found in the arms and hands, and in some cases can be very extensive, leading to upper-limb swelling.

REPORTING

Appropriate images should be recorded with an accompanying report. Dual- or split-screen imaging can be useful for comparison with one side showing the vein with no compression and the other with compression. The report should indicate the scan to be normal or abnormal, and if abnormal, the level and extent of the

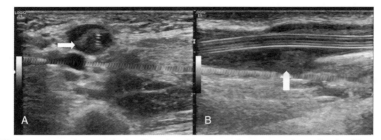

Fig. 14.33 (A) A transverse image of a basilic vein with a central venous catheter in situ. The reflection from the catheter is clearly seen and there is evidence of surrounding thrombus *(arrow)*. (B) A longitudinal image clearly demonstrates the catheter and surrounding thrombus *(arrow)*.

thrombosis should be stated. The report should also clearly specify which veins were examined and which were omitted or not assessed due to technical limitations. This avoids any confusion or assumption that veins not referenced on the report are normal. Other pathologic conditions that may mimic the symptoms of DVT should also be reported. The report of a positive DVT should be brought to the attention of the appropriate medical staff as soon as possible so that appropriate management can be implemented.

15

Graft Surveillance and Preoperative Vein Mapping for Bypass Surgery

OUTLINE

INTRODUCTION

Providing they are fit enough for treatment, patients with significant lower-limb ischemia or threatened limb loss usually require arterial bypass surgery if no other option is available to improve blood flow in the leg. Vascular surgeons are able to perform an extensive range of arterial bypass procedures to restore circulation to the extremities. Bypass surgery can also be combined with angioplasty and stenting as part of a hybrid procedure. Bypass grafts can be made of synthetic materials, such as polytetrafluoroethylene (PTFE), or constructed from native vein, which can be assessed and marked preoperatively as described at the end of this chapter. Failure of a bypass graft due to the development of a graft stenosis is a serious complication that can result in amputation if it is not possible to unblock the graft. It is therefore common practice for vascular laboratories to perform regular graft surveillance scans to detect the development of graft defects. The majority of surveillance scans are performed for native vein bypass grafts below the groin (infrainguinal grafts). The surveillance of synthetic grafts is equivocal, and benefits are less clear-cut (Lane et al. 2011). Ultrasound can also be used to image areas of potential infection following graft surgery, to see if the region of infection is in contact with the graft. The emphasis of this chapter will be on infrainguinal vein graft surveillance.

ANATOMY

The routes of grafts vary considerably and depend on the level and extent of the native arterial disease that has been bypassed. Synthetic grafts are mainly used to bypass inflow disease (aortoiliac segment), whereas vein grafts are frequently used for distal procedures below the inguinal ligament. The different types of graft frequently encountered in the graft surveillance clinic are shown in Fig. 15.1.

Vein Grafts

Whenever possible, native vein is used for femoral distal bypass surgery, as it offers good long-term patency rates and there is less risk associated with infection compared to synthetic grafts. The great saphenous vein is the vein of choice for infrainguinal bypass surgery, although an arm vein or the small saphenous vein can also be used if the great saphenous vein is unsuitable in part or all of its length. The proximal anastomosis of a vein graft is usually located at the common femoral artery, although the position can vary and it may be sited at the superficial femoral artery or, less commonly, at the popliteal artery if a calf artery bypass is being performed. The position of the distal anastomosis can be variable and depends on the distal extent of the native arterial disease. In some cases this can be to pedal arteries in the foot. The geometry of the distal anastomosis can vary but most are end of graft to side of native artery (end to side) or, more rarely, end of graft to end of native artery when an interposition graft is performed. The distal anastomosis may lie very deep in the leg, particularly if the graft is anastomosed to the tibioperoneal trunk or peroneal artery. Vein grafts composed of more than one segment of vein are known as autogenous composite vein grafts.

Femoral distal bypass surgery is performed using three common types of surgical procedure (see Fig. 15.2).

The first is the in situ technique, in which the great saphenous vein is exposed but left in its native position and side branches are ligated to prevent blood shunting from the graft to the venous system. As the vein contains valves that would prevent blood flow toward the foot, they have to be removed or disrupted using a device called a valvulotome. The main body of an in situ vein graft lies superficially along the medial aspect of the thigh. In the second technique, called a non-reversed vein graft, the vein is removed from its bed and can be tunneled or positioned elsewhere in the leg. The natural taper of the vein along the leg matches the naturally decreasing diameter of the arteries as they run to the periphery.

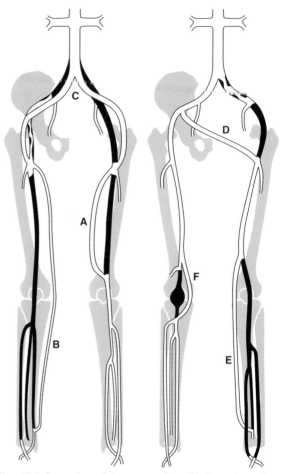

Fig. 15.1 Examples of bypass grafts. *(A)* Above-knee femoropopliteal graft. *(B)* Femoroposterior tibial artery graft. *(C)* Aortobifemoral graft. *(D)* Iliofemoral cross-over graft. *(E)* Superficial femoral artery to peroneal artery graft. *(F)* Popliteal artery bypass graft for a thrombosed popliteal aneurysm.

In the third type of procedure, the great saphenous vein is completely removed and turned through 180° so that the distal end of the vein will form the proximal anastomosis. This is called a reversed vein graft. One particular advantage of this technique is that, in this orientation, the valves will not prevent blood flow toward the foot and do not need to be removed (Fig. 15.2B). Reversed vein grafts are often tunneled deep in the thigh beneath the sartorius muscle, which can make imaging difficult. As the vein is reversed, the diameter of the proximal segment of the graft is usually smaller than the distal segment. This can result in a size mismatch between the proximal inflow artery and proximal graft that is evident on the scan. When there is insufficient length of native vein available, a combination of synthetic material and vein may be used to form a composite graft.

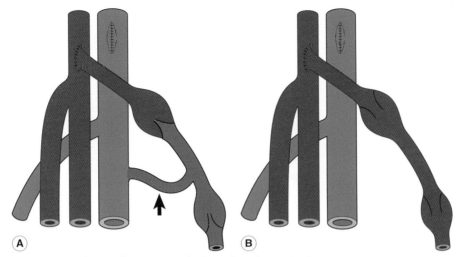

Fig. 15.2 Diagrams of two different types of vein graft at the proximal anastomosis to the common femoral artery. (A) An in situ vein graft. Blood will not flow beyond the first valve, and therefore the valves in the great saphenous vein have to be removed (see text). The tributaries must be ligated to prevent blood flowing directly back into the femoral vein *(arrow)*. (B) A reversed vein graft. The valves will open in the direction of flow.

Synthetic Grafts

Synthetic grafts are used for aortobifemoral, iliofemoral, axillofemoral, and femorofemoral cross-over grafts. Synthetic PTFE grafts are also used for femoropopliteal bypass, but the long-term patency rates are not as good as grafts constructed from native vein (Klinkert et al. 2003). Vein cuffs or collars are sometimes used to join the distal end of a synthetic femoral distal graft to the native artery. They produce a localized dilation at the anastomosis, which is thought to reduce the risk of a stenosis occurring.

PURPOSE OF GRAFT SURVEILLANCE

Vein Grafts

The development of an intrinsic vein graft stenosis is a major source of vein graft failure (Davies et al. 2005). An angiogram demonstrating a graft stenosis is shown in Fig. 15.3. Early graft failure, within the first 30 days, is attributed to technical defects or poor patient selection. Such an example would be a patient with very poor run-off below the graft, resulting in increased resistance to flow and eventual graft thrombosis, or the use of small or poor-quality vein. Graft failure beyond this period is attributed to the development of intimal hyperplasia that can occur when there is damage to the endothelium of the vessel wall. This causes smooth-muscle proliferation into the vessel lumen and subsequent narrowing. Stenoses can occur at any point along the graft and can sometimes be

extremely short, web-like lesions. Incomplete removal of valve cusps during in situ bypass surgery can also cause localized flow disturbance and narrowing. Late graft failure, beyond 12 months, can also be due to progression of atherosclerotic disease in the native inflow or outflow arteries, above and below the graft (see Fig. 15.12).

Patients are normally scanned at regular intervals in the first 12 months following bypass surgery (Zierler et al. 2018). An example surveillance program, from our experience, is shown in Box 15.1. Some vascular units also continue to scan patients indefinitely beyond the first year, at 6-month or yearly intervals, to detect late graft problems. The time interval between scans is shortened to 1–2 months if a patient shows signs of developing a moderate stenosis. Patients requiring angioplasty or surgical revision of a significant graft defect recommence the surveillance program from the beginning. It can be seen that graft surveillance programs require considerable commitment from the vascular laboratory and many departments have developed local protocols.

Synthetic Grafts

The surveillance of synthetic grafts remains debatable, as many synthetic graft occlusions occur due to spontaneous graft thrombosis. Some vascular centers perform surveillance of iliofemoral and femorofemoral cross-over grafts and aortobifemoral grafts, particularly if there have been problems with disease in the inflow

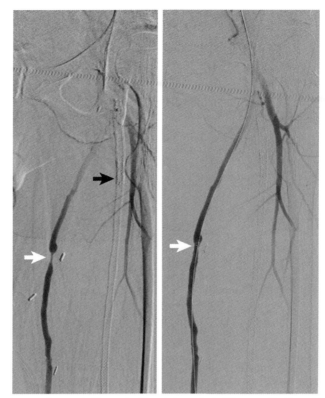

Fig. 15.3 (A) An angiogram demonstrating a significant stenosis *(white arrow)* in the mid-segment of a femoropopliteal vein graft (common femoral artery to popliteal artery). Note, the presence of an occluded superficial femoral artery stent in the image *(black arrow)*. (B) The stenosis has been successfully dilated by balloon angioplasty *(arrow)*.

BOX 15.1 Suggested Program for Graft Surveillance Following Discharge From Hospital (Time Intervals Are Shown in Months [M])

Program If No Significant Abnormality Is Detected, Peak Systolic Velocity (PSV) Ratio < 2

1 M, 3 M, 6 M, 9 M, 12 M, 18 M, and 24 M then the patient is discharged from the surveillance program

If a stenosis is detected, surveillance intervals can be shortened or intervention undertaken dependent on the significance (see Tables 15.2 and 15.3).

---

or outflow arteries. Synthetic grafts are more likely to become infected, and fluid collections or pus are sometimes found surrounding the graft at the site of infection, which frequently occurs at the groin. Graft infection is a serious complication and can cause the breakdown of the graft anastomosis, leading to false aneurysm and the possibility of uncontrollable hemorrhage. Duplex scanning can be used in the investigation and monitoring of potential graft infections.

SYMPTOMS AND TREATMENT OF GRAFT STENOSIS OR FAILURE

ADVICE

Issue the patient with an information card giving the details of their graft and appropriate phone numbers to contact if problems or symptoms are encountered, such as the vascular laboratory and vascular ward.

Most patients experience no symptoms in the presence of a developing graft stenosis, and grafts may fail without any prior warning. However, symptoms that can be attributable to imminent graft failure are the sudden onset of severe claudication or a sensation of coldness or color change involving the foot. Urgent intervention is required in this situation to prevent graft occlusion. Most graft stenoses are treated successfully by balloon angioplasty. However, recurrent stenoses sometimes require surgical revision involving local patching of a defect or partial graft replacement using a new segment of vein. Early graft occlusion can be treated by thrombolysis or graft thrombectomy. There is often an underlying cause for the occlusion that requires correction, such as a graft stenosis, inflow stenosis, or run-off occlusion. Conversely, some grafts develop a local aneurysm that may become so large that a segment of graft has to be replaced.

PRACTICAL CONSIDERATIONS FOR SCANNING BYPASS GRAFTS

What Does the Clinician Want to Know?

- Is the graft patent?
- Is there a graft stenosis and where is it located?
- What is the peak systolic velocity (PSV) across the stenosis?
- What is the PSV ratio across the stenosis?
- Estimate the degree of stenosis
- Does flow appear compromised in the graft (damped flow, low-velocity flow, or very high-resistant flow)?
- Is there evidence of inflow or outflow obstruction?
- Are there any graft aneurysms? Measure their size and position
- Is there evidence of graft entrapment? State the position
- Are there abnormal fluid collections associated with the graft? State the position
- Are there any significant changes since the previous scan? If so, what are they?

If a significant problem is suspected, it is advisable to seek senior medical advice before letting the patient go home as this can make arrangements for admission or treatment easier.

Problems Finding the Graft?

Beware: in some situations the great saphenous vein is removed and tunneled elsewhere in the leg and may follow an unusual anatomic route. It can save a lot of time by having access to a copy of the operation and procedure notes before starting the scan.

No special preparation is required for the examination, and the vast majority of graft scans can be completed within half an hour. The majority of bypass scans are performed with the patient lying supine or semisupine. When scanning vein grafts, the leg should be externally rotated and the knee gently flexed and supported. It is sometimes necessary to roll the patient over to one side in order to scan the posterior lower thigh, popliteal fossa, or upper posterior calf if the graft is anastomosed to the popliteal artery. Positions for scanning the tibial arteries are discussed in Chapter 9. The scanner should be configured for a graft scan, or in the absence of a specific preset, a lower-limb arterial investigation. Adjustment of the controls is frequently necessary, especially if there is low-volume flow in the graft (see Ch. 7).

Before beginning the scan, it is important to know the position and type of graft that is to be examined. The examination request card or operation notes should indicate this information. A potentially confusing situation can occur if a previous graft has been inserted and this has since occluded. An old, thrombosed graft might be mistakenly identified as the new graft, which would then be reported as occluded. A combination of mid- and high-frequency, flat linear array transducers are most suited for graft surveillance in the thigh and calf. A low-frequency probe is required for imaging grafts above the inguinal ligament or for grafts that have been tunneled very deep in the thigh. A hockey-stick transducer is useful for scanning the distal sections of grafts anastomosed to distal calf or pedal arteries.

SCANNING TECHNIQUES

ADVICE

Do not apply excessive probe pressure when scanning superficial grafts, as it is possible to compress the graft, especially if more pressure is applied to one end of the transducer, giving the false impression of a stenosis or narrowing. This is particularly important if the graft is close to or running over a bony surface.

In Situ Vein Graft

An ultrasound montage of an in situ vein graft is shown in Fig. 15.4. The main body of an in situ vein graft remains superficial in the leg and runs along the medial aspect of the thigh (Fig. 15.5). It is often easier to locate

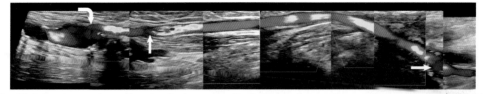

Fig. 15.4 A color montage of an in situ femoropopliteal vein graft from the proximal anastomosis *(curved arrow)*, where the proximal section of the occluded superficial femoral artery can be seen, to the distal anastomosis *(horizontal arrow)*. An area of color flow aliasing and flow disturbance within the body of the graft may indicate a graft stenosis *(vertical arrow)* and should be closely checked with spectral Doppler.

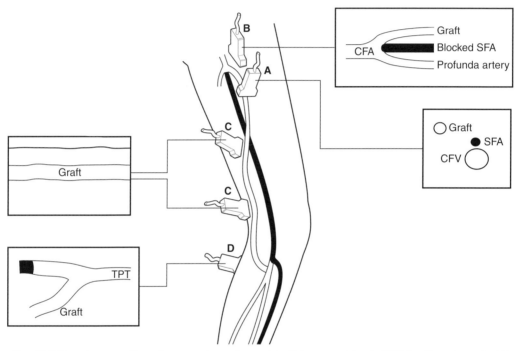

Fig. 15.5 Transducer positions for assessing a femoral to tibioperoneal trunk *(TPT)* in situ vein graft. *(A)* Proximal graft, transverse section. *(B)* Proximal anastomosis, longitudinal section. *(C)* Main body of the graft, longitudinal section. *(D)* Distal anastomosis below the popliteal fossa, longitudinal section. Scanning from a medial position below the knee may also provide a good image of the distal anastomosis. *CFA,* Common femoral artery; *SFA,* superficial femoral artery.

the graft in the upper medial thigh using a transverse imaging plane and then to follow the graft up to the proximal anastomosis (Fig. 15.5A). A virtual convex setting in B-mode is useful for imaging a wider region of the anatomy.

The transducer is rotated into a longitudinal scan plane at the proximal anastomosis (Fig. 15.5B). Ideally, a minimum 5 cm length of the inflow artery above the graft origin should be examined to exclude any disease. For instance, damped waveforms at this level are likely to indicate significant inflow disease that should be

investigated further. The proximal anastomosis should be carefully interrogated using color flow imaging and spectral Doppler for any signs of stenosis.

The graft is then carefully followed in longitudinal section along the thigh (Fig. 15.5C) with the color pulse repetition frequency (PRF)/color scale optimized to demonstrate any flow disturbances. Typically, a color scale between 20 and 30 cm/s is a good starting point for a normally functioning graft. A high-frequency transducer provides the best image of the main body of an in situ graft. Spectral Doppler measurements should be

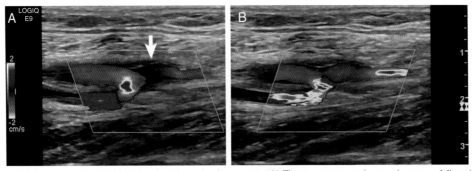

Fig. 15.6 The importance of optimizing the color box steer. (A) There appears to be an absence of flow in a region at the distal anastomosis *(arrow)* that could represent a stenosis or thrombus. (B) The color box steer angle has been optimized to the direction of flow and flow is now clearly demonstrated across the anastomosis.

made along the length of the graft, looking for waveform changes, especially in areas demonstrating color flow changes. It is often difficult to obtain good Doppler angles when scanning superficial vein grafts, and gentle "heel-toeing" of the transducer may be required. A wedge of ultrasound gel can help if a specific region needs close examination.

The distal portion of many in situ vein grafts run deep to join a native artery at the distal anastomosis (Fig. 15.5D). This is especially true for grafts joined to the popliteal or peroneal arteries. It is often necessary to use a mid-frequency transducer in this region. The distal anastomosis should be scrutinized very closely with color flow imaging and spectral Doppler, and it can be necessary to use a range of Doppler angles to demonstrate flow (see Fig. 15.6). Grafts that are anastomosed to the anterior tibial artery are commonly tunneled through the interosseous membrane (Fig. 15.7). The graft is imaged on the medial or posteromedial aspect of the calf, where it is seen to drop away very sharply and disappear through the membrane. The graft can then be relocated by scanning over the anterolateral aspect of the calf, where it will be seen to rise toward the transducer and followed distally to locate the anastomosis. There should be a longitudinal scar on the anterior aspect of the calf in the region of the anastomosis. Transducer positions for locating the distal anastomosis are shown in Table 15.1.

Reversed and Non-Reversed Vein Grafts

The imaging techniques are similar to those for in situ grafts, but reversed and non-reversed vein grafts are frequently tunneled deep in the thigh and, consequently, are more difficult to image. A mid-range transducer is

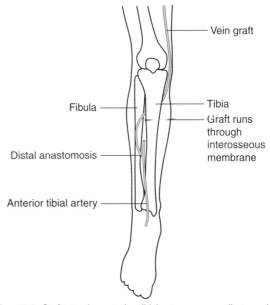

Fig. 15.7 Grafts to the anterior tibial artery are usually tunneled through the interosseous membrane between the tibia and fibula.

usually required for imaging such grafts. The graft is best located in transverse section as it divides from the native artery. The graft may drop away deeply from the proximal anastomosis. If the proximal anastomosis is located at the common femoral artery, the graft can be mistaken for the profunda femoris artery, or vice versa. If the graft lies deep, it may be very difficult to follow from the medial aspect of the thigh, and it can be easier to image from a posterior thigh position. If the graft is proving very difficult to locate in the thigh, attempt to find a more distal segment around the level of the knee in the popliteal fossa and work upward. In some cases, it may be necessary to use a low-frequency transducer to locate a deep segment of graft in the thigh or calf (see Fig. 15.8).

Synthetic Grafts

The majority of problems occurring in synthetic grafts are located at the proximal or distal anastomosis. It is rare for problems to develop in the main body of the

graft, and a surveillance scan can often take the form of a spot check for patency combined with a more detailed assessment of the anastomosis. It is necessary to perform a detailed assessment of the inflow and outflow of the graft when abnormal graft flow is recorded in the absence of any obvious graft defect.

For inflow grafts anastomosed to the common femoral arteries, the proximal profunda artery and superficial femoral artery should be checked for any stenoses or occlusions that might compromise flow in the graft due to increased outflow resistance.

Femoropopliteal PTFE Grafts

These are scanned in a similar fashion to vein grafts. The graft is often tunneled deep in the leg.

Aortobifemoral Grafts

These are imaged by locating the graft at the level of the groin and following it proximally to the aorta. A combination of low- and mid-frequency transducers is required for this examination.

Femorofemoral Cross-Over Grafts

These can be imaged by starting at either groin and following the graft across the pubic region to the

TABLE 15.1 Common Transducer Positions for Imaging the Distal Anastomosis of an Infrainguinal Graft	
Level of Anastomosis	**Transducer Position**
Above-knee popliteal artery	Medial aspect of lower thigh or posterior lower thigh just above popliteal fossa
Below-knee popliteal artery and tibioperoneal trunk	Popliteal fossa or posterior, lateral, and medial aspects of upper calf
Posterior tibial artery	Medial aspect of calf
Peroneal artery	Medial aspect of calf or from a lateral posterior position
Anterior tibial artery	Anterolateral aspect of calf

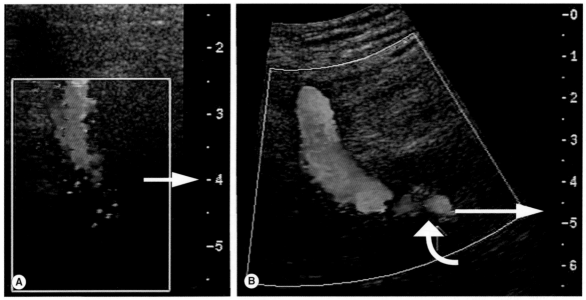

Fig. 15.8 Two images of the same graft toward the distal anastomosis, located in the lower thigh of a patient with healing wounds. (A) A mid-range transducer is unable to show flow in the distal section of the graft below 4 cm depth *(arrow)*. (B) A low-frequency transducer demonstrates flow to the anastomosis *(curved arrow)*, which is located at a depth of 4.5 cm. This will allow for interrogation with spectral Doppler.

opposite side. This can normally be achieved with a mid-frequency transducer.

Iliofemoral Cross-Over Grafts

These grafts are easier to scan by starting at the distal anastomosis at the level of the femoral artery and following the graft back to the proximal anastomosis in the contralateral iliac artery. A combination of mid-frequency linear and low-frequency curvilinear transducers is needed for this assessment. It is useful to scan the iliac artery above the proximal anastomosis to identify any inflow disease.

Axillobifemoral Grafts

These usually remain relatively superficial along their length. The cross-over section of the graft can be scanned starting from the distal anastomosis at the femoral artery and following it to its bifurcation from the main segment of the graft on the opposite side of the body. The remainder of the graft is then imaged from the ipsilateral groin, along the lateral wall of the abdomen and chest, to the infraclavicular fossa, where the anastomosis to the axillary artery can be imaged.

B-MODE IMAGES

Normal Appearance

Vein Grafts

The graft lumen should be clear and of a reasonably even caliber. Some gentle tapering is often seen in the lower portion of an in situ vein graft or non-reversed graft, as the native great saphenous vein is smaller in the lower leg. In contrast, the proximal lumen of a reversed vein graft may be smaller in caliber than the distal graft. It is common to see slight areas of dilation along a vein graft at points corresponding to valve sites. The proximal and distal anastomoses are sometimes difficult to image clearly, due to surrounding scar tissue or depth. It may be difficult to image a deep reversed vein graft without color flow imaging.

Synthetic Grafts

Synthetic grafts made of PTFE produce a characteristic image, with the anterior and posterior walls displaying a "double line" appearance due to the strong reflection of ultrasound (Fig. 15.9). Some PTFE grafts are externally supported by rings that can be seen on the image (see Fig. 2.36). The corrugated structure of Dacron grafts,

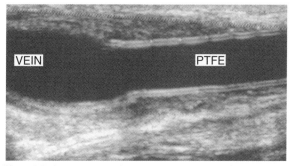

Fig. 15.9 An example of a composite polytetrafluorethylene *(PTFE)* and vein graft.

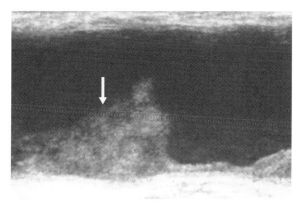

Fig. 15.10 In this magnified B-mode image, a large area of intimal hyperplasia *(arrow)* is seen in a vein graft.

used mainly for aortobifemoral bypass surgery, is usually easy to see. Vein cuffs or collars are sometimes used to join the graft to the distal native artery, and these are often seen as a short dilation at the anastomosis.

Abnormal Appearance

Many vein graft stenoses are difficult to identify with B-mode imaging alone, as they can be short or web-like and poorly echogenic. Larger areas of hyperplasia can appear as moderately echogenic regions in the vessel lumen (Fig. 15.10). It is sometimes possible to see remnant valve cusps flapping in the lumen of in situ vein grafts due to inadequate stripping with the valvulotome. Areas of vein grafts may become tortuous and dilated over time, and changes in graft diameter should be recorded. In some cases, large areas of thrombus or hyperplasia can be seen in aneurysmal segments, and the B-mode image may show partial stagnation or stasis of blood flow in these areas. This will be visualized as strong specular reflections in the dilated region, swirling in time with arterial pulsation. True and false aneurysms of vein or synthetic grafts can be easily seen and are discussed later in this chapter.

COLOR DOPPLER IMAGES

Normal Appearance of Vein Grafts

The color flow image often demonstrates areas of flow disturbance and flow reversal at the proximal anastomosis due to the size, geometry, and orientation of the graft origin from the native artery. This may also be seen at the level of the distal anastomosis and should not be considered abnormal unless spectral Doppler recordings demonstrate significant velocity changes. Beyond the proximal anastomosis, the color flow image should demonstrate an undisturbed flow pattern. Grafts with well-established biphasic or triphasic flow will display normal reversal of flow (from red to blue or vice versa) during the diastolic phase. New grafts may demonstrate hyperemic flow due to peripheral dilation and the flow requirements of healing tissue, exhibited as constant forward flow throughout the cardiac cycle. If the graft has a large lumen, the flow velocity may be very low, and the PRF/color scale may have to be significantly lowered to demonstrate color filling. Some areas of flow reversal may be seen in areas of vein grafts corresponding to valve sites. In rare instances in which the vein is found to be bifid for a short segment, it is possible to see two flow lumens. The distal anastomosis of a femoral distal graft is usually easier to identify with color flow imaging than with B-mode imaging. It is common to see the graft supplying a patent segment of the native artery above the anastomosis as well as distally, and retrograde flow will be seen in the native vessel above the anastomosis, producing a Y-shaped junction (Fig. 15.11). There is often a considerable size discrepancy between the distal end of a vein graft, which can be quite large, and the outflow artery, which may be a smaller tibial vessel. This will cause a natural velocity increase due to the change in vessel diameter, possibly producing color aliasing at the position of the anastomosis and proximal run-off vessel, but this should not be assumed to indicate a significant stenosis without close interrogation with spectral Doppler. In some case the graft may be widely patent, but there may be calcified disease of the run-off vessels beyond the graft (Fig. 15.12).

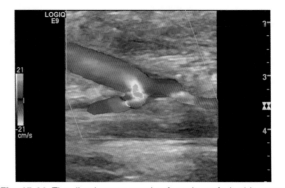

Fig. 15.11 The distal anastomosis of a vein graft. In this example of an end to side anastomosis the graft is also supplying a patent segment of the native vessel above the distal anastomosis (retrograde flow, *coded blue*).

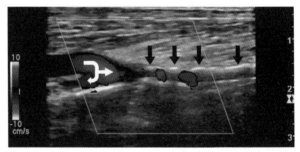

Fig. 15.12 There is evidence of calcified disease in the tibial artery beyond the distal anastomosis *(black arrows)* leading to poor color filling with a beaded appearance. The *white arrows* show direction of flow.

Normal Appearance of Synthetic Grafts

Flow in synthetic grafts can sometimes be difficult to demonstrate using color flow imaging, as the graft material attenuates the Doppler signal, requiring an increase in the color gain. Significant flow disturbance can be seen at the origins and ends of synthetic iliofemoral or femorofemoral cross-over grafts, as the graft is often joined at a 90° angle to the native artery (see Fig. 15.19).

Abnormal Appearance of Vein Grafts

A significant graft stenosis will produce marked flow disturbance, which is usually associated with aliasing on the color flow image (Figs. 15.13 and 15.14), and there may be considerable flow disturbance beyond the stenosis. Failing grafts may demonstrate very low-volume flow, which can sometimes be difficult to demonstrate with color flow imaging, and the graft may be mistakenly reported as occluded. If no flow is detected in the

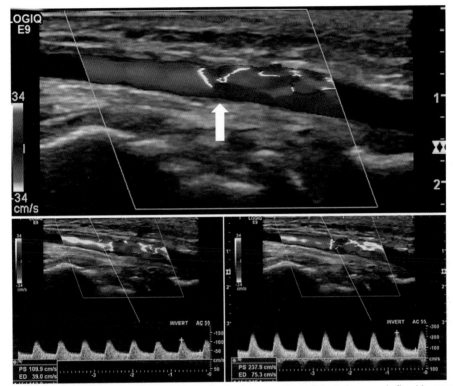

Fig. 15.13 A moderate stenosis is indicated in the body of a new vein graft (note hyperemic flow) by an area of color aliasing *(arrow)*. Spectral Doppler measurements show a moderate velocity increase across the stenosis from 110 to 238 cm/s, equivalent to 2.2 times velocity ratio. This should be monitored for any progression.

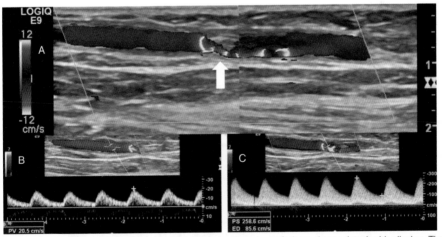

Fig. 15.14 (A) A severe stenosis in the main body of an in situ vein graft *(arrow)* associated with aliasing. The peak systolic velocity (PSV) ratio is used to estimate the degree of narrowing across a graft stenosis. (B) The PSV just proximal to the stenosis is 20.5 cm/s. (C) The PSV at the stenosis is 258 cm/s, associated with marked spectral broadening. This represents a 12.6 times velocity ratio, indicating a critical stenosis. In this example it is also apparent that there is a proximal problem above this region, as the Doppler waveform in the pre-stenotic section (B) demonstrates marked damping with increased systolic rise time, as compared to the hyperemic flow seen in Fig. 15.13.

graft, the color PRF and high-pass filter setting should be reduced to confirm the occlusion, which should also be checked with spectral Doppler. Arteriovenous fistulas and aneurysms are other graft abnormalities that are visible with color flow imaging, as discussed later.

SPECTRAL DOPPLER WAVEFORMS

Normal Appearance

> **CAUTION**
>
> Remember, when comparing peak systolic velocities in adjacent segments of a vessel with differing diameters, the respective velocities will be different even in the absence of a stenosis as flow velocity is inversely proportional to cross-sectional area (Fig. 15.16).

The waveform shapes in normal vein grafts can vary considerably depending on the age of the graft. New grafts may demonstrate a hyperemic monophasic flow profile because of sustained peripheral vasodilation that can be due to a combination of the previous ischemia and healing tissue (Fig. 15.15A). Over time, the flow pattern should become pulsatile, and biphasic or triphasic waveforms are usually recorded (Fig. 15.15B). It is good practice to take spectral Doppler measurements at regular intervals along a graft, even in the presence of a normal color flow display, as changes in the waveform shape can indicate an approaching problem. Disturbed flow, including areas of flow reversal, is usually encountered around the proximal anastomosis, but there should be no significant increase in systolic velocity (Fig. 15.15C). Natural changes in the diameter of the graft will produce changes in the peak systolic velocity (PSV), which should not automatically be assumed to represent a

stenosis. In this situation, velocities should be compared in adjacent areas of similar vessel diameter. Perhaps the most difficult assessment to make during graft surveillance is the estimation of the degree of narrowing at the distal anastomosis, where there is often a large-diameter vein graft joined to a smaller outflow artery, producing a natural velocity increase. In this situation, it is possible to see a significant increase in the PSV in the absence of a stenosis. However, flow velocities just below the distal anastomosis should be similar to those several centimeters downstream, provided that the vessel diameter is the same. A significant stenosis would be indicated if the velocities at the anastomosis were found to be substantially higher (i.e., three to four times) than distal velocities (Fig. 15.16). It is also important to ensure that the spectral Doppler angle is set correctly at the distal anastomosis, as flow is not always parallel to the vessel walls, and this can lead to errors in velocity measurements.

Abnormal Appearance

Graft stenoses are categorized using a similar method to that for grading lower-limb arterial disease. The PSV in the stenosis is divided by the PSV in a normal segment of graft just proximal to the stenosis (Figs. 15.13 and 15.14). There have been different criteria published for grading graft stenoses as shown in Tables 15.2 and 15.3 (London et al. 1993; Armstrong et al. 2004; Bandyk 2007). In addition, a PSV in a stenosis of >300 cm/s is also considered hemodynamically significant (Armstrong et al. 2004). It is important to validate criteria locally to determine when intervention by angioplasty or surgical revision is undertaken. Stenoses producing a PSV ratio of >2 but below the thresholds for intervention are kept under closer surveillance to monitor any progression. Conversely, a low graft PSV has been suggested as possible indicator of a failing graft. A study by Gibson

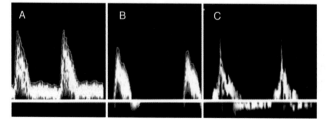

Fig. 15.15 Doppler waveforms can exhibit different patterns in the absence of disease. (A) Hyperemic flow is often seen in the early postoperative period. (B) Over time, the flow normally assumes a bidirectional flow pattern. (C) A Doppler waveform taken from the origin of a vein graft indicates a slightly disturbed flow pattern with systolic spikes due to the geometry of the anastomosis but there is no evidence of stenotic flow.

et al. (2001) found that a mean graft PSV (MGV) of <50 cm/s associated with a graft stenosis having a PSV ratio of >3.5 is a potential indicator for graft repair. The MGV is calculated by averaging the PSVs measured at several points along the entire graft excluding the velocities at any stenotic areas or at the proximal or distal anastomosis. However, grafts where the MGV was less than 50 cm/s and no detectable inflow, outflow, or graft lesions can be identified may be safely followed as the incidence of graft thrombosis in these grafts was low.

Damped flow in the artery proximal to the proximal anastomosis often indicates an inflow stenosis, and this should be examined with duplex, as poor inflow can lead to graft occlusion. A stenosis of the outflow artery below the distal anastomosis can also dramatically reduce flow in the graft by increasing distal resistance. For this reason, it is important to scan the run-off artery below the graft. However, it is interesting to note that some grafts remain patent for years, despite occlusion of the run-off vessel. This is due to retrograde flow into a patent segment of artery above the anastomosis, filling collateral vessels (Fig. 15.17).

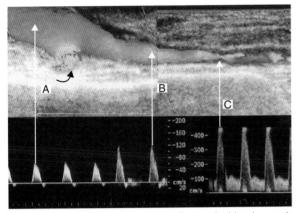

Fig. 15.16 Problems in interpreting flow velocities in a vein graft anastomosed to the posterior tibial artery. At point *A*, the peak systolic velocity (PSV) in the distal graft is 65 cm/s. At point *B* the PSV in the posterior tibial artery, just distal to the anastomosis, is 120 cm/s. This represents a near doubling in velocity, suggesting a stenosis. However, the diameter of the posterior tibial artery is significantly smaller than that of the distal graft, leading to a natural increase in systolic velocity, as flow velocity is inversely related to cross-sectional area, and in this example no narrowing is indicated. However, at point *C*, a significant stenosis is demonstrated in the posterior tibial artery, 2 cm distal to the anastomosis, by color flow aliasing and there is a significant increase in the PSV, >400 cm/s. In this image there is some retrograde filling of the native vessel above the anastomosis *(curved arrow)*.

TABLE 15.3 Spectral Doppler Criteria for Grading a Graft Stenosis

Peak Systolic Velocity (PSV) and PSV Ratio	Outcome
PSV < 150 cm/s and PSV ratio < 3.4	Normal surveillance follow-up. Use caution if PSV is ≥2.5
PSV ≥ 150 cm/s but <300 cm/s PSV ratio < 3.5	Reduced surveillance interval to 4–8 weeks
PSV ratio ≥ 3.5 PSV ≥ 300 cm/s	Hemodynamically significant stenosis. Consider intervention

Based on Armstrong et al. (2004) and Bandyk (2007).

TABLE 15.2 Spectral Doppler Criteria for Grading a Graft Stenosis

Diameter Reduction	Spectral Doppler Criteria
<50%	PSV ratio < 2
50%–69%	PSV ratio 2–2.9; increased spectral broadening and turbulence just beyond the stenosis; waveform becomes more monophasic Reduce surveillance interval to 4–8 weeks
70%–99%	PSV ratio ≥ 3; marked turbulence distal to the stenosis; waveform may be monophasic
Occlusion	No flow signal present

Based on London et al. (1993).

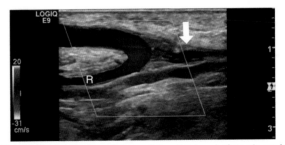

Fig. 15.17 A color flow image of the distal end of a vein graft demonstrates occlusion of the posterior tibial artery *(arrow)* at the distal anastomosis. However, the graft remains patent due to retrograde flow *(R)*, filling a segment of native vessel above the anastomosis.

GRAFT FAILURE AND OCCLUSION

Despite the most aggressive surveillance programs, some grafts will occlude for a variety of reasons. Occluded vein grafts can be difficult to identify by B-mode imaging, especially if the graft lies deep, as it may merge into the tissue planes. When it is possible to identify the graft, there is usually thrombus seen within the lumen. An occluded graft is usually easiest to identify by scanning at the level of the proximal anastomosis. The most obvious signs of graft occlusion are an absence of color flow and spectral Doppler signals. Ankle–brachial pressures will also be reduced and demonstrate audibly damped waveforms. A thrombosing graft may contain clot at the distal end, and spectral Doppler will demonstrate a characteristic low-volume, high-resistance flow pattern in the patent lumen above this area with no net forward flow (Fig. 15.18). In this situation the B-mode image may demonstrate slight backward and forward pulsation of the blood, exhibited as motion of the speckle pattern. This indicates imminent graft occlusion and should be reported immediately. Conversely, a low-volume damped waveform in the proximal graft would indicate an inflow stenosis. It is normally easy to identify occlusions of synthetic grafts as the synthetic walls are normally prominent, but no color filling is recorded (Fig. 15.19). The only caution is with newly implanted grafts as the fabric takes a few days to become porous to blood before adequate color and spectral Doppler signals can be recorded across the wall. In this situation good pulsatile flow should still be observed in the run-off vessels.

COMMONLY ENCOUNTERED PROBLEMS

Patients with a high body mass index can be difficult to examine, and it may be necessary to use a lower-frequency transducer (Fig. 15.8). Early postoperative scans can be difficult if the wounds are still healing and scanning over a sterile transparent plastic dressing is useful in this situation. Having no prior knowledge of the type and position of graft can lead to considerable problems. For example, a popliteal to pedal vein bypass graft may require the great saphenous vein to be harvested from the thigh, as it is larger at this level. Therefore, a large scar will be seen in the thigh, but the graft will not be located at this level; however, the sonographer may automatically assume that this corresponds to

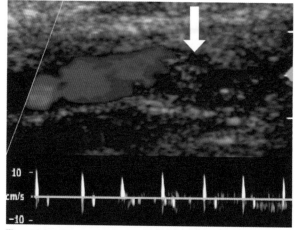

Fig. 15.18 Extremely low-volume flow recorded from an in situ vein graft indicates imminent graft occlusion. In this example the distal end of the graft had already thrombosed *(arrow)* and the Doppler waveform recorded from the graft coded red demonstrates no net forward flow.

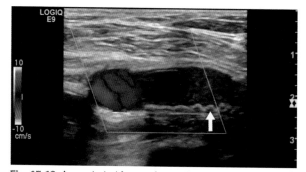

Fig. 15.19 An occluded femorofemoral cross-over graft is seen at the anastomosis to the right common femoral artery. Thrombus is seen within the graft. Note the corrugated appearance of the graft material *(arrow)*. It can also be seen that the anastomosis is at right angles to the femoral artery, which is common for this type of procedure.

the position of the proximal graft. A copy of the operation notes is a useful aid to locating the graft. If no operation details are available, it can also be very informative asking the patient about their surgical history, or even if they have had any cardiac surgery resulting in removal of a vein.

It is also possible for grafts to be routed in unusual directions, such as across the anterolateral thigh to join the anterior tibial artery in the calf. Some patients may have had a previous graft that has since occluded, and this could be mistaken for the new graft, which may still be patent. It is also possible for segments of native vessels to be patent, such as the superficial femoral artery, and this may cause some confusion or may even be mistaken for the graft.

TRUE AND FALSE ANEURYSMS

Vein grafts can develop true aneurysmal dilations over time, particularly at valve sites or at the anastomoses (Fig. 15.20). This can occur if the vein wall becomes structurally weak. A localized doubling in the graft diameter indicates the development of an aneurysm, and this should be reported and kept under regular surveillance to monitor progression. It is not uncommon to see thrombus in aneurysmal areas. Color flow imaging and spectral Doppler usually demonstrate areas of flow reversal in the aneurysmal regions. Large true aneurysms are repaired surgically by replacing the aneurysmal area with a new segment of vein.

False aneurysms are caused by blood flowing into and out of a defect in the vessel wall (see Ch. 11). They are typified as swirling areas of flow in a contained cavity outside the true flow lumen and may contain thrombus. They can occur if the suture line at the anastomosis fails or as a complication of balloon angioplasty, due to splitting of the graft wall following high-pressure balloon inflation (Fig. 15.21). False aneurysms also occur at catheter puncture sites (see Ch. 11).

ENTRAPMENT OF GRAFTS

Entrapment of grafts can occur around the knee level, especially where in situ vein grafts run from superficial to deep, through a tunnel in the muscles. In this situation, normal flow may be recorded with the leg extended, but mild-to-moderate flexion of the knee joint produces pinching of the graft between muscle groups, causing a temporary stenosis (see Fig. 15.22). Conversely, some grafts become temporarily obstructed during full knee extension. This is a relatively rare problem, but it will be seen from time to time in a busy laboratory. If the problem is significant, the muscle can be divided or the graft rerouted.

ARTERIOVENOUS FISTULAS

Arteriovenous fistulas occur in in situ vein grafts where there has been incomplete ligation of a great saphenous vein side branch, allowing blood to short-circuit from the graft directly into the venous system. Arteriovenous

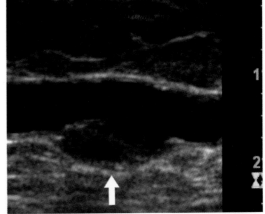

Fig. 15.20 An aneurysmal area in a vein graft corresponding to a valve site. Note the area of hyperplasia or thrombus *(arrow)* in the area of dilation.

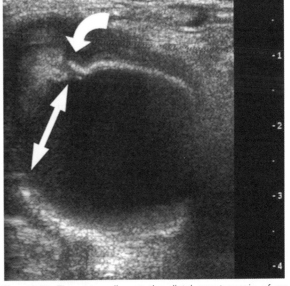

Fig. 15.21 The suture line at the distal anastomosis of an aortobifemoral graft has failed and a large gap is now visible between the graft material *(double-headed arrow)*, creating a false aneurysm, which in this case mainly contains thrombus *(curved arrow)*.

fistulas are characterized by hyperemic or high-volume flow in the graft proximal to the fistula, with an area of marked color flow disturbance at the site of the fistula. Spectral Doppler also demonstrates turbulent high-volume flow with a low-resistance waveform at this site. The veins leading from the fistula also demonstrate a high-volume flow pattern. Flow in the graft distal to the

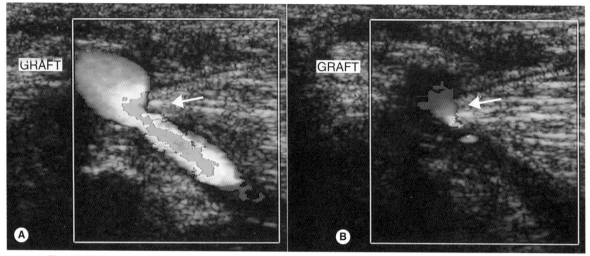

Fig. 15.22 An example of graft entrapment. (A) A vein graft is running between two muscles in the lower thigh, and a moderate stenosis is seen *(arrow)*. (B) During leg flexion the graft is compressed between the muscles, causing a virtual occlusion *(arrow)*.

fistula is usually lower in volume and more pulsatile. In some circumstances, the graft below the site of the fistula may be totally occluded. Arteriovenous fistulas can be ligated or embolized. It is useful to mark the level of the defect using duplex so that the surgeon can easily locate the fistula.

SEROMAS, FLUID COLLECTIONS, AND GRAFT INFECTIONS

Seromas are serous fluid collections that can occur following surgery, and they are occasionally seen adjacent to vein grafts, particularly at the level of the groin. They can be mistaken for false aneurysms on B-mode imaging, but color flow imaging will demonstrate an absence of flow (Fig. 15.23). Fluid collections around synthetic grafts can be due to local reaction of the surrounding tissues, but they can also be due to graft infection (Fig. 15.24). Graft infections are a serious complication and are more frequently associated with synthetic grafts. The outcome for patients with synthetic graft infections is often poor (Siracuse et al. 2013). Infections at the level of the groin are common due to the rich source of bacteria in this region, and aortobifemoral, iliofemoral, and axillobifemoral grafts are especially at risk. Complications of infection can lead to the disintegration of a graft anastomosis, resulting in false aneurysm or severe

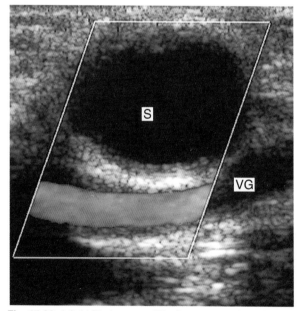

Fig. 15.23 A fluid-filled seroma *(S)* adjacent to a vein graft *(VG)*.

hemorrhage. Failure of wound healing is also a frequent complication. Ultrasound imaging can be useful for investigating wound infections, as the B-mode image can show whether the graft is in direct contact with suspected areas of infection, especially if the suspected region tracks to discharging wounds or openings on the

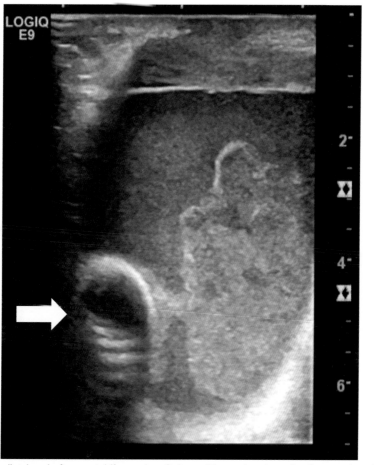

Fig. 15.24 The distal end of an aortobifemoral graft *(arrow)* is running through a large region of echogenic fluid that is tracking to the skin surface and is suspicious for a region of infection.

skin surface. It is essential to image any suspected area of graft infection in cross-section to see how it relates to the graft and surrounding structures. It can be difficult to differentiate areas of infection from simple hematomas. Computed tomography and magnetic resonance imaging are also commonly used for investigating graft infections, especially in the abdomen where the use of duplex is very limited. Antimicrobial-resistant infections such as methicillin-resistant *Staphylococcus aureus* (MRSA) are now endemic in most hospitals. Graft infections caused by bacteria resistant to antibiotics are difficult to treat, requiring prolonged use of powerful antibiotics. In some cases, graft removal is necessary to remove the focus of infection, but this may lead to inevitable amputation of the limb due to poor blood flow. In extreme situations, the patient may be overwhelmed by the infection and die.

REPORTING

As well as a written report, supported by images, a useful method of reporting the scan results is by the use of diagrams. The graft position can be drawn onto the diagram with velocity measurements and other relevant information recorded (Fig. 15.25). It is also useful to keep a file for each patient in the graft surveillance program

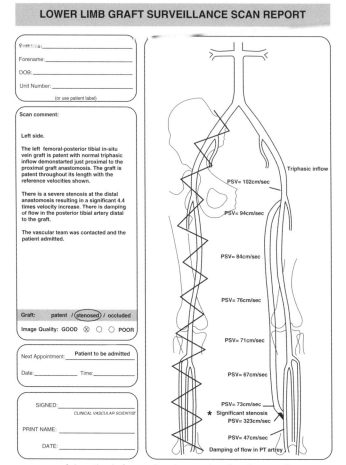

LOWER LIMB GRAFT SURVEILLANCE SCAN REPORT

Surname: _____

Forename: _____

DOB: _____

Unit Number: _____

(or use patient label)

Scan comment:

Left side.

The left femoral-posterior tibial in-situ vein graft is patent with normal triphasic inflow demonstarted just proximal to the proximal graft anastomosis. The graft is patent throughout its length with the reference velocities shown.

There is a severe stenosis at the distal anastomosis resulting in a significant 4.4 times velocity increase. There is damping of flow in the posterior tibial artery distal to the graft.

The vascular team was contacted and the patient admitted.

Graft: patent / (stenosed) / occluded

Image Quality: GOOD ⊗ ○ ○ POOR

Next Appointment: **Patient to be admitted**

Date: _____ Time: _____

SIGNED: _____
CLINICAL VASCULAR SCIENTIST

PRINT NAME: _____

DATE: _____

Triphasic inflow

PSV= 102cm/sec

PSV= 94cm/sec

PSV= 84cm/sec

PSV= 76cm/sec

PSV= 71cm/sec

PSV= 67cm/sec

PSV= 73cm/sec
★ Significant stenosis
PSV= 323cm/sec

PSV= 47cm/sec

Damping of flow in PT artrey

Fig. 15.25 Diagrams are a useful method of reporting the results of graft surveillance scans. It is easy to mark the area of stenosis. *PSV,* Peak systolic velocity.

in the vascular laboratory, as this makes comparison of serial follow-up scans easier. Any significant graft problems must be reported to the appropriate medical staff immediately. In addition, many vascular units combine the duplex assessment with a measurement of the ankle–brachial pressure index (ABPI). An ABPI <1 can indicate a problem. A serial reduction <0.15 in ABPI readings can be indicative of a significant problem (Nielsen 1996).

SUPERFICIAL VEIN MAPPING FOR ARTERIAL BYPASS SURGERY

A preoperative duplex scan can determine the suitability of a superficial vein for use as a bypass graft (Linni et al. 2012). Careful marking of its path avoids undermining of skin flaps during surgery and possible wound necrosis. The great saphenous vein is the most commonly used vein for arterial

bypass surgery, due to its length. Arm veins and the small saphenous vein can also be used for bypass grafts, provided that their lumens are of sufficient diameter. Preoperative marking can also be performed prior to coronary bypass surgery and the GSV in the calf is the main site for harvest.

Technique for Assessing the Great Saphenous Vein

OBSERVATION

Normal non-varicose great saphenous veins having a borderline diameter (2.5–3 mm) in younger patients can be relatively compliant and will dilate to a larger diameter when exposed to arterial pressure. Try examining the leg in a dependent position. Any doubts about vein suitability should be discussed with the surgeon.

The patient should be positioned with the feet tilted down to distend the veins. A high-frequency, flat linear array or hockey-stick transducer should be used to image the veins unless the vein is lying deep in a large leg. A venous preset is selected, but it is also useful to have a reasonable amount of contrast in the image and decreasing dynamic range can help to distinguish the vein from surrounding tissue. Starting at the top of the leg, the great saphenous vein should be identified in transverse section at the level of the saphenofemoral junction and followed distally down the thigh and into the calf. Scanning the vein in transverse section is important, because it is easier to assess its diameter and to identify any large tributaries dividing from the vein, or duplicated or bifid systems. The diameter of the vein should be recorded at frequent intervals throughout its length. Ideally, the diameter should be greater than 3 mm to be suitable as a graft. Veins of less than 2 mm in diameter are regarded as too small to be used for femoral distal bypass grafting. Veins that become excessively large (0.8–1 cm diameter) or grossly varicose may also be unsuitable, and this should be drawn to the attention of the surgeon. The common femoral vein, femoral vein, and popliteal vein should be examined when vein mapping to ensure deep venous patency, as the great saphenous vein can act as an important collateral pathway if the deep veins have been obstructed and, in such circumstances, should not be harvested for a graft. In this situation, other sources of vein can be assessed.

For mapping calf veins for coronary bypass surgery, a high-frequency flat linear array or hockey-stick transducer should be used. The depth setting should be in the region of 3 cm. The vein is easiest to locate in the lower calf in cross-section and then tracked proximally to the knee.

Arm Vein Mapping

It is not uncommon to find that part or all of the great saphenous vein is unsuitable for use as a graft because it is too small, because it is varicose, or because the deep veins are obstructed. In addition, the great saphenous vein may have already been removed for coronary artery bypass surgery. The cephalic or basilic veins of the arm can be harvested for bypass grafts provided they are of adequate diameter. The cephalic vein is the vein of choice, as it is longer than the basilic vein, and the anatomy of the basilic vein is more variable in its proximal segment. To image the veins, the arm should be in a comfortable dependent position with the palm facing upward. The cephalic vein can be located in transverse section along the outer aspect of the forearm 2 to 3 cm above the wrist, lateral to the radial artery and followed proximally. Alternatively, it can be located in the anterior aspect of the upper arm, lying superficial to the biceps muscle and then followed proximally toward the shoulder and then distally into the forearm (Fig. 15.26A). The vein can be difficult to follow as it crosses the antecubital fossa, as there are a number of superficial veins crossing this area.

The basilic vein is easiest to locate with the arm extended outward (abducted) and the palm facing upward. The probe is placed on the medial aspect of the arm 2 to 3 cm above the elbow joint. Imaging in cross-section, the basilic vein should be seen as separate from the brachial vein and artery (Fig. 15.26B). The vein can then be followed proximally, where it is usually seen to course toward the proximal brachial vein or the axillary vein, although there can be anatomical variation of the veins in this region. Following the basilic vein distally into the forearm can be confusing, as it sometimes joins the cephalic vein in the forearm via the median cubital vein, but it usually runs toward the medial (ulnar) aspect of the wrist. One potential pitfall of mapping the basilic vein is accidentally confusing it with the brachial artery or brachial vein but use of probe compression to collapse the vein and color flow imaging to identify arterial flow should avoid this error.

Technique of Marking the Vein

There are two techniques for marking leg or arm veins (Fig. 15.27). Using the first method, the vein is imaged in transverse section with the vein appearing in the center of the image. Using a marker pen, a dot is then placed on the skin surface against the middle of the probe. It is easier to start by marking the vein in the upper thigh, rather than at the level of the saphenofemoral junction, and then to work toward the saphenofemoral junction. The vein should be marked with a dot at frequent intervals along the thigh and calf. Finally, the gel is completely removed and the dots joined up with a continuous line using a permanent felt-tipped marker pen.

The second technique involves assessing the vein in transverse section for its size and position, and then marking the vein with the transducer turned into a longitudinal plane and the vein imaged in this direction. A dot is placed against the end of the transducer to correspond to the position and direction of the vein. This technique is more difficult in terms of imaging,

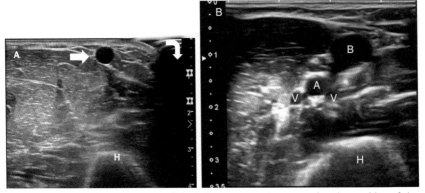

Fig. 15.26 (A) A transverse B-mode image of the left upper arm demonstrating the position of the cephalic vein *(arrow)*. The humerus *(H)* can be seen. It can be very easy to lose contact with the skin surface *(arrow)* due to the curvature of the arm. (B) A transverse image showing the basic vein *(B)* and brachial artery *(A)* and veins *(V)*. The arm was positioned with the palm facing up. The humerus is also seen *(H)*.

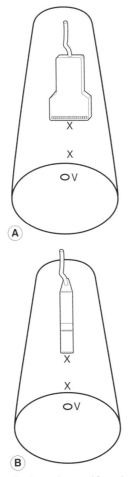

Fig. 15.27 Two methods can be used for vein mapping. (A) The vein *(V)* can be marked *(X)* in the transverse plane. (B) The vein can also be marked in a longitudinal plane.

as it is easy to "slip off" the image of the vein and follow a tissue plane, but it does seem to produce a more accurate map of the vein. When the position of the vein has been marked using this technique, it is wise to run down the length of marking with the transducer in transverse section to ensure that the dots follow the main trunk, in case a smaller side branch in the lower leg may have accidentally been followed using this method.

Problems Encountered During Vein Mapping

One major practical problem of vein mapping is trying to mark the position of the vein with a felt-tipped pen through the ultrasound gel, as the pen quickly becomes clogged with gel and no longer works. Many vascular units have their own personal preferences for overcoming this problem. A charcoal pencil can be useful for dotting in the position of the vein and the dots joined up later with a felt-tipped pen once the gel has been removed. Alternatively, using small amounts of gel and frequently wiping the gel away from the probe edge before marking prevents the pen tip from becoming saturated in ultrasound gel. It is also useful to place a nonsterile probe cover over the transducer when vein mapping, as this prevents the probe from becoming covered in ink from the marker pen.

If the patient has very poor muscle volume and the superficial tissues are baggy, it can be very difficult to ensure that the marking is accurate. If in any doubt, tell the surgeon. In obese patients, the vein may be very deep, and it can be difficult to mark it in the correct incision plane.

Ultrasound of Hemodialysis Access

INTRODUCTION

Ultrasound has an important role in planning temporary and permanent hemodialysis access, for examining permanent access fistulas and grafts prior to first use, and in the investigation of complications in these fistulas and grafts. Ultrasound has been proposed as a means for surveillance of hemodialysis access although its effectiveness in this role is controversial.

Portable ultrasound scanners may be used by dialysis units to aid needling where access is difficult. For a more detailed examination of the access, radiology departments and vascular laboratories are equipped to undertake ultrasound investigation of the whole access circuit. The high flows, unusual hemodynamics, and anatomy of fistulas and grafts can make this a challenging investigation but it is potentially a rewarding one. Ultrasound is a quick, safe, and effective means to identify existing and impending problems, enabling early radiological or surgical intervention to prolong the use of the existing access and to plan effective alternatives.

HEMODIALYSIS ACCESS

Hemodialysis requires high blood flow, from 250 to 400 mL/min, to the extracorporeal dialyzer. Hemodialysis is required in the following.

Acute Renal Failure

Following a sudden loss of renal function, dialysis or hemofiltration is usually via a central venous catheter. Ultrasound is used to examine central neck and arm veins and to guide catheter placement. In patients with reversible failure, renal replacement therapy is discontinued as the kidneys recover. In kidneys with irreversible failure, permanent access is planned, since venous catheters have a limited life.

Chronic Renal Failure

Once chronic end-stage renal failure is identified, measurement of the patient's creatinine levels and estimated glomerular filtration rate (eGFR) are used to determine the impending need for dialysis. Ideally, as the prospect of dialysis approaches, permanent access is planned and surgery undertaken so that the access is ready in time for first use.

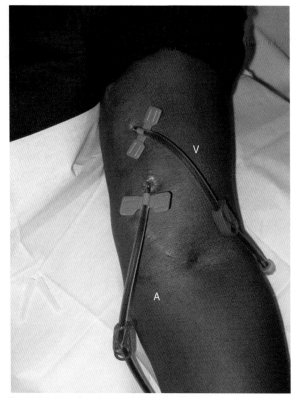

Fig. 16.1 Needles inserted into the basilic vein of a brachial artery/transposed basilic vein fistula prior to dialysis. The distal, upstream, needle is referred to as the arterial needle *(A)* from which blood is drawn for dialysis. Blood is returned through the venous needle *(V)*.

Permanent access, through a fistula or graft, requires high flows through a superficial vein or graft that can be repeatedly needled (Fig. 16.1), is easy to keep clean, and is comfortable for the patient during their periods of dialysis—typically three times a week each of around 4 hours' duration. American and European reviews and guidelines (NKF-K/DOQI, EBPG—European Best Practice Guidelines; Lok et al. [2019]; Tordoir et al. [2007]) have been produced and are updated to foster good hemodialysis practice. Both contain comprehensive bibliographies.

Access Sites

Permanent hemodialysis accesses can be either an arteriovenous fistula where the vein is used for needle access or a prosthetic graft between an artery and vein. Fistulas generally have a lower incidence

> **BOX 16.1   Main Sites for A-V Fistulas and Grafts in Approximate Order of Preference**
>
> - Radiocephalic fistula
> - Brachiocephalic fistula
> - Brachial artery–transposed basilic vein fistula
> - Forearm graft from radial artery to cubital fossa vein or looped graft from brachial artery to cubital fossa vein
> - Upper-arm graft brachial artery to axillary vein
> - Femoral–femoral loop graft
> - Axillary artery–contralateral axillary vein graft

of complications than grafts (0.2 events/patient/year cf 0.8–1.0 events/patient/year, EBPG) and superior long-term patency. Grafts can be used earlier following surgery whereas fistulas need more time for the vein to develop and diameter to increase, typically 6 weeks postoperatively. Recommendations are to use fistulas where possible initially.

There are several possible sites for fistulas and grafts in the arms. Once arm accesses are exhausted, femoral artery to femoral vein grafts may be used. Several unusual variations of grafts and veins are possible where access is difficult, depending on the preference of the surgeon and the availability and access of suitable arteries and veins.

The main sites for fistulas and grafts are listed in Box 16.1 and shown diagrammatically in Fig. 16.2. The non-dominant arm is generally used initially. The list shows an approximate order of preference; the choice for an individual patient depends on many factors. For example, a young patient with good peripheral arm vessels may be a better candidate for a radiocephalic fistula, whereas an elderly patient with diabetes and known peripheral vascular disease might start dialysis with a more proximal access. A major advantage of a peripheral fistula is that it may leave more proximal vessels available for future accesses.

Temporary Access—Role of Ultrasound

Ultrasound is useful to assess central veins to ensure patency for emergency central dialysis catheter placement in patients with acute renal failure of failed permanent access. The patient should be lying flat so that the central veins are not collapsed. The internal and external jugular veins are examined using a low-frequency (4–8 MHz) linear array in B-mode and with color and pulsed

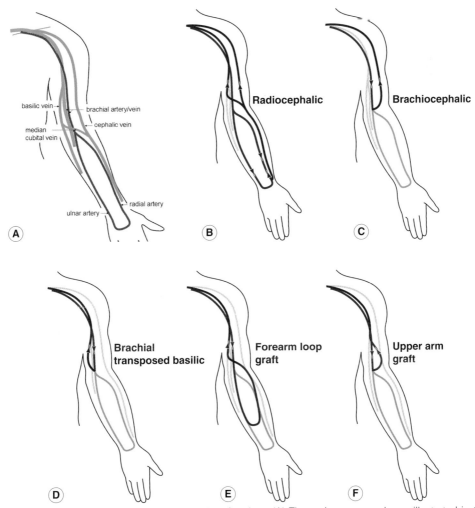

basilic vein

brachial artery/vein

cephalic vein

median cubital vein

radial artery

ulnar artery

(A)

Radiocephalic

(B)

Brachiocephalic

(C)

Brachial transposed basilic

(D)

Forearm loop graft

(E)

Upper arm graft

(F)

Fig. 16.2 Diagram of common arm fistula and grafts sites. (A) The main arm vessels are illustrated in the upper left image. In the other images, the arterial supply and venous drainage for the high-flow dialysis access circulation are shown in *bold*.

Doppler to ensure patency and normal venous flow patterns. The subclavian veins may be imaged in long section either supraclavicularly or infraclavicularly (Fig. 16.3). The subclavian vein often collapses during the cardiac cycle or in response to breathing or sniffing. The R and L proximal internal jugular vein and subclavian veins may be difficult to image with a linear array due to clavicle, sternum, and ribs that restrict ultrasound access. A small footprint phased or tightly curved array (Fig. 16.4) aids in color flow imaging of these veins (Fig. 16.5) and the brachiocephalic veins, although B-mode images are poor and compression of all these veins, to rule out deep venous thrombosis (DVT), is impossible.

If central stenosis or occlusion is suspected, venography is usually performed.

PERMANENT ACCESS

Preassessment

A successful dialysis access requires good inflow and outflow. Poor selection of vessels for permanent access is associated with high failure rates. As dialysis is increasingly offered to older patients and those with diabetes and arterial disease, ultrasound has an important role to complement physical examination in identifying the most suitable site for access surgery. Trials have shown

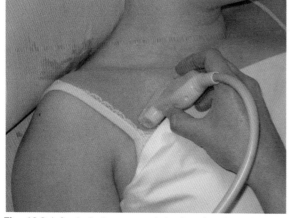

Fig. 16.3 Infraclavicular approach for imaging the subclavian vein with a linear array.

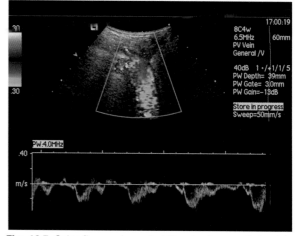

Fig. 16.5 Color flow and spectral Doppler image of the right brachiocephalic vein. The B-mode image is poor but contiguous color flow and venous waveform fluctuations indicate normal venous return.

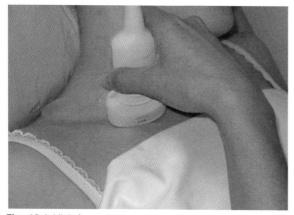

Fig. 16.4 High-frequency curvilinear array used to image the brachiocephalic vein.

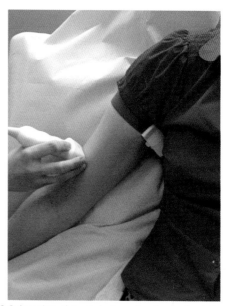

Fig. 16.6 Imaging the cephalic vein. A proximal tourniquet causes the vein to enlarge.

that ultrasound measurement of arterial and venous diameters can be predictive of likely success of a radiocephalic fistula. In reviewing the results of published investigations, European recommendations are that the minimum diameter of radial artery and cephalic vein at the wrist level should be 2 mm, although 2.5 mm is also used as a threshold (ACR 2016).

Technique for Assessing Arm Veins and Arteries

The arm to be imaged is supported comfortably with the palm of the hand uppermost (Fig. 16.6). For the superficial veins, a high-frequency (for example, 8–14 MHz) linear array is used. A tourniquet is applied proximal to the measurement sites to occlude venous return, and the veins are allowed to expand (Fig. 16.7).

It is important to use very light pressure; even with a tourniquet, veins are readily compressed and the diameter may be underestimated. Vein diameter can be affected by temperature and the patient's state of hydration. The veins are measured in transverse section and are scanned through their length to check for patency, narrowing, particularly near confluences/bifurcations,

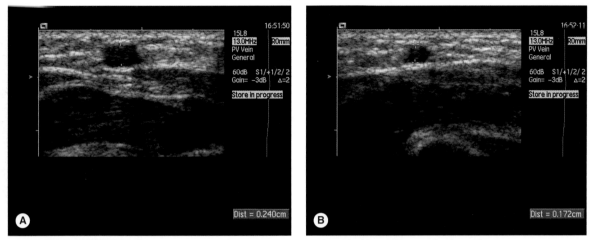

Fig. 16.7 Transverse image of cephalic vein with (A) and without (B) a proximal tourniquet.

anatomical variations (for example, large veins communicating with the deep veins), and continuity of flow. The proximal cephalic vein may be compressed extrinsically by surrounding tissue just before its insertion to the axillary vein. This is sometimes relieved by relaxation of the arm. Measurements of the internal diameter of the cephalic vein in the forearm and upper arm are recorded, as is the diameter of the basilic vein in the upper arm. It is important to ensure that there is a sufficient length of basilic vein (>4 cm) before its confluence with the brachial vein, since formation of a brachial artery–transposed basilic vein fistula requires a sufficient length of straight vein for successful needling.

The deep veins are imaged to ensure patency for the outflow of the fistula. For the proximal arm veins, axillary, and subclavian veins, a lower-frequency transducer may be required. Color filling of the deep veins is helpful where compression is impossible (Fig. 16.5). Flow waveforms in the proximal veins should show phasicity with respiration (Fig. 16.8). Lack of or reduced phasicity is an indication of possible proximal occlusion or stenosis; compare the waveforms with those on the contralateral side. A phased or curvilinear array may be helpful to determine central vein patency, but if there are suggestions or concerns of central vein stenosis or occlusion, alternative imaging is essential.

The arteries should be examined for normal pulsatile flow to wrist level. Radial artery internal diameter should be measured and note is taken of arterial disease, including general calcification in the arm arteries. Even moderate stenoses should be noted, as they can become

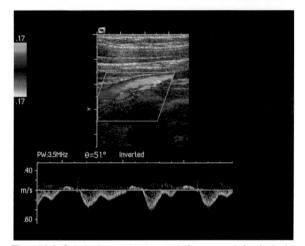

Fig. 16.8 Subclavian vein imaged from an infraclavicular approach. The flow waveform is phasic with changes in right atrial pressures, indicative of unimpeded venous return.

more hemodynamically significant with the larger flow volumes after fistula creation. It is important to identify the brachial bifurcation level if surgery in the cubital fossa is contemplated. For patients with evidence of arterial disease, measurement of right and left brachial artery blood pressure may reveal proximal disease.

A checklist of observations and measurements made is listed in Box 16.2.

Postoperative Assessment of Dialysis Access

Postoperatively, a fistula establishes a direct low-resistance path from artery to vein, bypassing the normal resistance vessels of the arm and hand. This leads

---

BOX 16.2   Measurements and Checklist for Arm Preassessment Scan for Hemodialysis Access

- Cephalic vein diameter upper arm/lower arm*
- Basilic vein diameter upper arm/lower arm*
- Anomalies (thrombus/stenosis/unusual anatomy) of superficial veins
- Patency of deep veins including brachial, axillary, subclavian, and brachiocephalic veins
- Radial artery internal diameter at wrist
- Normal flow waveforms in major arm arteries (including radial/ulnar/brachial)
- Level of brachial artery bifurcation
- Anomalies (calcification/occlusion/unusual anatomy) of arm arteries

Note: It should be stated whether the * measurements of superficial vein diameter are made with or without a proximal tourniquet.

---

to high flows through the supplying artery and draining fistula vein with a large pressure gradient at the fistula site leading to turbulence as the high-velocity blood flow turns though a large angle. The artery may expand slightly with time. The high flows and raised pressure in the vein (typically 30–40 mmHg) cause it to enlarge and the wall to thicken over time (Corpataux et al. 2002; Dixon 2006).

There is an initial large increase of flow into the vein followed by a gradual further increase for several weeks. The fistula is examined clinically to determine its readiness for dialysis, which occurs typically from about 6 weeks postoperatively onward. It is our practice to measure flow by duplex ultrasound at 6 weeks postoperatively and to record the size and depth of the fistula vein as a baseline record. This early scan also shows potential difficulties including multiple venous returns, venous occlusions, and abnormal flows, particularly low flows. The "rule of sixes" is a guide for satisfactory venous cannulation of a fistula; the flow should be at least 600 mL/min, the vein diameter at least 6 mm, and the depth of the vein should not exceed 6 mm. In practice, skilled dialysis nurses can needle veins as little as 4 mm diameter, and radiocephalic fistulas may be successfully used with lower flows, although early postoperative flows <400 mL/min have a high incidence of nonmaturation and failure (Tordoir et al. 2003).

If the fistula fails to mature at this stage or the dialysis staff have concerns, then a full ultrasound investigation is completed. Complications can include use of

inappropriate vessels, stenosis in the vein adjacent to the anastomosis from hyperplasia, stenosis in the supplying arteries or draining veins, thrombosis, or venous return through communicating veins to deep veins.

Grafts have a higher initial flow and can be used earlier. An early scan can confirm adequate flows and provide baseline values for flow and peak systolic velocities (PSVs) in the circuit.

Once in use, later complications of fistulas and grafts include:

- Stenosis. In fistulas this occurs most commonly in the vein close to the anastomosis or at needling sites and in the more central veins but may also occur in the artery or anastomosis. In grafts the most common site is at the venous anastomsosis
- Thrombosis
- Aneurysms/pseudoaneurysms
- Infection, which may lead to poor dialysis access function
- Steal
- Venous hypertension
- Congestive heart failure, which may require revision of the fistula or graft.

In grafts the most common complication is thrombosis, and in fistulas the most common is reduced flow from stenosis. Stenosis in the access circuit is commonplace even in fistulas and grafts with good function. The presence of a stenosis without other clinical or hemodynamic anomalies is not sufficient to classify the access as a dysfunctional access. These stenoses can usually be left untreated but can be monitored clinically and by ultrasound.

Ultrasound Investigation of Dialysis Access

The health of dialysis access is monitored by clinical examination and by the success of a patient's dialysis. If concerns are raised, then ultrasound is often used to image the access and make measurements of flow and vein diameter and any causes of poor access performance. The use of ultrasound depends on its availability and local practice.

Prior to starting the scan, it is important to get complete details for the patient's referral; good communication with the dialysis nursing staff is essential. For example, the cause of steal in the hand distal to fistula is more likely to be from arterial insufficiency, possibly due to proximal stenosis. The reason for high venous pressures is more likely to be a venous complication. Nurses' experience of the most recent dialysis sessions may be helpful and, for scans booked several days in advance, discussion with the patient can sometimes reveal that a problem has now resolved.

Volume Flow

Volume flow is an important indication of the health of the access. The ultrasound examination should always include a measurement of flow through the fistula or graft. Flows may range from 300–400 to 3000 mL/min, although most fall in the range 600 to 1500 mL/min.

Other techniques are available to measure flow at the time of dialysis, and there is a close correlation of these methods with duplex ultrasound. Volume flow is affected by severe stenoses anywhere in the access circuit. There is a high risk of thrombosis if flow falls below 300 mL/min in a fistula or 600 mL/min in a graft. Low flows lead to recirculation where blood leaving the dialyzer is drawn back into, it leading to inefficient dialysis (see Fig. 16.9). Recommendations are that investigations for the cause of low or reduced flow should be made if flows fall below a certain level or show a reduction in consecutive scans. Recommended criteria are given in Box 16.3.

Ultrasound measurement of volume flow is fraught with possible technical errors. There is also normal variation in measured flow in an access in individual patients, for example, pre- and post-dialysis. Despite this, the high flows in dialysis accesses and large changes in a failing access make this a practical and useful measurement in clinical practice.

The volume flow is calculated by:

$$\text{Volume flow (mL/min)} = \text{cross- sectional area}(cm^2) \times \text{mean velocity (cm/s)} \times 60.$$

The cross-sectional area is obtained from the diameter (area = diameter^2 × π/4) and mean velocity by obtaining the weighted time-averaged velocity over several cardiac cycles (see Fig. 16.10).

Flow should be measured in the supplying subclavian or brachial artery even for wrist fistulas for the following reasons:

- The subclavian and brachial arteries have a circular cross-section, enabling measurement of area to be obtained from diameter. Flow velocities are predominantly axial in the direction of the vessel, allowing good approximation of mean velocity to be measured. The arteries are relatively straight, permitting accurate Doppler angle correction.

- Most of the flow through the brachial artery is to the fistula/graft with only a small proportion supplying the forearm and hand. If measurements are obtained from the same position at subsequent visits, the change in flow reflects changes in the access circuit.

- In radiocephalic fistulas, flow to the fistula is usually both from the radial artery and ulnar artery via the arch (see Fig. 16.2). Measuring flow in the subclavian or brachial artery accounts for all of the flow to the fistula/graft.

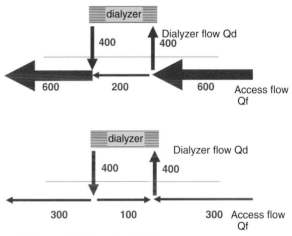

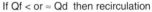

If Qf < or ≈ Qd then recirculation

Fig. 16.9 Diagram of adequate *(above)* and inadequate *(below)* access flow. If access flow falls to less or close to dialyzer flow, recirculation of blood from the venous needle back into the arterial needle leads to inefficient dialysis.

BOX 16.3 Criteria for Further Investigation/Intervention of Access

EBPG recommendations	
Grafts	<600 mL/min
	>20% reduction in flow/month
Forearm fistulas	<300 mL/min
NFK/DOQI guidelines	
Grafts	<600 mL/min
	Flow 1000 mL/min with decrease >25% over 4 months
Fistulas	No absolute measure recommended. Flows should be considered for individuals. It is noted that levels of <400 mL/min and 650 mL/min have been proposed.

DOQI, Kidney Disease Outcomes Quality Initiative Guidelines; *EBPG,* European Best Practice Guidelines; *NFK,* National Kidney Foundation.

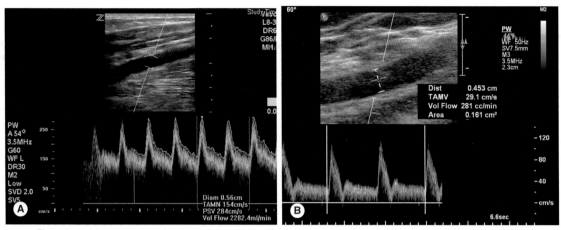

Fig. 16.10 Measurement of volume flow. (A) The flow waveform is regular, the sample volume spans the artery. The scanner uses the measured diameter and mean velocity (*TAMN* in this scanner), to calculate flow as 2282 mL/min. (B) Measurement of volume flow shows low flow, 281 mL/min. The arterial flow waveform is more pulsatile than that in (A) with low diastolic flow, indicating downstream high resistance, in this case a severe venous stenosis.

- Measurements in the vein are prone to error from turbulent nonaxial flow velocities and noncircular cross-sectional area (Fig. 16.11).

When making measurements of diameter and mean velocity, ensure the following:

- Obtain a longitudinal image of the artery, scanning through the plane of maximum diameter, and measure the diameter in B-mode from inner edge to inner edge (Fig. 16.12). Some users recommend a transverse scan where area can be measured directly but the site may not be identical to that for the Doppler measurement of velocity.

- When measuring mean velocity, scan longitudinally where there is a straight portion of artery. Ensure that the sample volume covers the entire width of the artery and that the beam/vessel angle is 60° or less (Fig. 16.13). If the sample volume only insonates the center of the vessel, mean velocity is overestimated with consequent errors in volume flow (see Ch. 6).

- Ensure that the flow waveform is regular and that it does not contain evidence of flow disturbances or low-frequency bruits. Ensure that the spectrum only displays signal from the artery; venous velocities below the baseline may subtract from the arterial signals and reduce the calculated mean velocity in the spectrum. Ensure that the Doppler filter does not remove significant low velocities, thereby falsely raising the mean velocity measurement. Measure the time-averaged velocity over several cardiac cycles.

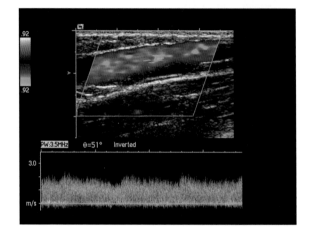

Fig. 16.11 Flow in the cephalic vein in a fistula. The irregular "feathered" peaks are indicative of velocity fluctuations in the center of the vessel. Flow is unlikely to be completely axial along the vessel direction and mean velocity measurements will be inaccurate.

- Ensure that the patient is resting. Experience has shown us that flow is stable within 3 minutes of a change of posture.

It is worth repeating flow measurements to determine/ascertain the reproducibility of your technique. We routinely take three separate measurements to ensure consistency.

Scanning the Access

Ensure that the patient is comfortable with the arm supported to allow ultrasound access to the major arteries and veins from neck to wrist level. Use an appropriate

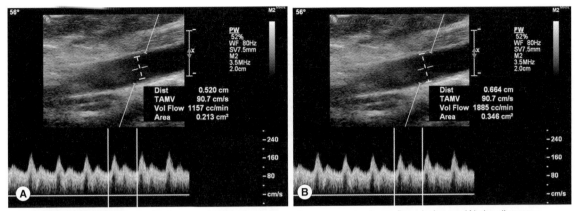

Fig. 16.12 Slight errors in diameter lead to large errors in measured volume flow. In image (A) the diameter calipers are inside the artery wall, measured diameter is 5.2 mm, and the flow 1157 mL/min. In image (B) the calipers are placed on the artery wall, diameter is 6.6 mm, and the calculated flow is 1885 mL/min.

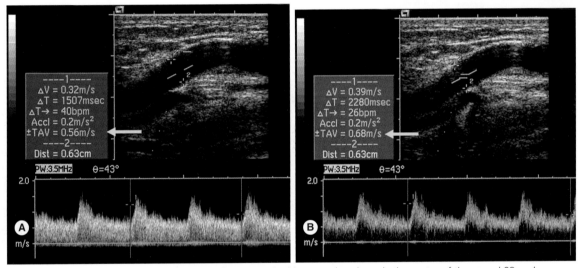

Fig. 16.13 Mean velocity (TAV arrowed) measured with a sample volume in the center of the vessel 68 cm/s (B) and across the vessel 56 cm/s (A). By omitting lower velocities near the vessel wall the mean velocity value is artificially raised when the sample volume only insonates the center of the artery.

linear array. For access work there is a compromise to be made between the need for good B-mode imaging in the near field, for which a high-frequency linear array (7–15 MHz) is best, and the need to image very high velocities where lower Doppler frequencies, resulting from lower-frequency transducers (3–8 MHz), are less prone to aliasing (see Ch. 3).

Measure volume flow as described earlier. If flow has decreased significantly since the last scan, then it is imperative to identify possible causes.

The entire circuit is scanned for evidence of abnormality. An initial rapid transverse scan of the vessels with color flow can identify major anomalies including aneurysms, partial thrombus, and collections and can ascertain the presence of multiple unsuspected venous returns or venous occlusions. PSVs are measured in longitudinal scanning. Angle correction is used for the artery and vein, but care must be taken when measuring velocities at the anastomosis, since the flow direction changes markedly over small distances and using angle correction at the anastomosis can lead to errors, overestimating the already high velocities and leading to alarm. One way of avoiding this is to use no angle correction (angle 0°) and to maneuver the transducer and the beam to image along

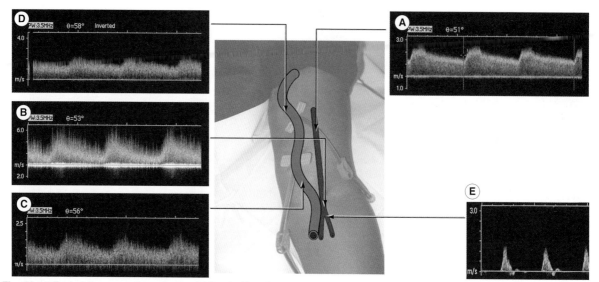

Fig. 16.14 Typical flow waveforms in arterial fistula. The sites are:
A Arterial supply, high velocities, low resistance.
B Fistula site. High flows with turbulence and changes in flow direction.
C Fistula vein close to the fistula, flow disturbances from the fistula site are evident.
D Fistula vein. The flow becomes more ordered downstream. Damped arterial-like waveforms are evident.
E Distal arteries exhibit normal triphasic flow waveforms.

the velocity jet at the anastomosis without angle correction. High-frequency transducers can be used to image the anastomosis directly in B-mode.

Normal Characteristics

Typical flow waveforms in the circuit are illustrated in Fig. 16.14. Flow in the supplying artery is characterized by high-velocity, low pulsatility flow with a resistive index (RI) < 0.5. At the site of a fistula, velocities are usually very high with sudden changes in direction (Fig. 16.15). Close to the anastomosis, venous flows may be turbulent and exhibits nonaxial flow (Fig. 16.14C), which reorganize more proximally downstream. The vein normally exhibits arterial-like pulsations up to axillary/subclavian vein level. More proximally, venous pulsations may become more evident. Pressure in the vein at the needling site is high (typically), and light pressure from the transducer should not cause visible compression. The vein diameter should be adequate for repeated needling; diameters of at least 5 mm are recommended, 6 mm is preferred.

In radiocephalic fistulas, flow to the vein is commonly from antegrade flow in the radial artery and retrograde flow from the radial artery distal to the anastomosis from the ulnar artery via the palmar arches (Fig. 16.16).

Abnormalites and Complications

Thrombosis. Occlusive thrombosis most commonly occurs in the vein or graft at the site of needling. In grafts, thrombosis rapidly extends along the entire length of the graft. In veins the length of thrombosis depends on collateral flow, which may keep sections of the vein patent. In cases of vein and graft thrombosis, flow in the supplying artery shows a high distal resistance, usually triphasic, flow waveform (Fig. 16.17A). Thrombus is evident in the vein, and there may be small channel of flow around it (Fig. 16.17B). Thrombosis may occur in the artery leading to the fistula; for example, in the radial artery in radiocephalic fistulas. It is important to determine the site and length of thrombus so that the clinical team can plan for surgical or radiological intervention. Venous diameter must be reported, as aneurysms can affect management strategy for the thrombosed native fistula. It is also helpful to establish the age of the thrombus if possible, for example, if the thrombus is still "fresh" such that it is still partially compressible. The patient may be able to give a useful guide as to when the access stopped "buzzing," a vibration at the site of the fistula caused by the high-velocity hemodynamics.

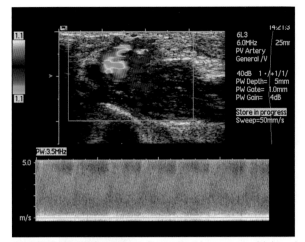

Fig. 16.15 At the fistula site, flow velocities are very high and change directions over a short distance. Accurate measurement of velocity is difficult. In this example there is no angle correction made and measured velocities are at least 5 m/s. Aliasing and noise in the color flow image and spectral trace are evident. Measurements here should be placed in the context of overall flow and hemodynamics throughout the access circuit.

Stenoses, aneurysms, pseudoaneurysms. Accesses frequently contain stenoses, aneurysms, pseudoaneurysms, or hybrid aneurysms/pseudoaneurysms. By themselves they do not necessarily preclude successful dialysis. Older fistulas can develop multiple aneurysms at the needling sites yet still be viable for dialysis (Fig. 16.18). These pose challenges for imaging and Doppler measurement, not least from maintaining good transducer contact (Fig. 16.19). Other anomalies can include partial thrombus, which may be evident particularly at the needling site. Aneurysms, stenoses, and the presence of partial thrombus give rise to complex flows with turbulence and areas of recirculation, which may promote thrombus formation around the dialysis needle. Aneurysms and pseudoaneurysms are visible on B-mode and color flow imaging. The lumen, size of the aneurysm/pseudoaneurysm, and the presence of thrombus can be imaged and measured (Figs. 16.20 and 16.21).

Stenoses may be evident on B-mode but are determined by their PSV and the PSV ratio of prestenotic or poststenotic flow to in-stenosis flow. High PSVs are indicative of pressure loss at the stenosis. Typical criteria used are PSVs >400 cm/s and/or PSV ratios of >3:1 (Older et al. 1998; ACR Guidelines 2019) for both fistulas and grafts. The following points are useful when considering stenoses:

- When reporting stenoses we combine measurement of PSV ratios with absolute measure of PSV to give an assessment of the anatomy and severity and functional importance of the stenosis (Figs. 16.22 and 16.23). The PSV ratio reflects the anatomical severity of a stenosis but the absolute PSV gives an indication of the degree of pressure loss through the narrowing.
- It is essential to view the stenosis in the context of the flow measurement or changes in flow from a previous scan and from the clinical indications for the scan. Moderate stenoses (for example, ×2 PSV increase, maximum velocity 200 cm/s) may be incidental findings and even more severe stenoses may be found in fistulas with good function.
- The cephalic vein is often narrowed close to its insertion to the axillary vein and may be compressed by pressure from the transducer. True stenoses have high velocities with little extrinsic pressure, in a range of arm positions.
- The presence of bruits can obscure the color flow image of a stenosis. Severe bruits and very elevated velocities are indicative of pressure reducing and flow-limiting stenoses (Fig. 16.24).
- Flow waveform changes are useful in identifying severe stenosis with more pulsatile flow upstream of a narrowing and damped flow downstream and turbulent flow in the poststenotic region.
- A qualitative measure of venous pressure can be gained by observing the ease of vein compression with pressure from the transducer. Low-pressure veins are indicative of upstream stenosis. High-pressure veins with low flow are indicative of downstream stenosis. Pressure loss across the stenosis in a fistula vein may be evident as a marked difference in compressibility of the vein prestenosis and poststenosis.
- Do not overcall the high velocities at the site of the anastomosis. There are generally high velocities here (see earlier), and criteria applicable in the rest of the circuit do not apply to the specific anatomy and hemodynamics of the anastomosis.
- In grafts, the most common site of narrowing is at the venous anastomosis. There is usually a PSV change as the caliber changes from the graft to the vein. Several thresholds for PSV and PSV ratios have been used to characterize stenoses here. It is important to record the values at the baseline scan and to record any changes to these in the context of clinical indications and changes to flow.

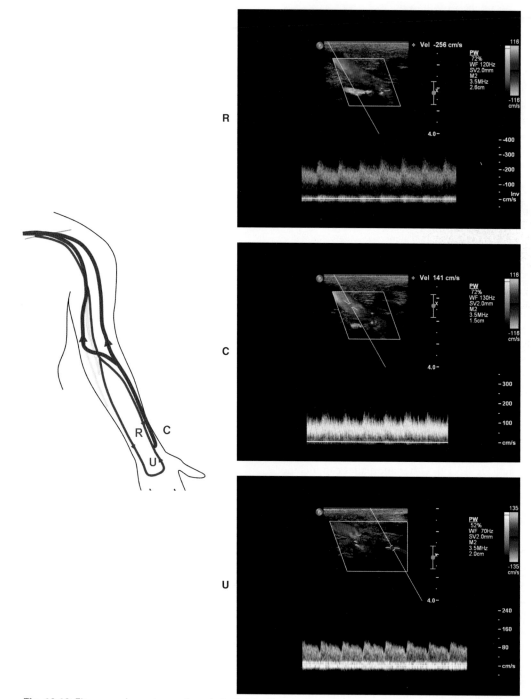

Fig. 16.16 Flow waveforms in a radiocephalic fistula. Flow in the radial artery distal to the fistula shows flow back toward the fistula from the ulnar artery and palmar arch. *C*, cephalic vein; *R*, radial artery; *U*, flow from ulnar artery via palmar arch.

Steal

Steal may occur in hemodialysis with inadequate flow to distal tissue, resulting in pain in the hand and fingers and, if severe, tissue changes associated with ischemia. Ultrasound can be used to determine vascular anatomy, vessel patency, and qualitative evaluation of the circulation in the arm and hand. It has been shown that steal is associated with a high incidence of arterial stenosis in the arterial supply to the hand (Leon & Asif 2007). Ultrasound is effective in identifying this and as an aid to planning therapy through angioplasty or surgical revision.

Other Findings

Collections and hematoma should be noted. These can lead to difficulties when needling fistulas and can cause extrinsic compression of the access circuit (Fig. 16.25). Very high-volume flows are possible and can lead to cardiac problems. Ultrasound can be used to quantify the flow and monitor therapy (Fig. 16.26).

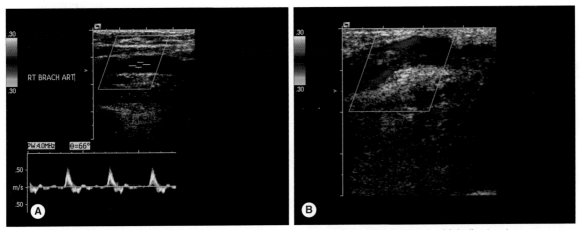

Fig. 16.17 Flow waveform in the brachial artery leading to an occluded fistula showing high distal resistance (A). Color flow imaging shows a vein with thrombus almost completely occluding the lumen (B).

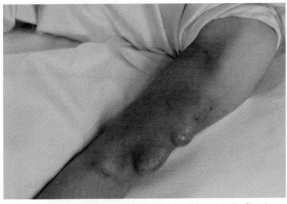

Fig. 16.18 Aneurysms visible in a brachiocephalic fistula.

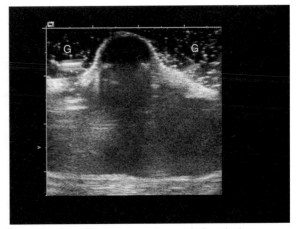

Fig. 16.19 Superficial aneurysm in a cephalic vein. Large quantities of ultrasound gel *(G)* are needed to maintain ultrasound contact with the skin.

A protocol for postoperative imaging of permanent access is given in Box 16.4.

REPORTING

The report should describe the flow and any significant changes to flow when compared with previous investigations. PSVs through stenoses should be described and ratios calculated. If diameters are clear on B-mode, then these can also be used to describe the stenosis. The presence of thrombus, aneurysms/pseudoaneurysms, and collections should be noted and

dimensions recorded. The diameter of the vein should be determined and, in cases where needling is difficult, its depth. If the fistula flow returns through more than one pathway then this should be described. It is important to report unusual flow pathways and flow in unsuspected directions.

We use diagrams of the access to aid dialysis staff where needling is difficult or as a guide for planning radiological intervention or surgery (Fig. 16.27).

SURVEILLANCE

Preserving a functional dialysis access is enormously beneficial for the patient. Several surveillance methods are used to complement clinical monitoring (Koirala et al. 2016). Ultrasound has been advocated for surveillance for its ability to measure flow and also image the circuit for causes of changes in flow and dialysis performance. However, its efficacy is controversial (Tessitore & Poli 2019; Moist & Lok 2019). Among challenges are the differences in reported success and criteria between grafts and fistulas, normal fluctuations in volume flow in individual patients, the rapidity of stenosis progression, and the relationship between this and a recognizable fall in flow, selecting the optimum interval for surveillance and the risk of over-intervention on stenoses identified. The future of ultrasound in routine surveillance may advance with the wider availability

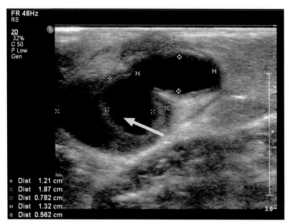

Fig. 16.20 Transverse image of a fistula vein with pseudoaneurysm partially filled with thrombus *(arrowed)*.

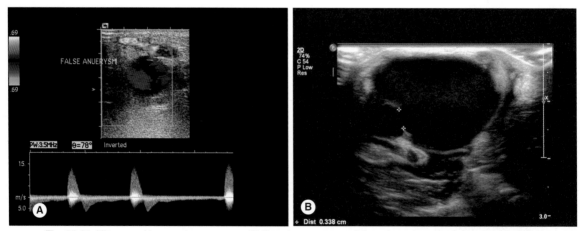

Fig. 16.21 Ultrasound in pseudoaneurysms. (A) Doppler spectrum of flow through a tract into a pseudoaneurysm, caused by needling through the deep wall of the vessel. (B) Ultrasound measurement of the size of the breach in the vein wall can help in planning intervention.

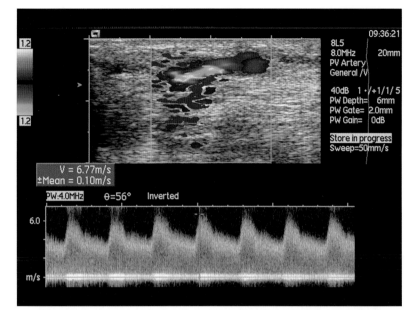

Fig. 16.22 Severe stenosis in a cephalic vein. Color flow and spectral Doppler show severe narrowing. Peak velocities exceed 6 m/s, at the upper limit of velocities possible in the circulation and indicative of low pressures at this point.

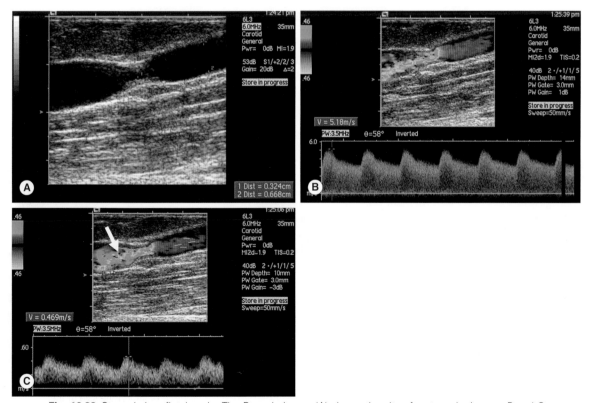

Fig. 16.23 Stenosis in a fistula vein. The B-mode image (A) shows the site of a stenosis. Images B and C show velocity changes through the stenosis, note the disordered turbulent flow downstream of the stenosis (arrow). Peak velocities obtained in the stenosis (B) exceed 5 m/s and are over 10 times that in the pre-stenosis vein (C).

lower-cost ultrasound devices within dialysis centers, improved reproducibility of measurements, and selection of high-risk patients and accesses in whom the additional resources required are justified.

However, there remains a need for high-quality vascular ultrasound imaging and measurement of dialysis accesses in the hands of expert ultrasound practitioners.

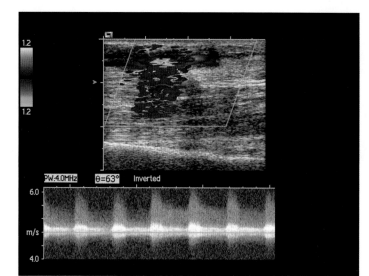

Fig. 16.24 High velocities through a stenosis lead to a bruit, vibration of the tissue that is evident as color flow noise, and high-intensity low-velocity spectral traces.

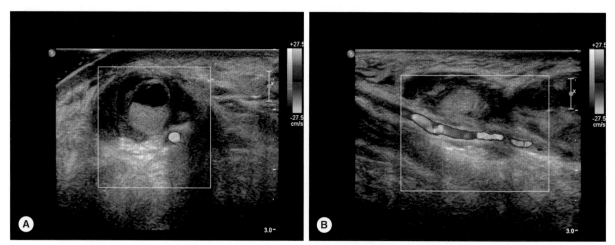

Fig. 16.25 Transverse (A) and longitudinal (B) image of a cephalic vein compressed by hematoma in the immediate postoperative period following fistula formation.

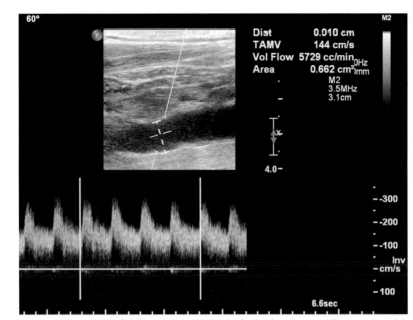

Fig. 16.26 Measured flow in this fistula exceeds 5.5 L/min, indicating the need for urgent revision to reduce flow.

BOX 16.4 Protocol for Evaluating Hemodialysis Arm Access Postoperatively

- Measure flow in the brachial or subclavian artery supplying the access
- Scan the circuit from subclavian artery through the fistula/graft to the draining veins to central veins
- Note any abnormality (thrombus, aneurysms, pseudoaneurysms, collections)
- Note any abnormal flows (unusual flow velocities or pulsatility, flow direction in veins)
- It there are multiple venous paths, draw them and state approximately the flow through each. Note where flow returns to the deep veins
- Measure vein diameter and depth, especially if there are needling problems. Note any sudden change in vein direction and the presence of thrombus/intimal flaps, etc., in the needling area
- Note any stenoses and measure them on B-mode and with peak systolic velocity and ratios of stenosis to pre/poststenosis velocities

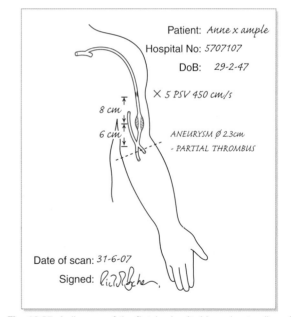

Fig. 16.27 A diagram of the fistula circuit aids understanding of the ultrasound examination and is helpful when planning intervention. *PSV*, peak systolic velocity.

Transcranial Doppler Ultrasound

INTRODUCTION

Transcranial Doppler ultrasound (TCD) enables investigation of flow in major intracranial arteries and, to a lesser extent, veins. Since its first reported use in 1982 (Aaslid et al. 1982), it has been developed and utilized for several applications including assessment of intracranial stenoses, investigation of physiological changes, and monitoring of emboli as an indication of stroke risk. Many different specialities use TCD; the equipment itself is specialized and can be found in neurology and stroke units, critical care units, hematology units, radiology departments, and vascular laboratories. Applications continue to be developed, and while the technique is now integral to a few clinical pathways, other applications may be found in centers where there is enthusiasm for the development of tests or particular interest in using its unique capabilities.

This chapter provides a brief overview of equipment and techniques and highlights a few key applications the reader may find in clinical practice. There is a wealth of literature on these and other applications, and further reading is recommended for those wishing to develop their knowledge of the technique and specific applications.

ANATOMY AND SCANNING WINDOWS

Anatomy of the Intracranial Arteries Examined by Transtemporal TCD

The internal carotid artery (ICA) terminates where it divides into the anterior (ACA) and middle cerebral arteries (MCA). The MCA is divided into a number of segments, but for TCD it is normally the M1 segment, from the bifurcation running laterally, that is insonated. The posterior communicating artery (PcomA) branches from the ICA just proximal to the point where it terminates. The ACA is also divided into segments, the proximal segment A1 is from the terminal ICA bifurcation running to the anterior communicating artery (AcomA) between the left and right ACAs. The A2 segment extends anteriorly beyond the AcomA.

The vertebral arteries join to form the basilar artery that terminates into the left and right posterior

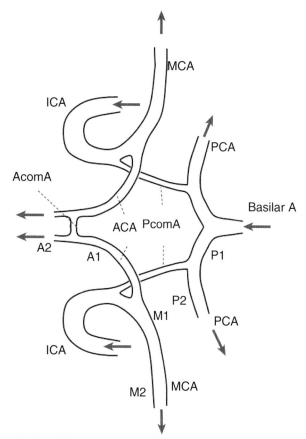

Fig. 17.1 Diagram of the major intracranial arteries investigated by TCD. The orientation is with anterior to the left of the image. The terminal ICA rises to the ACA/MCA bifurcation. The basilar rises to the division of the right and left PCAs. The named segments are shown, *M2* of the MCA is where the MCA turns superior in the head. *ACA,* Anterior cerebral artery; *ICA,* internal carotid artery; *MCA,* middle cerebral artery; *PCA,* posterior cerebral artery; *TCD,* transcranial Doppler.

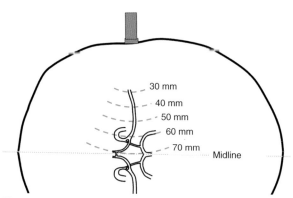

Fig. 17.2 Approximate distance of the major intracranial arteries in adults from the transcranial Doppler probe from a transtemporal approach.

TABLE 17.1 **Dimensions of Major Intracranial Arteries.**		
	Diameter (mm)	**Length (mm)**
ACA A1 segment	1.6–2.1	12.7–13.5
MCA M1 segment	2.2–2.8	
PCA P1 segment	1.9–2.1	6.3–7.0
Basilar artery	2.6–3.5	32.0

ACA, Anterior cerebral artery; *MCA,* middle cerebral artery; *PCA,* posterior cerebral artery.
Saver & Feldman (1993).

cerebral arteries (PCAs). The P1 segment of the PCA runs from the basilar bifurcation to the PcomA branch. The P2 segment then arcs posteriorly around the peduncles.

Fig. 17.1 demonstrates this, with the approximate depths of these vessels from a transtemporal approach illustrated in Fig. 17.2.

The proximal PCAs, ACAs, and the PcomAs and the AcomA form the circle of Willis, which allows collateral flow where a major artery is narrowed or occluded. For example, in the presence of a left ICA occlusion, flow from the right ICA can maintain left hemisphere circulation via the AcomA. It is also possible for flow from the posterior circulation to supply the anterior circulation or vice versa via the PcomAs. The dimensions of the major arteries and depths from the TCD probe are described in Table 17.1 (Saver & Feldman 1993). A standard circle of Willis is present in less than half of subjects; common variants include hypoplasia of the P1 segment of a PCA, hypoplasia of one A1 segment of the ACAs, and hypoplasia of one or both PcomAs.

Scanning Windows

There are three "acoustic windows" in the skull through which major cerebral arteries can be investigated. These are:

Transtemporal: In most patients there are regions of the temporal bone that allow sufficient transmission and reception of ultrasound to and from major vessels. The transtemporal window can normally be located by placing a finger adjacent to front of the ear in its mid-section and running the finger upward where a small depression will indicate the position of the transtemporal window. In some subjects it may

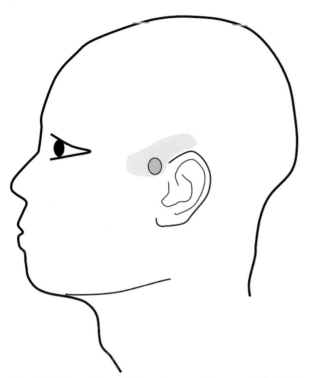

Fig. 17.3 Range of area for transtemporal transcranial Doppler investigation and imaging. The usual position is just anterior to the ear, but in some patients better acoustic windows are found from other approaches.

not be evident. The bone structure causes refraction from the cortical bone surfaces depending on its geometry and scattering and attenuation from the internal spongy diploe bone, which can distort and attenuate the ultrasound beam. The most usual location for good transmission is anterior to the ear and cephalad (above) the zygomatic arch, but other locations may provide better images (see Fig. 17.3). In some patients there is no adequate transtemporal window (reported as approximately 10%). The incidence of poor windows is worse in older patients and in women. The transtemporal approach gives good access to the major arteries and branches of the circle of Willis, particularly the MCA, which courses toward the transducer. Most of the applications described in this chapter are undertaken with the transtemporal approach.

Transorbital: This approach is used for examination of the ophthalmic artery and its branches. It can also be used to examine the ICA at the level of the carotid siphon. Safety guidelines for transorbital scanning state that the beam power should be limited and the mechanical index, MI, should not exceed 0.23. Thermal index (TIS) should not exceed 1.0.

Suboccipital approach: By pointing up into the foramen with neck flexed, the confluence of the two vertebral arteries and the basilar artery can be insonated and imaged. The basilar artery is normally located with the probe in the mid-line, and the vertebral arteries can be located by shifting the probe slightly laterally.

In addition to the acoustic windows of the skull, a submandibular approach can be used to examine the extracranial ICA. By placing the TCD probe submandibularly, the entire length of the distal cervical ICA may be insonated or imaged using depths of 40 to 60 mm. This complements more conventional imaging of the ICA using linear array transducers.

Equipment

Two distinct types of TCD equipment are available, nonimaging and imaging TCD.

Nonimaging TCD

In nonimaging TCD, a circular 2 MHz pulsed-wave (PW) single-element focused transducer (Fig. 17.4) is used to obtain the Doppler spectrum of vessels at specific sample volumes along the path of the beam chosen by the operator. The probe provides a circular section beam profile along its length and is focused for optimal performance at around 40 to 60 mm depth (see Fig. 17.5). Once placed on an acoustic window, the probe can be manipulated to direct the beam and the sample volume depth adjusted to identify or target specific intracranial vessels. Power output, gain, pulse repetition frequency (scale), sample volume length, flow direction, and baseline also need to be optimized using a control panel on the device. This requires skill, practice, and a knowledge of anatomy and the expected dimensions and depth of intracranial vessels.

Many of the applications require measurement of the maximum velocity along the length of the arteries insonated. Audio clues as to the strength and maximum Doppler frequency are used to optimize the beam direction for the vessel under examination. Because there is no imaging, there is no correction made for the angle between the ultrasound beam and the vessel. Inevitably there will be errors depending on the vessel to the beam angle, but studies have ascertained normal and abnormal velocity and waveform values for a range

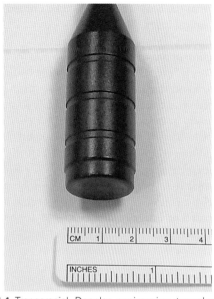

Fig. 17.4 Transcranial Doppler nonimaging transducer. The pulsed-wave Doppler probe is optimized to investigate arteries at 40- to 60-mm depth.

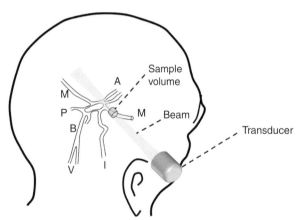

Fig. 17.5 Nonimaging transcranial Doppler. The beam is directed by the operator in the direction of the intracranial arteries. The size and depth of the sample volume is controlled by the operator to insonate specific arteries. *A,* anterior cerebral artery; *B,* basilar artery; *I,* internal carotid artery; *M,* middle cerebral artery; *P,* posterior cerebral artery; *V,* vertebral arteries.

of applications. The transducers are light and can be mounted in a headband to allow measurement of long-term changes in cerebral circulation.

Most of the early studies in the application of TCD techniques were done using nonimaging TCD, and reference velocities for normal values and diagnostic values

specific to applications are based on these dedicated systems where no angle correction is made.

Another nonimaging Doppler modality, power M-mode Doppler (sometimes referred as power-motion mode Doppler), has the advantage of demonstrating the intensity and direction of blood flow Doppler signals along the path of the beam over a distance of several centimeters by using multiple sample volumes. The display is normally coded red and blue for direction. In this way, several sections of arteries may be displayed (Fig. 17.6). This aids understanding of anatomy and optimal placement of the PW Doppler sample volume. It can also aid in the tracking of emboli through the vessel.

Imaging TCD

In imaging TCD (TCDI), also sometimes described as transcranial color Doppler (TCCD), conventional ultrasound scanners are used to image the brain using low-frequency—typically 1 to 4 MHz—phased arrays to penetrate the bone. A two-dimensional color map of vessels (Fig. 17.7) aids in placement of the PW Doppler sample volume to investigate flow at specific locations (Fig. 17.8). Focusing in the plane of the image is achieved through timing of the different elements for transmit and receive beams. Focusing in the elevation plane is by an acoustic lens so that the beam profile is not circular as it is in nonimaging systems. Transducers used are those usually used for cardiac applications and may not be optimized for TCD applications. Nevertheless, and despite the challenges of transmitting and receiving through bone, most ultrasound systems now have dedicated TCD software and settings to provide diagnostic color flow images and satisfactory Doppler sensitivity.

Doppler velocity criteria for TCD applications have been based on nonimaging TCD measurements. When using imaging TCD, beam/vessel angle correction should not normally be made. As in nonimaging TCD, the sonogram should be optimized by moving the transducer and aligning the beam optimally with the major vessels.

Measurements

The Doppler spectrum permits measurement of velocities, indices of flow waveform shape, and the detection of emboli.

Velocities

The main measurement of velocity used in TCD is the TCD mean velocity. This is the mean of the maximum of

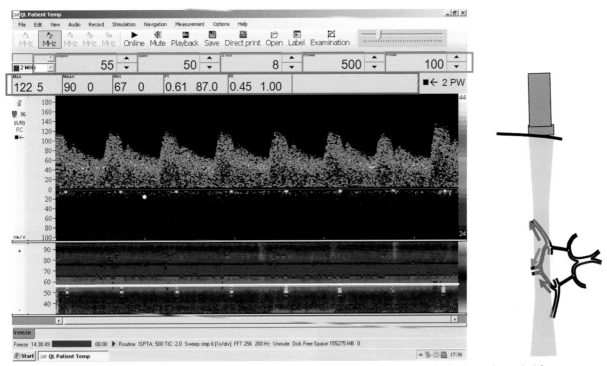

Fig. 17.6 Color M-mode TCD. The lower part of the display shows flow along the beam, color coded for direction. The scale *(left)* shows the depth of the color flow signal, in this case flow in a MCA, and two ACAs are seen from 50 to 87 mm from the probe. The depth of the sample volume for PW spectral analysis in the upper part of the display is shown by the white horizontal line in the lower red M-mode display at a depth of 55 mm. Scanning parameters are shown within the *green rectangle*, recorded values in the *red rectangle*. *ACA*, Anterior cerebral artery; *MCA*, middle cerebral artery; *PW*, pulsed-wave; *TCD*, transcranial Doppler.

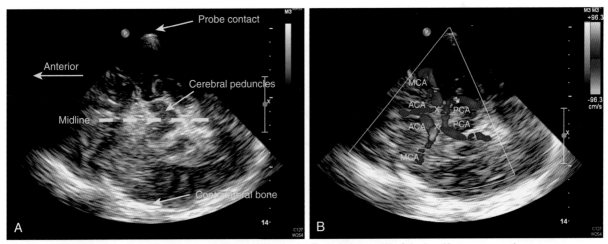

Fig. 17.7 B-mode and color flow of TCD imaging. In the B-mode image (A) of the head in transverse, the opposite bone is seen. The cerebral peduncles are displayed as a dark butterfly-shaped symmetrical area. In this scan the color flow image (B) shows the proximal MCAs, ACAs, and PCAs on both sides. The color is reversed on opposite sides. Location *X* shows where the terminal ICA rises to the bifurcation of the MCA/ACA. The PCAs are not always seen in the same plane as the MCA and ACA. *ACA*, Anterior cerebral artery; *ICA*, internal carotid artery; *MCA*, middle cerebral artery; *PCA*, posterior cerebral artery; *TCD*, transcranial Doppler.

the sonogram over one or more cardiac cycles (Fig. 17.8). This was chosen early in TCD studies to be most representative of changes in flow in an artery. Increases in velocity do reflect increases in flow provided that the artery itself does not change diameter. Conversely, changes in diameter will lead to changes in velocity if flow is unchanged. Velocity increases may be used to quantify stenoses.

The use of the term *mean velocity* can cause confusion for those used to the nomenclature of ultrasound scanners where mean velocity usually refers to a weighted mean such as that used to measure volume flow. For scanners,

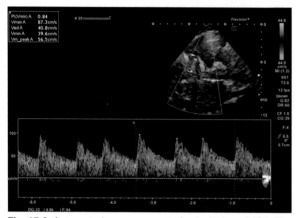

Fig. 17.8 Automated measurement of velocity in an MCA. The TCD mean velocity is the mean of the maximum trace, in this scanner described as V_m_peak A with a value of 56.5 cm/s. Pulsatility index (PI) is 0.84. *MCA*, Middle cerebral artery; *TCD*, transcranial Doppler.

TCD mean is usually referred to as time-averaged maximum velocity (TAMX) or time-averaged mean maximum velocity (TAMMV), although other descriptions are used (see Fig. 17.8). Most scanners provide an automated measurement of the outline of the velocity trace, for example, as used in the calculation of pulsatility index (PI), but others use alternative ways of calculating TCD mean; for example, one scanner we use measured it as 1/3 of peak systolic velocity + 2/3 of end-diastolic velocity.

As in other velocities measured by Doppler, the value depends on the accuracy of the trace around the maximum velocities. In weak Doppler sonograms, automated measurements may be inaccurate. Altering gain or the threshold on which to measure the Doppler envelope will also affect measured velocities (Fig. 17.9). Manual tracing of faint sonograms or an estimate of the mean maximum may be a pragmatic way of estimating mean velocity (Fig. 17.10).

Normal values for mean velocity in the major branches of the circle of Willis for adults and children, including normal pulsatility indices for adults, are shown in Tables 17.2A–C.

Flow Waveform Indices

PI is an indication of changes in cerebrovascular resistance (Figs. 17.8 and 17.11) but is also affected by proximal changes, for example, in severe carotid artery stenoses or occlusion, which can result in damping of distal waveforms, particularly if there is poor collateral contribution (see Fig. 17.12).

Normal adult values for PI are shown in Table 17.2B.

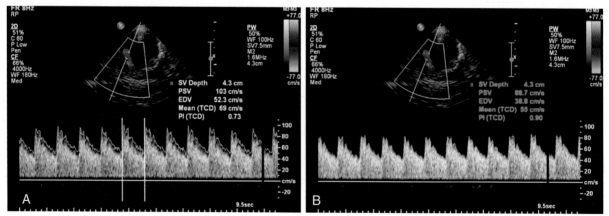

Fig. 17.9 MCA mean velocity measured automatically with the spectrum maximum threshold set at two different levels to include or exclude weaker Doppler frequencies. The TCD mean values range from 69 cm/s (A) to 55 cm/s (B). Pulsatility index measurements also reflect the change in velocities, measured as 0.73 and 0.9. *MCA*, Middle cerebral artery; *TCD*, transcranial Doppler.

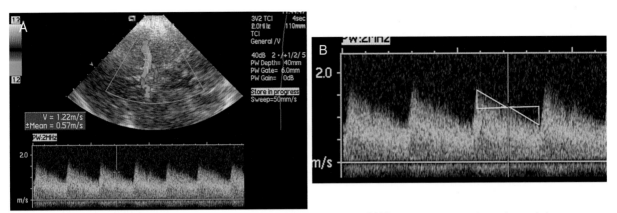

Fig. 17.10 Manual estimation of the transcranial Doppler mean. (A) The sonogram contains noise and the cursor has been placed using an estimation of the mean height of the waveform. (B) By estimating that the area above the cursor in systole matches the area below it in diastole, the cursor is placed. Manual tracing of noisy sonograms is also possible but this is also prone to error. The choice of method and the precision and accuracy of measurements made are dependent on the application and constraints of the scan.

TABLE 17.2A   Mean and SD Adult Normal Intracranial Mean Velocities (cm/s)

	<40 years	40–59 years	>60 years
MCA (M1)	58.4 ± 8.4	57.7 ± 11.5	44.7 ± 11.1
ACA (A1)	47.3 ± 13.6	53.1 ± 10.5	45.3 ± 13.5
PCA (P1)	34.2 ± 7.8	36.6 ± 9.8	29.9 ± 9.3
VA/BA	34.9 ± 7.8	36.4 ± 11.7	30.5 ± 12.4

TABLE 17.2B   Mean and SD Adult Normal Intracranial Pulsatility Indices

Arteries	Pulsatility Index (PI)
R MCA	0.90 ± 0.24
L MCA	0.94 ± 0.27
R ACA	0.78 ± 0.15
L ACA	0.83 ± 0.17
R PCA	0.88 ± 0.23
L PCA	0.88 ± 0.20

Hennerici et al. (1987).

TABLE 17.2C   Mean and SD Children Normal Intracranial Mean Velocities (cm/s)

	1.0–2.9 years	3.0–5.9 years	6.0–9.9 years	10–18 years
MCA (M1)	85 ± 10	94 ± 10	97 ± 9	81 ± 11
ACA (A1)	55 ± 13	71 ± 5	65 ± 13	56 ± 14
PCA (P1)	50 ± 17	56 ± 13	57 ± 9	50 ± 10
VA/BA	51 ± 6	58 ± 6	58 ± 9	46 ± 8

ACA, Anterior cerebral artery; *MCA,* middle cerebral artery; *PCA,* posterior cerebral artery.
Bode & Wais (1998).

Embolus Detection

Blood-borne small emboli produce short high-intensity reflections as they pass through the sample volume. Emboli can be air or particulate; in general, higher-intensity signals are reflected from air emboli. These high-intensity transient signals (HITS) have a characteristic "blip" sound. The importance of microemboli has been extensively studied to assess, for example:

- To try and distinguish air from particulate emboli
- Whether microemboli are precursors of larger emboli
- The prevalence of microemboli in certain applications, for example, distal to symptomatic and asymptomatic carotid stenoses
- The optimum duration of investigation to capture examples of microemboli and the associated risk posed

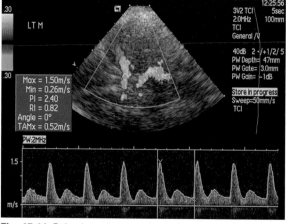

Fig. 17.11 Raised cerebrovascular resistance results in pulsatile flow waveforms with reduced diastolic flow, in this case with a pulsatility index of 2.4 and a mean velocity of 52 cm/s.

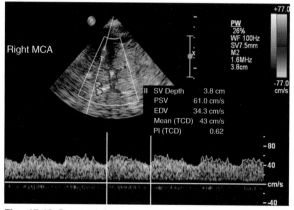

Fig. 17.12 Damped flow (PI 0.62) and low velocities (TCD mean 43 cm/s) downstream of an ICA severe stenosis. *ICA*, Internal carotid artery; *PI*, pulsatility index; *TCD*, transcranial Doppler.

- How best to detect the distinctive spectral fingerprint of emboli, how they sound and appear on the sonogram (Fig. 17.13)

Technique and Optimization for Transtemporal TCD

Nonimaging Doppler

Typical depths of the major arteries are shown in Table 17.1 and Fig. 17.2. To detect flow in the MCA, the sample volume is typically set at a depth of around 50 mm and the probe orientated slightly upward and anteriorly (Fig. 17.5). A sample volume of 6 to 7 mm improves sensitivity to flow. Once flow is detected, the probe can be moved to best align the beam with the flow direction. The pitch (frequency) of the Doppler sonogram and the displayed velocities will be at maximum when beam and artery are best aligned. The sample volume depth can be reduced to insonate the distal MCA and is increased to sample the bifurcation of the ACA/MCA and the terminal ICA. The probe is dipped inferiorly to insonate the terminal ICA. The ACA can be followed by angling the probe anteriorly and increasing the sample volume depth. The PCA can be insonated by angling the probe posterior to the MCA by angling toward the ear.

Transtemporal TCD Imaging

The scan starts with a transverse B-mode image of the brain locating the cerebral peduncles (Fig. 17.7) as a dark butterfly-like shape. If a good B-mode image is visible, then Doppler images should be clear, and poor B-mode images are indicative of problems to come (Fig. 17.14). The major arteries of the circle of Willis can often be detected as pulsing structures. Color flow imaging is selected in order to demonstrate the circle of Willis and

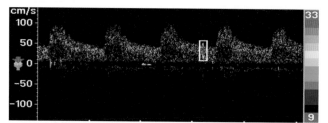

Fig. 17.13 Doppler sonogram from a transcranial Doppler nonimaging system showing a high-intensity transient signal *(highlighted in white box)*. The scale to the right of the sonogram shows the intensity of echoes, and the embolic signal causes much higher intensity echoes than blood.

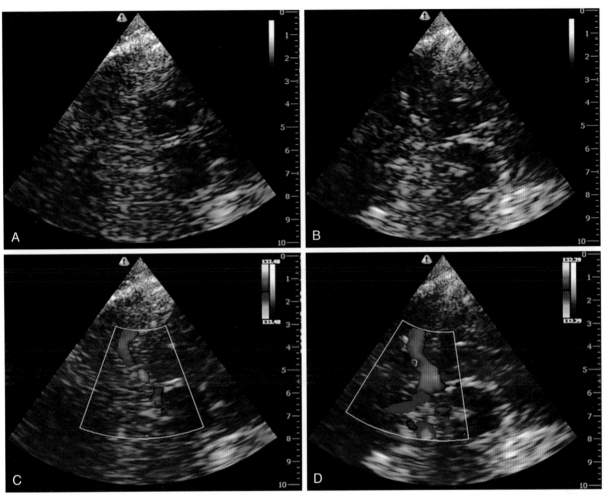

Fig. 17.14 B-mode images (A and B) from a transtemporal approach show differences in clarity of the cerebral peduncles, better defined in image (B) where the transducer has been moved slightly. The corresponding color flow images (C and D) reflect the improvement, there is better sensitivity to flow in image (D).

branches (Figs. 17.7 and 17.14). By tilting the probe, arteries from the terminal ICA to the MCA and ACA and PCA may be identified and velocities measured from them. The appearance and clarity of the images is dependent on the anatomy and the distortion of the ultrasound beam through the skull. As in nonimaging TCD, it is essential to move the transducer to optimize the image and to align the Doppler beam to the artery direction as best as is possible. The color flow image may demonstrate aliasing, especially in the MCA, due to its direction toward the transducer, and the color scale or pulse repetition frequency can be increased to overcome the aliasing so that peak systolic flow along the vessel is toward the upper end of the color bar. Discrete areas of stenosis will

still be visible as areas of aliasing. It is important to use a large sample volume (typically 4–6 mm) to improve the Doppler sonogram signal through the bone. Small sample volumes produce noisy sonograms that are difficult to measure velocities from (Fig. 17.15).

Major Applications

The American Academy of Neurosciences has drawn up guidelines of applications based on proven evidence of clinical effectiveness. This was last updated in 2004 (Sloan et al. 2004), and the guidelines were retired in 2018. The two applications for which there was evidence-based established clinical value were the screening of children aged 2 to 16 with sickle cell

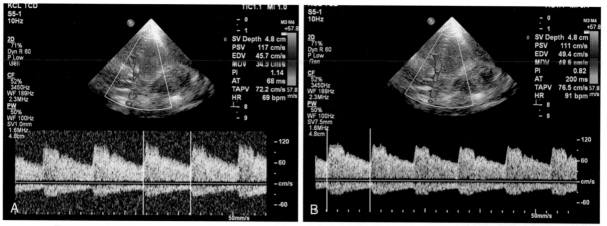

Fig. 17.15 Doppler sonograms with a sample volume of 1 mm (A) and 7.5 mm (B). A large sample volume produces a clearer display of velocities.

disease (SCD) for stroke risk and the detection and monitoring of angiographic vasospasm after spontaneous subarachnoid hemorrhage (SAH). These continue to be applications with robust evidence as to their effectiveness.

The American College of Radiology (ACR), American Institute of Ultrasound in Medicine (AIUM), Society of Pediatric Radiology (SPR), and Society of Radiologists in Ultrasound (SRU) list the following clinical applications in 2017:

- Evaluation of SCD to determine stroke risk,
- Detection and follow-up of stenosis or occlusion of major intracranial artery in the circle of Willis of vertebrobasilar system,
- Detection of cerebral vasculopathy,
- Detection and monitoring of vasospasm in patients with spontaneous or traumatic SAH,
- Evaluation of collateral pathways of intracranial blood flow, including after intervention,
- Detection of circulating cerebral microemboli or HITS,
- Detection of right-to-left shunts,
- Assessment of cerebral vasomotor reactivity (VMR),
- As an adjunct to the clinical diagnosis of brain death,
- Intraoperative and periprocedural monitoring to detect cerebral thrombosis, embolization, hypoperfusion, and hyperperfusion,
- Assessment of arteriovenous malformations, before and after treatment,
- Detection and follow-up of intracranial aneurysms,
- Evaluation of positional vertigo.

The following is an introduction to representative applications of which the authors have experience.

TCD in Pediatric Sickle Cell Disease

Children with SCD have a high risk of stroke. Untreated, overt stroke is reported in 6% to 8% of 2- to 10-year olds, and silent stroke has been reported in 30%. The risk of stroke is complex over the lifetime of patients with ischemic and hemorrhagic causes. In children, vasculopathy affects the major intracranial cerebral arteries by causes that continue to be studied (Connes et al. 2013) but may involve damage to the vessel endothelium, inflammation, and coagulopathy. In the 1990s it was established that investigation of the terminal intracranial ICA, MCA, ACA, and PCA by TCD identified children at risk of stroke by identifying raised velocities related to stenosis (Fig. 17.16) and permitted therapeutic blood transfusions, significantly reducing the number of children with strokes. Work culminated in the Stroke Prevention in Sickle Cell Disease (STOP) trial (Adams et al. 1998) in which children identified with risk of stroke had a markedly improved outcome if transfused compared with those who were not. This has established standards for investigation and treatment that form the basis of screening programs in those countries with effective provision for transfusion therapy.

The risk is higher in early years (2–8) and diminishes thereafter. Children are screened annually from the age of 2 and stratified into risks depending on the velocities in the major cerebral arteries (see Table 17.3).

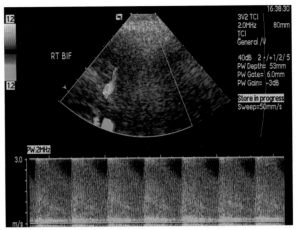

Fig. 17.16 High MCA velocities in a child with sickle cell indicative of a severe stenosis. Aliasing prevents accurate velocity measurements but TCD mean exceeds 250 cm/s. *MCA*, Middle cerebral artery; *TCD*, transcranial Doppler.

TABLE 17.3 TCD Pediatric Sickle Cell—STOP Criteria

Category	Arteries	Values
Normal	MCA, distal ICA, ACA, PCA, basilar artery	<170 cm/s
Conditional	MCA, distal ICA, ACA, PCA, basilar artery	≥170 cm/s < 200 cm/s
Abnormal	MCA, distal ICA	≥200 cm/s

Low MCA velocities (<70 cm/s) or asymmetric velocities (MCA <50% of contralateral) are also cause for concern and merit further imaging or investigation.
ACA, Anterior cerebral artery; *ICA*, internal carotid artery; *MCA*, middle cerebral artery; *PCA*, posterior cerebral artery; *TCD*, transcranial Doppler.

Children in the conditional range have early repeated scans to review development or resolution. Children with velocities in the abnormal range have repeated scans usually within 2 weeks and will advance to therapy based on TCD results, clinical findings, and MRI of the brain. TCD velocities vary in an individual dependent on the hematocrit level, important in this group, since children with a low hematocrit will generally have higher velocities as result of low blood viscosity, increased cardiac output, and vasodilation. Children should be awake and calm (good luck) during the examination; sleep causes changes to velocities. The examination can be

challenging in young children. If time is limited due to patient noncompliance, it is best to image the terminal ICA and MCA.

In the early implementation of STOP criteria, several studies compared nonimaging and imaging TCD values. Results were mixed, TCDI velocities were reported to be lower than TCD by 10%, other studies showed no difference. TCD mean velocities can be affected by alignment to the vessel, gain, and the software to trace around the Doppler spectrum envelope (Fig. 17.9), but careful optimization and measurement can resolve discrepancy between these techniques.

More recent evidence suggests that extracranial carotid arteries may also be affected in SCD and that they may play a role in the development of cerebral infarction (Bernaudin et al. 2015). No trials have been conducted into the importance of extracranial artery stenosis screening, but imaging of these vessels has now been included in many centers.

TCD in Vasospasm

Vasospasm following SAH is a major cause of ischemic neurologic deficit and death. TCD can be used to monitor increases in velocity occurring from constriction of the MCA and basilar artery. Measurement of mean velocity can be complemented by assessment of the Lindegaard ratio (LR), defined as the ratio of the mean velocity in the MCA to that in the ICA, measured by the TCD probe from a submandibular approach (Fig. 17.17). The ratio helps distinguish hyperemic changes to those resulting from vasospasm since in hyperemic changes, velocities are elevated in the MCA and ICA.

Vasospasm usually occurs 4 days following SAH. In those patients in whom vasospasm is a risk, daily monitoring can aid in treatment planning. MCA velocities of >120 cm/s are indicative of vasospasm and >200 cm/s of severe vasospasm. LRs (MCA/ICA velocity) of 3 to 6 are indicative of moderate vasospasm and >6 of severe vasospasm. A high velocity with LR less than 3 is suggestive of a hyperemia (Kirsch et al. 2013). Rises of 65 cm/s or >20% at days 3 to 7 are indicative of poor outcome (Tsivgoulis et al. 2009).

TCD and Raised Intracranial Pressure

Raised intracranial pressure (ICP) and a reduction of cerebral perfusion pressure (CPP) are important parameters in critical care, for example, in traumatic brain injury or hepatic encephalopathy where severe intracranial hypertension may lead to a catastrophic reduction

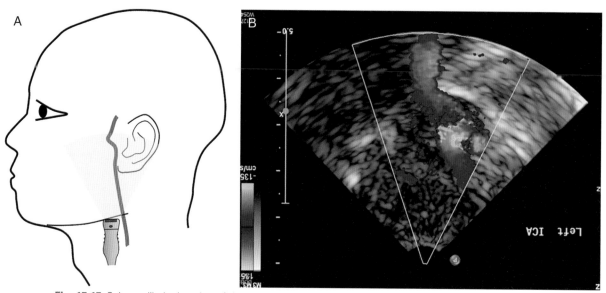

Fig. 17.17 Submandibular imaging of the extracranial internal carotid artery. The probe is directed to image along the artery. This can be done with nonimaging systems, and by convention, in this approach, no angle correction is made. The color flow image shows arterial flow as blue away from the transducer.

in cerebral blood flow. ICP is measured invasively, but this poses risks to the patient. Early studies using TCD indicated that changes in flow waveform reflect changes in ICP and that measurement of PI might reduce the need for direct invasive measurement or allow estimates of ICP where invasive measurement was not appropriate. Measurement of diastolic flow has been used to estimate CPP. Subsequent studies have shown that accuracy is variable and that the complex causes of changes to ICP and CPP and the response of flow to changes in blood pressure and ICP might require more sophisticated modeling and use of TCD parameters. A review of nearly 100 studies (Cardim et al. 2016) is a useful reference of work to date and outlines the complexity and effectiveness of TCD for these applications.

Cerebral Circulatory Arrest/Brain Stem Death

TCD can be used to confirm the absence of perfusion in circulatory cerebral arrest. Measurement of flow is made in the MCAs and basilar artery and indications of no flow are characterized by:

- Sharp initial systolic forward flow followed by flow reversal demonstrating no net flow (Fig. 17.18)
- Small systolic short spikes (<200 m/s) with no diastolic flow

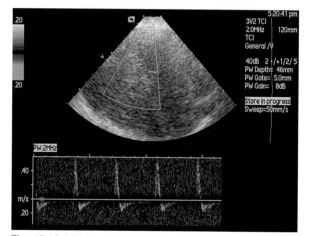

Fig. 17.18 Middle cerebral artery flow waveform in patient with cerebral circulatory arrest. The short early systolic forward spike of flow in the artery is followed by reverse flow. There is no net flow in the artery.

- Absent intracranial flow with flow reversal in the extracranial circulation.

Reported sensitivity is high, although poor temporal windows in a small percentage of patients is a limitation. It is recommended that two sets of readings taken 30 minutes apart be recorded to confirm the status.

INTRAOPERATIVE MONITORING DURING CAROTID ENDARTERECTOMY

Nonimaging TCD can be used to monitor cerebral blood flow during carotid endarterectomy to ensure that the cerebral perfusion to the ICA territory in the brain is maintained. It can also be used for the detection of emboli, both air and particulate, during the procedure. Local protocols will vary but there are key points during the procedure where monitoring can be useful. These are:

- The dissection phase. If emboli are detected, they will be particulate, and the operating surgeon can be alerted to a potentially fragile plaque and avoid undue disturbance to the artery.
- The clamping phase to open the bifurcation and remove the plaque. If the velocity falls by more than half the preshunt value or less than 15 cm/s, the surgeon should be alerted.
- If a shunt is used, the shunt velocities can be monitored for any kinking or ingress of air.
- ICA flow restored. The velocity and presence of emboli can be recorded.
- Detection of emboli during wound closure. Some air emboli may be heard, but evidence of particulate embolization should be reported to the surgeon, as this could indicate thrombus within the artery.

In addition, TCD can be used to monitor the risk of hyperperfusion syndrome if the patient's blood pressure is high following the procedure or if there are high velocities >80 cm/s at the end of the procedure.

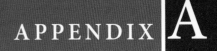
Decibel Scale

The decibel scale allows the large range of values of ultrasound intensities, or signal voltages, to be expressed by a smaller range of numbers, as shown in Table A.1. The decibel scale expresses the ratios of intensities, or voltages, using a logarithmic scale. The decibel scale is used to describe ultrasound attenuation and amplifier gain.

TABLE A.1 Decibel Scale Applied to Intensity and Voltage (or Echo Amplitude)

Intensity Ratio (I/I_0)	Decibel (dB)	Amplitude Ratio (V/V_0)
1 000 000	60	1000
10 000	40	100
100	20	10
10	10	3
2	3	1.4
0.5	−3	0.7
0.1	−10	0.3
0.01	−20	0.1
0.000 1	−40	0.01
0.000 001	−60	0.001

Intensity I (relative to I_0) in dB = $10 \log_{10}(I/I_0)$.
Gain in dB = $20 \log_{10}(V/V_0)$.

Sensitivity and Specificity

When a new test is developed, a threshold at which the results are considered to indicate the presence or absence of the disease has to be selected. To do this, the results of the test are compared to another method of detecting the disease, often known as the "gold standard." Unfortunately, there is usually an overlap between the results obtained in the presence of the disease and the results obtained in the absence of disease. This means that some patients will be falsely diagnosed as having the disease whereas others will be falsely diagnosed as not having the disease. Selecting the best threshold for the test depends partly on the prevalence of the disease within the group tested and also on the consequence of a false classification (i.e., missing the disease or incorrectly diagnosing disease in a normal patient). The performance of a diagnostic test can be measured by its sensitivity and specificity, which are defined as follows:

$$\text{Senstivity} = \frac{\text{Number of patients with the disease correctly diagnosed}}{\text{Number of patients with the disease}}$$

The number of patients with the disease includes people with a true positive result and those with a false-negative result.

$$\text{Specificity} = \frac{\text{Number of patients without the disease correctly diagnosed}}{\text{Number of patients without the disease}}$$

The number of patients without the disease includes people with a true negative result and those with a false positive result.

The value of the sensitivity and specificity will vary as the threshold of the test is altered. For example, if the threshold is changed to improve sensitivity, the specificity will fall. Altering the threshold and calculating the specificity and sensitivity can permit the selection of the optimal threshold and allow the value of the diagnostic test to be assessed. Other closely related qualities of a test often quoted in the literature are the positive predictive value (PPV) and negative predictive value (NPV). The PPV is the percentage of patients with a positive test who have the disease.

$$\text{PPV} = \frac{\text{Number of patients with the disease correctly diagnosed}}{\text{Total number of patients with positive results}}$$

The total number of patients with positive results includes people with true-positive results and false-positive results. A true-positive result is a result that is positive when it should be positive. A false-positive result is a result that is positive when it should be negative.

$$\text{NPV} = \frac{\text{Number of patients without the disease correctly diagnosed}}{\text{Total number of patient with negative results}}$$

The total number of patients with negative results includes people with true-negative results and false-negative results. A true-negative result is a result that is negative when it should be negative. A false-negative result is a result that is negative when it should be positive.

PPV and NPV are often more helpful to clinicians, as these are related to the prevalence of a specific disease in the population. For instance, PPV and NPV will provide information on how well a screening test will perform in a population with a known prevalence of a specific disease. It is important when determining the cost-effectiveness of commissioning a screening program, such as ultrasound screening for abdominal aortic aneurysms. If the prevalence of the disease in a population is high, it is likely that the PPV will be higher and the NPV lower, and vice versa. Sensitivity and specificity are related to the accuracy of a test compared to a reference test or gold standard and are independent of the prevalence of disease. Readers who require more detailed information about this subject and example calculations should consult an appropriate statistics text.

Summary of Scanner Controls

B-MODE CONTROLS			
Control	**Effect**		**Comment**
Overall gain and time gain compensation *Frequent adjustment*	**Increase** Increases the amplification and brightness of returning echoes	**Decrease** Decreases the amplification and brightness of returning echoes	Time gain compensation (TGC) sliders can be used to adjust the gain at discrete depths in the image. Can equalize the brightness of echoes returning from the near field and far field to compensate for attenuation. On most scanners the TGC sliders are positioned on a straight line one above the other at the start of the scan
Depth *Frequent adjustment*	**Increase** To display structures lying deeper in the body that are in the path of the beam. Will result in lower frame rate with increasing depth	**Decrease** If there is too much depth (several cm) in the image below the region or area of interest	Depth markings are shown on the side of the image display in centimeters and sometimes half or quarter centimeter marks or dashes
Focus *Frequent adjustment*	Position at the level of interest. If multiple focal zones are used, ensure that the area of interest is roughly in the middle of the zones		Adjusted by operator with a paddle, rotary knob, or touch screen. Newer scanners may not have transmit focus
Freeze *Frequent use*	Will freeze the image. Used to capture images and to make measurements with calipers such as vessel diameter		Scanners store images from the previous 10–30 seconds, which can be recalled for analysis
Zoom *Occasional use*	The zoom control selects an area of the image for display, enlarging the selected area on the screen. It may allow improved performance in this area (write zoom) or may just magnify the processed image (read zoom). Zooming on a frozen image is read zoom. Systems also have image sector width control for curvilinear and phased array transducers to concentrate the display on the center of the image.		Be aware that when using high zoom, it is possible to lose your orientation within the image and relationship to other tissues within the transducer scan plane. If this occurs, switch off the zoom, re-position the transducer, and switch the zoom back on

B-MODE CONTROLS

Control	Effect		Comment
Transmit frequency *Occasional adjustment depending on application*	On most systems the imaging frequency of the transducer can be adjusted. Lower frequency will enable better penetration but will result in a reduction in resolution. It is also possible to increase the imaging frequency to improve resolution but at the expense of penetration		Can be useful if the region being investigated is not clearly defined using the default frequency setting. Reducing the imaging frequency may help instead of switching to a lower-frequency transducer. The range of frequency options will vary between systems and transducers and will include harmonic options (see later)
Harmonic imaging on/off *Occasional adjustment*	Normally on by default in most presets. Decreases reverberation and side lobe artifacts. Improved signal-to-noise ratio		Many scanners display H or THI on the side of the screen when harmonic imaging is active
Compound imaging on/off *Infrequent adjustment*	Normally on by default in most presets. Decreases noise and speckle artifacts by acquiring images from a number of different angles. Can reduce shadows from the side walls of vessels and cysts, small areas of calcification, and catheters		The strength of beam compounding can be adjusted by the operator, although it is normally optimized in the preset for a specific examination. Too much compounding can reduce frame rate and lead to "over-smoothing" of some images
Adaptive processing *Infrequent adjustment*	Described and executed in different ways by different manufacturers. Adjusts image processing such as smoothing and edge enhancement depending on the content of the image		Different levels of processing produce changes in image appearance. High levels of adaptive processing can introduce new larger scale patterns in the image
Trapezoidal/wide screen *Occasional adjustment*	On linear arrays, the width of the image can be extended by beam steering at the edges of the image		Useful when measuring the length of superficial structures
Dynamic range (sometimes called compression) *Occasional adjustment*	**Increase** Increases the range of echo amplitudes displayed on the image. The overall image appears smoother	**Decrease** Decreases the range of echo amplitudes displayed in the image. Image has more contrast	Defined as the ratio of largest to smallest signal the system is capable of processing. Generally set to low to mid-level for vascular imaging
Gray-scale map *Occasional adjustment*	Grayscale maps modify the relationship between the level of echo received, following gain and compression, to the displayed level of gray/white/black. Some maps will enhance low level echoes, some mid-level, and some high level		The grayscale map function provides a range of map options, labeled by a letter or number. The operator manual may need to be consulted to determine how to change the grayscale map

B-MODE CONTROLS

Control	Effect		Comment
B-mode color maps *Infrequent adjustment*	B-mode color map can improve the contrast resolution by enhancing subtle soft-tissue differences. B-color images are created by converting grayscale information into various levels of color intensity. The advantage is that the human eye can only appreciate a limited number of gray shades but is able to distinguish a greater number of different color hues and tints		Operator preference
Edge enhancement *Infrequent adjustment*	Accentuates the appearances of edges in the image. Useful for scans where multiple diameter measurements are being undertaken, such as abdominal aortic aneurysm screening		Edge enhancement, also known as sharpness or enhance, is an algorithm that attempts to sharpen the image by identifying and enhancing the interfaces or boundaries between structures. Sharpening of the edges or borders of structures can enable easier placement of measurement calipers
Line density *Infrequent adjustment*	**Increase** Increases the number of scan lines used to create the image, improving spatial resolution, but can result in lower frame rate	**Decrease** Decrease the number of scan lines, leading to poorer spatial resolution but higher frame rate	Normally optimized by the preset. Increased line density will lead to a lower frame rate
Persistence or frame averaging *Infrequent adjustment*	**Increase** A number of frames are averaged to provide a single image, reducing noise, but objects that are moving within the image may be blurred. The image can also blur if the probe is moved rapidly	**Decrease** Can provide a more dynamic image in real time but can lead to more noise within the image	Normally optimized by the preset
Output power *Infrequent adjustment*	Increasing power increases the intensity of the beam (output of the scanner), increasing signal to noise in returning echoes. It can lead to increased heating of tissue in the path of the beam See the section on safety		Normally optimized by the preset. In many systems it is set at or near maximum in the preset, so in reality may not be possible to increase significantly. If the image is poor at depth, consider using a lower-frequency transducer rather than increasing the power

COLOR FLOW IMAGING CONTROLS

Control	Effect		Comment
Color gain *Frequent adjustment*	**Increase** Increase if there is poor color filling of a vessels. If it is increased too high, then noise can appear outside the vessel lumen	**Decrease** Decrease if there is excess color noise or the color flow signal "bleeds" outside the vessel	
Color box steer *Frequent adjustment*	Optimize the steering of the box to reduce the beam to flow angle for the vessel being investigated		Steer left, center, or right. Normally a paddle switch, rotary knob, or touch key
Color box size *Frequent adjustment*	**Increase** To interrogate a larger region of a vessel or tissue. This will decrease frame rate	**Decrease** To interrogate a small area of vessel or tissue. Can improve frame rate; the display can be less distracting	
Color scale *Frequent adjustment*	**Increase** To demonstrate higher velocity flow, such as arterial flow in nondiseased vessels without aliasing	**Decrease** To demonstrate lower velocity flow, such as venous flow or flow distal to significant arterial disease	A nominal color scale is set in specific presets. However, frequent adjustment may be needed. As a guide, scale for normal arterial flow is around 25 cm/s. For venous flow it is around 10 cm/s
Color invert *Frequent adjustment*	Inverts the colors on the two halves of the color bar. The color displayed above the baseline demonstrates flow that is toward the probe. Useful if venous flow is displayed in red, as it can be inverted to blue and vice versa for an artery		Some scanners may automatically invert when the steer angle is changed for right to left or left to right
Color transmit frequency *Occasional adjustment*	**Increase** More sensitive to low velocities. More susceptible to aliasing	**Decrease** Improved penetration to deep vessels	Particularly important in abdominal Doppler but also influences appearance in other applications
Color wall filter *Occasional adjustment*	**Increase** Removes low-velocity flow or low-velocity motion. However, may remove important information such as low-velocity diastolic flow or trickle flow beyond a critical stenosis	**Decrease** Enables low-velocity motion to be displayed, but this may be unwanted signals from wall motion	Normally optimized by the preset
Color write priority *Occasional adjustment*	A control that can be adjusted to determine if a pixel on the screen within the color box will be a displayed as color or B-mode gray scale. The threshold can be changed to give priority to writing color. This will enable color to be displayed on a bright B-mode image or within small vessels poorly visualized on B-mode		Normally optimized by the preset and not commonly changed if the B-mode gain is optimized at the start of the scan. The priority setting is normally shown as a horizontal line on the color bar

COLOR FLOW IMAGING CONTROLS

Control	Effect		Comment
Color map *Occasional adjustment*	Alters the color hues used to display different velocities. Can be used to highlight variation in flow velocities		Normally optimized by the pre-set to suit the sonographers' preferences
Line density *Infrequent adjustment*	**Increase** Increases the number of scan lines to create the image improving spatial resolution but can result in lower frame rate	**Decrease** Decreases the number of scan lines, leading to poorer resolution but higher frame rate	Normally optimized by the preset. Increased line density will lead to a slower frame rate but can lead to improved lateral spatial resolution in the color image
Ensemble length/color quality *Infrequent adjustment*	**Increase** Increases sensitivity to flow and quality of the color image	**Decrease** To enable a higher frame rate	Normally optimized by the preset
Persistence or frame averaging *Infrequent adjustment*	**Increase** Can enhance color sensitivity to low velocity flow	**Decrease** Leads to a more dynamic appearance of change	Normally optimized by the preset, arterial has low persistence, venous has higher persistence
Fast flow/slow flow (and variants) *Occasional adjustment*	One touch options selected to optimize several parameters for specific types of flow. For slow flow, this could be a lower transmit frequency, lower scale and filter, more frame averaging, and higher line density		Useful for applications where there are different flows to be imaged. For example, renal artery flow will be higher velocity and deep, but renal parenchymal flow will be lower velocity and more superficial

SPECTRAL DOPPLER CONTROLS

Control	Effect		Comment
Spectral Doppler gain *Frequent adjustment*	**Increase** The brightness of the spectrum is increased. Too much gain can result in signals appearing in the reverse channel, the appearance of increased spectral broadening, and increased noise	**Decrease** The brightness of the spectrum is decreased. If it is decreased too much, low-intensity flow signals may be missed	Spectral Doppler gain can result in errors when measuring peak velocity with measurement calipers or automated measurements. Too much gain can lead to broadening of the spectrum and an overestimation of velocity. Low gain can generate errors in automated velocity measurements
Spectral Doppler beam steering *Frequent adjustment*	The beam-to-vessel angle should be minimized to ensure that an adequate Doppler shift signal can be obtained and to reduce errors in velocity measurements		This should be undertaken with consideration to the angle correction cursor, as this will be the next stage of the process

continued

SPECTRAL DOPPLER CONTROLS

Control	Effect		Comment
Angle correction cursor *Frequent adjustment*	This is adjusted to measure the angle between the Doppler beam and direction of flow and is required in order for the system to calculate and display flow velocity in the path of the beam		The control can be a paddle, knob, or touch screen key to enable the cursor to be aligned with the flow. The angle should be less than 60° to reduce measurement errors
Spectral Doppler scale (PRF) *Frequent adjustment*	**Increase** The scale can be increased if aliasing is present, to accommodate the waveform within the display and enable accurate velocity measurement	**Decrease** Lower the scale so the waveform fills ¾ of the display	If blood flow velocity is very high, it may be impossible to avoid aliasing in the display. Try moving the baseline to the bottom of the display if no reverse flow is present
Spectral Doppler invert *Frequent adjustment*	This control will invert the spectral display. If the signal was displayed above the baseline, pressing invert will display the signal below the baseline		It is important to look at the figures on the velocity scale. They are shown as positive and negative numbers and will give an indication if flow is toward (positive number) or away (negative number) from the transducer
Baseline position *Frequent adjustment*	Adjusts the position of the baseline, representing zero velocity, on the spectral display. It can be set toward the bottom of the display if arterial flow in one direction is recorded to optimize the size of the Doppler waveform. When both forward and reverse flow are present, for instance biphasic/triphasic arterial flow, the baseline can be moved up in order to demonstrate the different directions of flow		The baseline position is normally adjusted by a rotary knob, paddle, or touch screen key. The baseline control is one of the controls that can be adjusted to overcome aliasing by moving it to the bottom of the image to try and accommodate the waveform
Sample volume size *Occasional* adjustment	**Increase** To sample flow across the entire vessel and for measurements of volume flow	**Decrease** To sample discrete areas within a vessel or flow across a stenosis	Normally optimized by the preset. Normally small for arterial investigations. Can be wider for venous studies
Transmit frequency *Occasional adjustment*	**Increase** More sensitive to low velocities	**Decrease** Improved penetration to deep vessels, delays requirement for HPRF in high-velocity deep Doppler applications	Useful in deep abdominal Doppler applications

SPECTRAL DOPPLER CONTROLS

Control	Effect		Comment
Sweep speed *Occasional adjustment*	The sweep speed is normally optimized by the preset but can be increased to provide more detail and separation of successive waveforms (they will move quickly across the display) or decreased, to display signals over a longer period within a complete sweep		Ideally, displaying four to eight arterial waveforms in one sweep is adequate for analysis and measurement
Doppler spectrum post-processing *Occasional adjustment*	Ascribes different gray or color levels to the Doppler spectrum, which can emphasize perception of spectral broadening		Normally optimized by the preset
Spectral Doppler filter (wall filter) *Occasional adjustment*	**Increase** Will filter out low-velocity motion such as wall thump but can remove low-velocity flow if set too high	**Decrease** Will enable low-velocity motion or flow to be displayed. However, wall thump or respiratory motion may be displayed	The wall filter is normally optimized by the preset

REFERENCES

Aaslid, R., Markwalder, T.-M., & Norris, H. (1982). Non-invasive transcranial Doppler ultrasound recording of flow velocity in basal cerebral arteries. *Journal of Neurosurgery*, *57*(6), 769–774. https://doi.org/10.3171/jns.1982.57.6.0769.

Aboyans, V., Ricco, J. B., Bartelink, M. L. E. L., Björck, M., Brodmann, M., Cohnert, T., et al. (2017). 2017 ESC guide-lines on the diagnosis and treatment of peripheral arterial diseases, developed in collaboration with the European Society for Vascular Surgery (ESVS). *European Heart Journal*, *39*(9), 763–816. https://doi.org/10.1093/eurheartj/ehx095.

Aboyans, V., Ricco, J. B., Bartelink, M. E. L., Björck, M., Brodmann, M., Cohnert, T., et al. (2018). 2017 ESC Guidelines on the diagnosis and treatment of peripheral arterial diseases, in collaboration with the European Society for Vascular Surgery (ESVS). *European Journal of Vascular and Endovascular Surgery*, *55*(3), 305–368. https://doi.org/10.1016/j.ejvs.2017.07.018.

AbuRahma, A. F. (2000). Segmental Doppler pressures and Doppler waveform analysis in peripheral vascular disease of the lower extremities. In A. F. AbuRahma, & J. J. Bergan (Eds.), *Noninvasive vascular diagnosis* (pp. 213–229). New York: Springer. https://doi.org/10.1007/978-1-4471-3837-2_15.

AbuRahma, A. F., Srivastava, M., Mousa, A. Y., Dearing, D. D., Hass, S. M., Campbell, J. R., et al. (2012). Critical analysis of renal duplex ultrasound parameters in detect-ing significant renal artery stenosis. *Journal of Vascular Surgery*, *56*(4), 1052–1060. https://doi.org/10.1016/j.jvs.2012.03.036.

AbuRahma, A. F., Stone, P. A., Srivastava, M., Dean, L. S., Keiffer, T., Hass, S. M., et al. (2012). Mesenteric/celiac duplex ultrasound interpretation criteria revisited. *Journal of Vascular Surgery*, *55*(2), 428–436. https://doi.org/10.1016/j.jvs.2011.08.052.

Adam, D. J., Bello, M., Hartshorne, T., & London, N. J. (2003). Role of superficial venous surgery in patients with combined superficial and segmental deep venous reflux. *European Journal of Vascular and Endovascular Surgery*, *25*(5), 469–472. https://doi.org/10.1053/ejvs.2002.1894.

Adams, R. J., McKie, V. C., Hsu, L., Files, B., Vichinsky, E., Pegelow, C., et al. (1998). Prevention of a first stroke by transfusions in children with sickle cell anemia and abnormal results in transcranial Doppler ultrasonography. *New England Journal of Medicine*, *339*(1), 5–11. https://doi.org/10.1056/NEJM199807023390102.

American College of Radiology. (Revised 2016). *ACR-AIUM-SRU Practice parameter for the performance of ultrasound vascular mapping for preoperative planning of dialysis access*. Retrieved from https://www.acr.org/-/media/ACR/Files/Practice-Parameters/US-PreOpDialysis.pdf.

American College of Radiology. (Revised 2019). *ACR-AIUM-SRU Practice parameter for the performance of vascular ultrasound for postoperative assessment of hemodialysis access*. Retrieved from https://www.acr.org/-/media/ACR/Files/Practice-Parameters/PostOpDialysis.pdf.

Anderson, F. A., Jr., & Spencer, F. A. (2003). Risk factors for venous thromboembolism. *Circulation*, *107*(23 Suppl. 1), I9–I16. https://doi.org/10.1161/01.CIR.0000078469.07362.E6.

Armstrong, P. A., Bandyk, D. F., Wilson, J. S., Shames, M. L., Johnson, B. L., & Back, M. R. (2004). Optimizing infrain-guinal arm vein bypass patency with duplex ultrasound surveillance and endovascular therapy. *Journal of Vascular Surgery*, *40*(4), 724–731. https://doi.org/10.1016/j.jvs.2004.07.037.

Asymptomatic Carotid Atherosclerosis Study Group. (1995). Carotid endarterectomy for patients with asymptomatic internal carotid artery stenosis. *Journal of the American Medical Association*, *273*, 1421–1428.

Baarslag, H. J., Van Beek, E. J., Koopman, M. M., & Reekers, J. A. (2002). Prospective study of color duplex ultraso-nography compared with contrast venography in patients suspected of having deep venous thrombosis of the upper extremities. *Annals of Internal Medicine*, *136*(12), 865–872. https://doi.org/10.7326/0003-4819-136-12-200206180-00007.

Bamford, J. M. (2000). The role of the clinical examination in the subclassification of stroke. *Cerebrovascular Diseases*, *10*(Suppl. 4), 2–4. https://doi.org/10.1159/000047582.

Bandyk, D. F. (2007). Surveillance after lower extremity arterial bypass. *Perspectives in Vascular Surgery and Endovascular Therapy*, *19*(4), 376–383. https://doi.org/10.1177/1531003507310460.

Baril, D. T., Rhee, R. Y., Kim, J., Makaroun, M. S., Chaer, R. A., & Marone, L. K. (2009). Duplex criteria for determi-nation of in-stent stenosis after angioplasty and stenting of the superficial femoral artery. *Journal of Vascular Surgery*, *49*(1), 133–138. https://doi.org/10.1016/j.jvs.2008.09.046.

Baxter, G. M., Ireland, H., Moss, J. G., Harden, P. N., Junor, B. J., Rodger, R. S., et al. (1995). Colour Doppler ultra-sound in renal transplant artery stenosis: Which Doppler index? *Clinical Radiology, 50*(9), 618–622. https://doi. org/10.1016/s0009-9260(05)83291-x.

Beckman, M. G., Hooper, W. C., Critchley, S. E., & Ortel, T. L. (2010). Venous thromboembolism: A public health concern. *American Journal of Preventative Medicine, 38*(Suppl. 4), S445–S450. https://doi.org/10.1016/ j.amepre.2009.12.017.

Beeman, B. R., Murtha, K., Doer, K., McAfee-Bennett, S., Dougherty, M. J., & Calligaro, K. D. (2010). Duplex ultrasound factors predicting persistent type II endoleak and increasing AAA sac diameter after EVAR. *Journal of Vascular Surgery, 52*(5), 1147–1152. https://doi.org/10.1016/j. jvs.2010.06.099.

Bernardini, E., De Rango, P., Piccioli, R., Bisacci, C., Pagliuca, V., Genovese, G., et al. (2010). Development of primary superficial venous insufficiency: The ascending theory. Observational and hemodynamic data from a 9-year experience. *Annals of Vascular Surgery, 24*(6), 709–720. https:// doi.org/10.1016/j.avsg.2010.01.011.

Bernaudin, F., Verlhac, S., Arnaud, C., Kamdem, A., Vasile, M., Kasbi, F., et al. (2015). Chronic acute anemia and extracranial internal carotid stenosis are risk factors for silent cerebral infarcts in sickle cell anemia. *Blood, 125*(10), 1653–1661. https://doi.org/10.1182/blood-2014-09-599852.

Beyer, J., & Schellong, S. (2005). Deep vein thrombosis: Current diagnostic strategy. *European Journal of Internal Medicine, 16*(4), 238–246. https://doi.org/10.1016/j. ejim.2005.04.001.

Bock, R. W., & Lusby, R. J. (1992). Carotid plaque morphology and interpretation of the echolucent lesions. In K. H. Labs, K. A. Jager, & D. E. Fitzgerald (Eds.), *Diagnostic vascular ultrasound* (pp. 225–236). London: Edward Arnold.

Bode, H., & Wais, U. (1988). Age dependence on flow velocities in basal cerebral arteries. *Archives of Disease Childhood, 63*(6), 606–611. https://doi.org/10.1136/ adc.63.6.606.

Bonfield, M., Cramp, F., & Robinson, T. (2012). Effect of patient positioning on the duration of venous reflux in duplex ultrasound for venous insufficiency. *Ultrasound, 20*(2), 92–97. https://doi.org/10.1258/ult.2012.011055.

Brake, M., Lim, C. S., Shepherd, A. C., Shalhoub, J., & Davies, A. H. (2013). Pathogenesis and etiology of recurrent varicose veins. *Journal of Vascular Surgery, 57*(3), 860–868. https://doi.org/10.1016/j.jvs.2012.10.102.

Brewster, D. C., Corniest, J. L., Hallett, J. W., Jr., Johnston, K. W., Krupski, W. C., & Matsumura, J. S. (2003). Guidelines for the treatment of abdominal aortic aneurysms. Report of a subcommittee of the Joint Council of the American Association for Vascular Surgery and Society for Vascular Surgery. *Journal of Vascular Surgery, 37*(5), 1106–1117. https://doi.org/10.1067/mva.2003.363.

British Medical Journal (BMJ) Best Practice. *Overview of Stroke.* Retrieved October 26, 2020 from https://bestpractice. bmj.com/topics/en-gb/1080.

Bromberg, J., Bøgsted, M., Lindholm, J. S., Behr-Rasmussen, C., Hørlyck, A., & Frøkjær, J. B. (2018). Superior reproducibility of the leading to leading edge and inner to inner edge methods in the ultrasound assessment of maximum abdominal aortic diameter. *European Journal of Vascular and Endovascular Surgery, 55*(2), 206–213. https://doi. org/10.1016/j.ejvs.2017.11.019.

Caggiati, A., Bergan, J. J., Gloviczki, P., Wendell-Smith, C. P., Partsch, H., & International Interdisciplinary Consensus Committee on Venous Anatomical Terminology. (2002). Nomenclature of the veins of the lower limbs: An international interdisciplinary consensus statement. *Journal of Vascular Surgery, 36*(2), 416–422. https://doi.org/10.1067/ mva.2002.125847.

Caggiati, A., Rippa Bonati, M., Pieri, A., & Riva, A. (2004). 1603–2003: Four centuries of valves. *European Journal of Vascular and Endovascular Surgery, 28*(4), 439–441. https://doi.org/10.1016/j.ejvs.2004.04.004.

Campbell, B. (2006). Varicose veins and their management. *British Medical Journal, 333*(7562), 287–292. https://doi. org/10.1136/bmj.333.7562.287.

Cardim, D., Robba, C., Bohdanowicz, M., Donnelly, J., Cabella, B., Liu, X., et al. (2016). Non-invasive monitoring of intracranial pressure using transcranial Doppler ultrasonography: Is it possible? *Neurocritical Care, 25*(3), 473–491. https://doi.org/10.1007/s12028-016-0258-6.

Caro, C. G., Pedley, T. J., Schroter, R. C., & Seed, W. A. (1978). *The mechanics of the circulation.* Oxford University Press.

Cavezzi, A., Labropoulos, N., Partsch, S., Ricci, S., Caggiati, A., Myers, K., et al. (2006). Duplex ultrasound investigation of the veins in chronic venous disease of the lower limbs – UIP consensus document. Part II. Anatomy. *European Journal of Vascular and Endovascular Surgery, 31*(3), 288–299. https://doi.org/10.1016/j.ejvs.2005.07.020.

Centers for Disease Control and Prevention. (2020). *Venous Thromboembolism (Blood Clots).* Retrieved September 21, 2020, from www.cdc.gov/ncbddd/dvt/data.html.

Chawla, L. S., Bellomo, R., Bihorac, A., Goldstein, S. L., Siew, E. D., Bagshaw, S. M., & Acute Disease Quality Initiative Workgroup 16., et al. (2017). Acute kidney disease and renal recovery: Consensus report of the Acute Disease Quality Initiative [ADQI] 16 workgroup. *Nature Reviews Nephrology, 13*(4), 241–257. https://doi.org/10.1038/nrneph.2017.2.

Clark, C. E., Taylor, R. S., Shore, A. C., Ukoumunne, O. C., & Campbell, J. L. (2012). Association of a difference in systolic blood pressure between arms with vascular disease and mortality: A systematic review and meta-analysis. *Lancet, 379*(9819), 905–914. https://doi.org/10.1016/ S0140-6736(11)61710-8.

Coffi, S. B., Ubbink, D. T., Zwiers, I., van Gurp, A. J., & Lege-mate, D. A. (2001). The value of the peak systolic velocity ratio in the assessment of the haemodynamic significance of subcritical iliac artery stenoses. *European Journal of Vascular and Endovascular Surgery*, 22(5), 424–428. https://doi.org/10.1053/ejvs.2001.1490.

Coleridge-Smith, P., Labropoulos, H., Partsch, H., Myers, K., Nicolaides, A., & Cavezzi, A. (2006). Duplex ultrasound investigation of the venous disease of the lower limbs – UIP consensus document. Part I. Basic principles. *European Journal of Vascular and Endovascular Surgery*, 31(1), 83–92. https://doi.org/10.1016/j.ejvs.2005.07.019.

Connes, P., Verlhac, S., & Bernaudin, F. (2013). Advances in understanding the pathogenesis of cerebrovascular vasculopathy in sickle cell anaemia. *British Journal of Haematology*, 161(4), 484–498. https://doi.org/10.1111/bjh.12300.

Conte, M. S., Bradbury, A. W., Kolh, P., White, J. V., Dick, F., Fitridge, R., et al. (2019). Global vascular guidelines on the management of chronic limb-threatening ischemia. *European Journal of Vascular and Endovascular Surgery*, 58(1S), S1–S109.e33. https://doi.org/10.1016/j.ejvs.2019.05.006.

Corpataux, J. M., Haesler, E., Silacci, P., Ris, H. B., & Hayoz, D. (2002). Low-pressure environment and remodelling of the forearm vein in Brescia-Cimino hemodialysis access. *Nephrology Dialysis Transplantation*, 17(6), 1057–1062. https://doi.org/10.1093/ndt/17.6.1057.

Cosmi, B. (2015). Management of superficial vein thrombosis. *Journal of Thrombosis and Haemostasis*, 13(7), 1175–1183. https://doi.org/10.1111/jth.12986.

Cossman, D. V., Ellison, J. E., Wagner, W. H., Carroll, R. M., Treiman, R. L., Foran, R. F., et al. (1989). Comparison of contrast arteriography to arterial mapping with color-flow duplex imaging in the lower extremities. *Journal of Vascular Surgery*, 10(5), 522–529. https://doi.org/10.1067/mva.1989.14963.

Cranley, J. J., Canos, A. J., & Sull, W. J. (1976). The diagnosis of deep vein thrombosis: Fallibility of clinical symptoms and signs. *Archives of Surgery*, 111(1), 34–36. https://doi.org/10.1001/archsurg.1976.01360190036005.

Criqui, M. H., & Aboyans, V. (2015). Epidemiology of peripheral artery disease. *Circulation Research*, 116(9), 1509–1526. https://doi.org/10.1161/CIRCRESAHA.116.303849.

Darwood, R., Theivacumar, N., Dellagrammaticas, D., Mavor, A. I., & Gough, M. J. (2008). Randomized clinical trial comparing endovenous laser ablation with surgery for the treatment of primary great saphenous veins. *British Journal of Surgery*, 95(3), 294–301. https://doi.org/10.1002/bjs.6101.

Davies, A. H. (2019). The seriousness of chronic venous disease: A review of real-world evidence. *Advances in Therapy*, 36(Suppl. 1), 5–12. https://doi.org/10.1007/s12325-019-0881-7.

Davies, A. H., Hawdon, A. J., Sydes, M. R., Thompson, S. G., & VGST Participants. (2005). Is duplex surveillance of value after leg vein bypass grafting? Principal results of the Vein Graft Surveillance Randomised Trial (VGST). *Circulation*, 112(13), 1985–1991. https://doi.org/10.1161/CIRCULATIONAHA.104.518738.

Deer, S. E., Ergul, E. A., Schermerhorn, M. L., Siracuse, J. J., Schanzer, A., Goodney, P. P., & Vascular Study Group of New England., et al. (2018). Aneurysm sac expansion is independently associated with late mortality in patients treated with endovascular aneurysm repair. *Journal of Vascular Surgery*, 67(1), 157–164. https://doi.org/10.1016/j.jvs.2017.06.075.

Dietzek, A. (2007). Endovenous radiofrequency ablation for the treatment of varicose veins. *Vascular*, 15(5), 255–261. https://doi.org/10.2310/6670.2007.00062.

Dixon, B. S. (2006). Why don't fistula mature? *Kidney International*, 70(8), 1413–1422. https://doi.org/10.1038/sj.ki.5001747.

Drieghe, B., Madaric, J., Sarno, G., Manoharan, G., Bartunek, J., Heyndrickx, G. R., et al. (2008). Assessment of renal artery stenosis: Side-by-side comparison of angiography and duplex ultrasound with pressure gradient measurements. *European Heart Journal*, 29(4), 517–524. https://doi.org/10.1093/eurheartj/ehm631.

Duck, F. A. (2019). Safety of diagnostic ultrasound. In Hoskins, P. R. Martin, K. & Thrush, A. (Eds.), *Diagnostic ultrasound: Physics and equipment* (3rd ed.) (pp. 305–324). Boca Raton, FL: CRC Press.

Earnshaw, J. J., & Lee, T. (2017). Update on screening for abdominal aortic aneurysm. *European Journal of Vascular and Endovascular Surgery*, 54(1), 1–2. https://doi.org/10.1016/j.ejvs.2017.04.002.

Easton, J. D., Saver, J. L., Albers, G. W., Alberts, M. J., Chaturvedi, S., Feldmann, E., & American Heart Association, American Stroke Association Stroke Council, Council on Cardiovascular Surgery and Anesthesia, Council on Cardiovascular Radiology and Intervention, Council on Cardiovascular Nursing, & Interdisciplinary Council on Peripheral Vascular Disease., et al. (2009). Definition and evaluation of transient ischemic attack: A scientific statement for healthcare professionals from the American Heart Association/American Stroke Association Stroke Council; Council on Cardiovascular Surgery and Anesthesia; Council on Cardiovascular Radiology and Intervention; Council on Cardiovascular Nursing; and the Interdisciplinary Council on Peripheral Vascular Disease. *Stroke*, 40(6), 2276–2293. https://doi.org/10.1161/STROKEAHA.108.192218.

Eifert, S., Villavicencio, J. L., Kao, T. C., Taute, B. M., & Rich, N. M. (2000). Prevalence of deep venous anomalies in congenital vascular malformations of venous predominance. *Journal of Vascular Surgery*, 31(3), 462–471.

Eklöf, B., Rutherford, R., Bergan, J., Carpentier, P. H., Gloviczki, P., Kistner, R. L., & American Venous Forum International Ad Hoc Committee for Revision of the CEAP Classification., et al. (2004). Revision of the CEAP classification for chronic venous disorders: Consensus statement. *Journal of Vascular Surgery*, *40*(6), 1248–1252. https://doi.org/10.1016/j.jvs.2004.09.027.

European Carotid Plaque Study Group. (1995). Carotid artery plaque composition – relationship to clinical presentation and ultrasound B-mode imaging. *European Journal of Endovascular Surgery*, *10*(1), 23–30. https://doi.org/10.1016/s1078-5884(05)80194-7.

European Carotid Surgery Trialists' Collaborative Group. (1998). Randomised trial of endarterectomy for recently symptomatic carotid stenosis: Final results of the MRC European Carotid Surgery Trial (ECST). *Lancet*, *351*(9113), 1379–1387.

Evans, C. J., Allan, P. L., Lee, A. J., Bradbury, A. W., Ruckley, C. V., & Fowkes, F. G. (1998). Prevalence of venous reflux in the general population on duplex scanning: The Edinburgh Vein Study. *Journal of Vascular Surgery*, *28*(5), 767–776. https://doi.org/10.1016/s0741-5214(98)70051-5.

EVAR Trial Participants. (2005). Endovascular repair versus open repair in patients with abdominal aortic aneurysm (EVAR trial 1): Randomized controlled trial. *Lancet*, *365*(9478), 2179–2186. https://doi.org/10.1016/S0140-6736(05)66627-5.

Filis, K. A., Arko, F. R., Johnson, B. L., Pipinos, I. I., Harris, E. J., Olcott, C. 4th, et al. (2002). Duplex ultrasound criteria for defining the severity of carotid stenosis. *Annals of Vascular Surgery*, *16*(4), 413–421. https://doi.org/10.1007/s10016-001-0175-8.

Fosse, E., Johnsen, S. H., Stensland-Bugge, E., Joakimsen, O., Mathiesen, E. B., Arnesen, E., et al. (2006). Repeated visual and computer-assisted carotid plaque characterization in a longitudinal population-based ultrasound study: The Tromso study. *Ultrasound in Medicine and Biology*, *32*(1), 3–11. https://doi.org/10.1016/j.ultrasmedbio.2005.09.006.

Gao, M., Hua, Y., Zhao, X., Jia, L., Yang, J., & Liu, B. (2018). Optimal ultrasound criteria for grading stenosis of the superficial femoral artery. *Ultrasound in Medicine and Biology*, *44*(2), 350–358. https://doi.org/10.1016/j.ultrasmedbio.2017.10.001.

Garcia-Criado, A., Gilabert, R., Nicolau, C., Real, M. I., Muntañá, X., Blasco, J., et al. (2005). Value of Doppler sonography for predicting clinical outcome after renal artery revascularization in atherosclerotic vascular disease. *Journal of Ultrasound Medicine*, *24*(12), 1641–1647.

Georgiev, M., Myers, K. A., & Belcaro, G. (2003). The thigh extension of the lesser saphenous vein: From Giacomini's observations to ultrasound scan imaging. *Journal of Vascular Surgery*, *37*(3), 558–563. Retrieved August 17, 2020, from https://ghr.nlm.nih.gov/condition/klippel-trenaunay-syndrome#genes.

Gibson, K. D., Caps, M. T., Gillen, D., Bergelin, R. O., Primozich, J., & Strandness, D. E., Jr. (2001). Identification of factors predictive of lower extremity vein graft thrombosis. *Journal of Vascular Surgery*, *33*(1), 24–31. https://doi.org/10.1067/mva.2001.112214.

Gordon, A. C., Wright, I., & Pugh, N. D. (1996). Duplication of the superficial femoral vein: Recognition with duplex ultrasonography. *Clinical Radiology*, *51*(9), 622–624. https://doi.org/10.1016/s0009-9260(96)80055-9.

Grant, E. G., Benson, C. B., Moneta, G. L., Alexandrov, A. V., Baker, J. D., Bluth, E. I., et al. (2003). Carotid artery stenosis: Gray-scale and Doppler US diagnosis. Society of Radiologists in Ultrasound Consensus Conference. *Radiology*, *229*(2), 340–346. https://doi.org/10.1148/radiol.2292030516.

Gray, C., Goodman, P., Herron, C. C., Lawler, L. P., O'Malley, M. K., O'Donohoe, M. K., et al. (2012). Use of colour duplex ultrasound as a first line surveillance tool following EVAR is associated with a reduction in cost without compromising accuracy. *European Journal of Vascular and Endovascular Surgery*, *44*(2), 145–150. https://doi.org/10.1016/j.ejvs.2012.05.008.

Gronholdt, M. L., Nordestgaard, B. G., Schroeder, T. V., & Sillesen, H. (2001). Ultrasound echolucent carotid plaques predict future strokes. *Circulation*, *104*(1), 68–73. https://doi.org/10.1161/hc2601.091704.

Haenen, J. H., Janssen, M. C., Wollersheim, H., Van't Hof, M. A., de Rooij, M. J., van Langen, H., et al. (2002). The development of postthrombotic syndrome in relationship to venous reflux and calf muscle pump dysfunction at 2 years after the onset of deep venous thrombosis. *Journal of Vascular Surgery*, *35*(6), 1184–1189. https://doi.org/10.1067/mva.2002.122886.

Hartshorne, T. C., McCollum, C. N., Earnshaw, J. J., Morris, J., & Nasim, A. (2011). Ultrasound measurement of aortic diameter in a national screening programme. *European Journal of Vascular and Endovascular Surgery*, *42*(2), 195–199. https://doi.org/10.1016/j.ejvs.2011.02.030.

Heine, G. H., Reichart, B., Ulrich, C., Köhler, H., & Girndt, M. (2007). Do ultrasound resistance indices reflect systemic rather than renal vascular damage in chronic kidney disease? *Nephrology Dialysis Transplantation*, *22*(1), 163–170. https://doi.org/10.1093/ndt/gfl484.

Hennerici, M., Rautenberg, W., Sitzer, G., & Schwarz, A. (1987). Transcranial Doppler ultrasound for the assessment of intracranial arterial flow velocity – Part 1 examination technique and normal values. *Surgical Neurology*, *27*(5), 439–448. https://doi.org/10.1016/0090-3019(87)90251-5.

House, M. K., Dowling, R. J., King, P., & Gibson, R. N. (1999). Using Doppler sonography to reveal renal artery stenosis: An evaluation of optimal imaging parameters. *American Journal of Roentgenology, 173*(3), 761–765. https://doi.org/10.2214/ajr.173.3.10470919.

Ikee, R., Kobayashi, S., Hemmi, N., Imakiire, T., Kikuchi, Y., Moriya, H., et al. (2005). Correlation between the resistive index by Doppler ultrasound and kidney function and histology. *American Journal of Kidney Disease, 46*(4), 603–609. https://doi.org/10.1053/j.ajkd.2005.06.006.

Illig, K. A., Donahue, D., Duncan, D., Freischlag, J., Gelabert, H., Johansen, K., et al. (2016). Reporting standards of the Society for Vascular Surgery for thoracic outlet syndrome. *Journal of Vascular Surgery, 64*(3), e23–e35. https://doi.org/10.1016/j.jvs.2016.04.039.

Jager, K. A., Ricketts, H. J., & Strandness, D. E., Jr. (1985). Duplex scanning for the evaluation of lower limb arterial disease. In E. F. Bernstein (Ed.), *Noninvasive diagnostic techniques in vascular disease* (pp. 619–631). Philadelphia: C V Mosby.

Johnston, K. W., Rutherford, R. B., Tilson, M. D., Shah, D. M., Hollier, L., & Stanley, J. C. (1991). Suggested standards for reporting on arterial aneurysms. Subcommittee on Reporting Standards for Arterial Aneurysms, Ad Hoc Committee on Reporting Standards, Society for Vascular Surgery and North American Chapter, International Society for Cardiovascular Surgery. *Journal of Vascular Surgery, 13*(3), 452–458. https://doi.org/10.1067/mva.1991.26737.

Jorgestrand, T., Lindqvist, M., & Nowak, J. (2002). Diagnostic performance of duplex ultrasonography in the detection of high grade internal carotid artery stenosis. *European Journal of Vascular and Endovascular Surgery, 23*(6), 510–518. https://doi.org/10.1053/ejvs.2002.1621.

Kawarada, O., Yokoi, Y., Takemoto, K., Morioka, N., Nakata, S., & Shiotani, S. (2006). The performance of renal duplex ultrasonography for the detection of hemodynamically significant renal artery stenosis. *Catheterization and Cardiovascular Interventions, 68*(2), 311–318. https://doi.org/10.1002/ccd.20837.

Kearon, C. (2003). Natural history of venous thromboembolism. *Circulation, 107*(23), I22–I30. https://doi.org/10.1161/01.CIR.0000078464.82671.78.

Khaw, K. (2002). The diagnosis of deep vein thrombosis. In J. D. Beard, & S. Murray (Eds.), *Pathways of care in vascular surgery* (pp. 161–169). Shrewsbury, UK: TFM Publishing.

Kirsch, J. D., Mathur, M., Johnson, M. H., Gunabushanam, G., & Scoutt, L. M. (2013). Advances in transcranial Doppler US: Imaging ahead. *Radiographics, 33*(1), E1–E14. https://doi.org/10.1148/rg.331125071.

Kleinjan, A., Di Nisio, M., Beyer-Westendorf, J., Camporese, G, Cosmi, B, Ghiradduzzi, A., et al. (2014). Safety and feasibility of a diagnostic algorithm combining clinical probability, d-dimer testing, and ultrasonography for suspected upper extremity deep venous thrombosis: a prospective management study. *Annals of Internal Medicine, 160*(7), 451–457. https://doi: 10.7326/M13-2056.

Klinkert, P., Schepers, A., Burger, D. H. C., van Bockel, J. H., & Breslau, P. J. (2003). Vein versus polytetrafluoroethylene in above-knee femoropopliteal bypass grafting: Five-year results of a randomized controlled trial. *Journal of Vascular Surgery, 37*(1), 149–155. https://doi.org/10.1067/mva.2002.86.

Kniemeyer, H. W., Kessler, T., Reber, P. U., Ris, H. B., Hakki, H., & Widmer, M. K. (2000). Treatment of ruptured abdominal aortic aneurysm, a permanent challenge or a waste of resources? Prediction of outcome using a multiorgan dysfunction score. *European Journal of Vascular and Endovascular Surgery, 19*(2), 190–196. https://doi.org/10.1053/ejvs.1999.0980.

Koirala, N., Anvari, E., & McLennan, G. (2016). Monitoring and surveillance of hemodialysis access. *Seminars in Interventional Radiology, 33*(1), 25–30. https://doi.org/10.1055/s-0036-1572548.

Kostas, T., Ioannou, C. V., Touloupakis, E., Daskalaki, E., Giannoukas, A. D., Tsetis, D., et al. (2004). Recurrent varicose veins after surgery: A new appraisal of a common and complex problem in vascular surgery. *European Journal of Vascular and Endovascular Surgery, 27*(3), 275–282. https://doi.org/10.1016/j.ejvs.2003.12.006.

Krueger, K., Zaehringer, M., Strohe, D., Stuetzer, H., Boecker, J., & Lackner, K. (2005). Postcatherization pseudoaneurysm: Results of US-guided percutaneous thrombin injection in 240 patients. *Radiology, 236*(3), 1104–1110. https://doi.org/10.1148/radiol.2363040736.

Labropoulos, N., Kang, S. S., Mansour, M. A., Giannoukas, A. D., Moutzouros, V., & Baker, W. H. (2002). Early thrombus remodelling of isolated calf deep vein thrombosis. *European Journal of Vascular and Endovascular Surgery, 23*(4), 344–348. https://doi.org/10.1053/ejvs.2002.1608.

Labropoulos, N., Tiongson, J., Pryor, L., Tassiopoulos, A. K., Kang, S. S., Ashraf Mansour, M., et al. (2003). Definition of venous reflux in lower extremity veins. *Journal of Vascular Surgery, 38*(4), 793–798. https://doi.org/10.1016/s0741-5214(03)00424-5.

Lal, B. K., Hobson, R. W., II, Tofighi, B., Kapadia, I., Cuadra, S., & Jamil, Z. (2008). Duplex ultrasound velocity criteria for the stented carotid artery. *Journal of Vascular Surgery, 47*(1), 63–73. https://doi.org/10.1016/j.jvs.2007.09.038.

Lane, T. R., Metcalfe, M. J., Narayanan, S., & Davies, A. H. (2011). Post-operative surveillance after open peripheral arterial surgery. *European Journal of Vascular and Endovascular Surgery, 42*(1), 59–77. https://doi.org/10.1016/j.ejvs.2011.03.023.

Legemate, D. A., Teeuwen, C., Hoeneveld, H., Ackerstaff, R. G., & Eikelboom, B. C. (1991). Spectral analysis criteria in duplex scanning of aortoiliac and femoropopliteal arterial disease. *Ultrasound in Medicine and Biology*, *17*(8), 769–776. https://doi.org/10.1016/0301 5629(91)90159-t

Leon, C., & Asif, A. (2007). Arteriovenous access and hand pain: The distal hypoperfusion ischemic syndrome. *Clinical Journal of the American Society of Nephrology*, *2*(1), 175–183. https://doi.org/10.2215/CJN.02230606.

Lindholt, J. S., Søgaard, R., & Laustsen, J. (2012). Prognosis of ruptured abdominal aortic aneurysms in Denmark from 1994-2008. *Clinical Epidemiology*, *4*, 111–113. https://doi.org/10.2147/CLEP.S31098.

Linni, K., Mader, N., Aspalter, M., Butturini, E., Ugurluoglu, A., Hitzl, W., et al. (2012). Ultrasonic vein mapping prior to infrainguinal autogenous bypass grafting reduces postoperative infections and readmissions. *Journal of Vascular Surgery*, *56*(1), 126–133. https://doi.org/10.1016/j.jvs.2011.10.135.

Lok, C. E., Huber, T. S., Lee, T., Shenoy, S., Yevzlin, A. S., Abreo, K., & National Kidney Foundation., et al. (2020). KDOQI Vascular Access Guideline Work Group. KDOQI clinical practice guideline for vascular access: 2019 update. *American Journal of Kidney Diseases*, *75*(4 Suppl. 2), S1–S164. https://doi.org/10.1053/j.ajkd.2019.12.001.

London, N. J. M., Sayers, R. D., Thompson, M., Naylor, A. R., Hartshorne, T., Ratliff, D. A., et al. (1993). Interventional radiology in the maintenance of infrainguinal vein graft patency. *British Journal of Surgery*, *80*(2), 187–193. https://doi.org/10.1002/bjs.1800800218.

Long, A., Rouet, L., Lindholt, J. S., & Allaire, E. (2012). Measuring the maximum diameter of native abdominal aortic aneurysms: Review and critical analysis. *European Journal of Vascular and Endovascular Surgery*, *43*(5), 515–524. https://doi.org/10.1016/j.ejvs.2012.01.018.

Luqmani, R., Lee, E., Singh, S., Gillett, M., Schmidt, W. A., Bradburn, M., et al. (2016). The role of ultrasound compared to biopsy of temporal arteries in the diagnosis and treatment of giant cell arteritis (TABUL): A diagnostic accuracy and cost-effectiveness study. *Health Technology Assessment*, *20*(90), 1–238. https://doi.org/10.3310/hta20900.

Macharzina, R. R., Schmid, S. F., Beschorner, U., Noory, E., Rastan, A., Vach, W., et al. (2015). Duplex ultrasound assessment of native stenoses in the superficial femoral and popliteal arteries: A comparative study examining the influence of multisegment lesions. *Journal of Endovascular Therapy*, *22*(2), 254–260. https://doi.org/10.1177/1526602815576094.

Makhoul, R. G., & Machleder, H. I. (1992). Developmental anomalies at the thoracic outlet: An analysis of 200 consecutive cases. *Journal of Vascular Surgery*, *16*(4), 534–545.

Malaterre, H. R., Kallee, K., Giusiano, B., Letallec, L., & Djiane, P. (2001). Holodiastolic reversal flow in the common carotid: Another indicator of the severity of aortic regurgitation. *International Journal of Cardiovascular Imaging*, *17*(5), 333–337. https://doi.org/10.1023/a:1011921501967.

McDicken, W. N. (1981). *Diagnostic ultrasonics: Principles and use of instruments* (2nd ed.). St. Louis, MO: Wiley.

McLafferty, R. B., Passman, M. A., Caprini, J. A., Rooke, T. W., Markwell, S. A., Lohr, J. M., et al. (2008). Increasing awareness about venous disease: The American Venous Forum expands the National Venous Screening Program. *Journal of Vascular Surgery*, *48*(2), 394–399. https://doi.org/10.1016/j.jvs.2008.03.041.

McLafferty, R. B., McCrary, B. S., Mattos, M. A., Karch, L. A., Ramsey, D. E., Solis, M. M., et al. (2002). The use of color-flow duplex scan for the detection of endoleaks. *Journal of Vascular Surgery*, *36*(1), 100–104. https://doi.org/10.1067/mva.2002.123089.

Millen, A., Canavati, R., Harrison, G., McWilliams, R. G., Wallace, S., Vallabhaneni, S. R., et al. (2013). Defining a role for contrast-enhanced ultrasound in endovascular aneurysm repair surveillance. *Journal of Vascular Surgery*, *58*(1), 18–23. https://doi.org/10.1016/j.jvs.2012.12.057.

Mills, Sr. J. L., Conte, M. S., Armstrong, D. G., Pomposelli, F. B., Schanzer, A., Sidawy, A. N., et al. (2013). The society for vascular surgery lower extremity threatened limb classification system: Risk stratification based on Wound, Ischemia, and foot Infection (WIfI). *Journal of Vascular Surgery*, *59*(1), 220–234. e1–e2. https://doi.org/10.1016/j.jvs.2013.08.003.

Moist, L., & Lok, C. E. (2019). Con: Vascular access surveillance in mature fistulas: Is it worthwhile? *Nephrology Dialysis Transplantation*, *34*(7), 1106–1111. https://doi.org/10.1093/ndt/gfz004.

Moneta, G. L., Yeager, R. A., Dalman, R., Antonovic, R., Hall, L. D., & Porter, J. M. (1991). Duplex ultrasound criteria for diagnosis of splanchnic artery stenosis or occlusion. *Journal Vascular Surgery*, *14*(4), 511–520. https://doi.org/10.1016/0741-5214(91)90245-P.

Monti, S., Floris, A., Ponte, C., Schmidt, W. A., Diamantopoulos, A. P., Pereira, C., et al. (2018). The use of ultrasound to assess giant cell arteritis: Review of the current evidence and practical guide for the rheumatologist. *Rheumatology*, *57*(2), 227–235. https://doi.org/10.1093/rheumatology/kex173.

Moran, C., & Butler, M. (2019). Contrast agents. In P. R. Hoskins, K. Martin, & A. Thrush (Eds.), *Diagnostic ultrasound: Physics and equipment* (pp. 239–256). Boca Raton, FL: CRC Press.

Mostbeck, G. H., Kain, R., Mallek, R., Derfler, K., Walter, R., Havelec, L., et al. (1991). Duplex Doppler sonography in renal parenchymal disease: Histopathologic correlation.

Journal of Ultrasound Medicine, 10(4), 189–194. https://doi.org/10.7863/jum.1991.10.4.189.

Mousa, Y. A., Morkous, R., Broce, M., Yacoub, M., Sticco, A., Viradia, R., et al. (2017). Validation of subclavian duplex velocity criteria to grade severity of subclavian artery stenosis. *Journal of Vascular Surgery, 65*(6), 1779–1785. https://doi.org/10.1016/j.jvs.2016.12.098.

Mühlberger, D., Morandini, L., & Brenner, E. (2008). An anatomical study of femoral vein valves near the saphenofemoral junction. *Journal of Vascular Surgery, 48*(4), 994–999. https://doi.org/10.1016/j.jvs.2008.04.045.

Mühlberger, D., Morandini, L., & Brenner, E. (2009). Venous valves and major superficial tributary veins near the saphenofemoral junction. *Journal of Vascular Surgery, 49*(6), 1562–1569. https://doi.org/10.1016/j.jvs.2009.02.241.

National Institute for Health and Care Excellence (NICE) clinical guidance (CG127). (2011). *Hypertension in adults: Diagnosis and management.* Retrieved June 22, 2020, from https://www.nice.org.uk/guidance/cg127.

National Institute for Health and Care Excellence (NICE). (2018). *Clinical guidance 147.* Peripheral arterial disease: Diagnosis and management. Retrieved June 22, 2020, from https://www.nice.org.uk/guidance/cg147/chapter/Recommendations#diagnosis.

National Institute for Health and Care Excellence. (2020). *How should I interpret ankle brachial pressure index (ABPI) results?* https://cks.nice.org.uk/topics/leg-ulcer-venous/diagnosis/interpretation-of-abpi/.

National Institute for Health and Care Excellence. (2020). *Varicose veins.* Retrieved August 16, 2020, from https://cks.nice.org.uk/varicose-veins#!scenario.

National Institute for Health and Care Excellence (NICE) clinical guidelines (NG89). (2018). Venous thromboembolism in over 16s: Reducing the risk of hospital-acquired deep vein thrombosis or pulmonary embolism. Last updated August 2020. Retrieved September 19, 2020, from www.nice.org.uk/guidance/ng89.

Naylor, A. R. (2008). Delay may reduce procedural risk, but at what price to the patient? *European Journal of Vascular and Endovascular Surgery, 35*(4), 383–391. https://doi.org/10.1016/j.ejvs.2008.01.002.

Naylor, A. R., Beard, J. D., & Gaines, P. A. (1998). Extracranial carotid disease. In J. D. Beard & P. A. Gaines (Eds.), *Vascular and endovascular surgery* (pp. 317–350). Philadelphia: WB Saunders.

Naylor, A. R., Ricco, J. –B., de Borst, G. J., Debus, S., de Haro, J., Halliday, A., et al. (2018). Management of atherosclerotic carotid and vertebral artery disease: 2017 Clinical Practice Guidelines of the European Society for Vascular Surgery (ESVS). *European Journal of Vascular and Endovascular Surgery, 55*(1), 3–81. https://doi.org/10.1016/j.ejvs.2017.06.021.

Needleman, L., Cronan, J. J., Lilly, M. P., Merli, G. J., Adhikari, S., Hertzberg, B. S., et al. (2018). Ultrasound for lower extremity deep venous thrombosis. Multidisciplinary recommendations from the Society of Radiologists in Ultrasound Consensus Conference. *Circulation, 137*(14), 1505–1515. https://doi.org/10.1161/CIRCULATIONAHA.117.030687.

National Institute for Health and Care Excellence (NICE) clinical guidelines (NG158). (2020). Venous thromboembolic diseases: Diagnosis, management and thrombophilia testing. Retrieved September 19, 2020, from www.nice.org.uk/guidance/ng158.

NICE guideline [NG158]. (Venous thromboembolic diseases: Diagnosis, management and thrombophilia testing Published date: 26 March 2020. Retrieved September 19, 2020, from www.nice.org.uk/guidance/ng158.

Nichols, W. N., & O'Rourke, M. F. (1990). *McDonald's blood flow in arteries.* London: Edward Arnold.

Nicolaides, A. N., Shifrin, E. G., Bradbury, A., Dhanjil, S., Griffin, M., Belcaro, G., et al. (1996). Angiographic and duplex grading of internal carotid stenosis: Can we overcome confusion? *Journal of Endovascular Surgery, 3*(2), 158–165. https://doi.org/10.1583/1074-6218(1996)003<0158:AADGIC>2.0.CO;2.

Nielsen, T. G. (1996). Natural history of infrainguinal vein bypass stenoses: Early lesions increase the risk of thrombosis. *European Journal of Vascular and Endovascular Surgery, 12*(1), 60–64. https://doi.org/10.1016/s1078-5884(96)80276-0.

Ninet, S., Schnell, D., Dewitte, A., Zeni, F., Meziani, F., & Darmon, M. (2015). Doppler-based renal resistive index for prediction of renal dysfunction reversibility: A systematic review and meta-analysis. *Journal of Critical Care, 30*(3), 629–635. https://doi.org/10.1016/j.jcrc.2015.02.008.

Norgren, L., Hiatt, W. R., Dormandy, J. A., Nehler, M. R., Harris, K. A., Fowkes, F. G., et al. (2007). Inter-Society consensus for the management of peripheral arterial disease (TASC II). *European Journal of Vascular and Endovascular Surgery, 33*(Suppl. 1), S1–S75. https://doi.org/10.1016/j.ejvs.2006.09.024.

North American Symptomatic Carotid Endarterectomy Trial Collaborators (NASCET). (1991). Beneficial effect of carotid endarterectomy in symptomatic patients with high-grade carotid stenosis. *New England Journal of Medicine, 325*(7), 445–453. https://doi.org/10.1161/HYPERTENSIONAHA.114.04183.

North American Symptomatic Carotid Endarterectomy Trial Collaborators. (1998). The final results of the NASCET trial. *New England Journal of Medicine, 339*, 1415–1425.

O'Neill, W. C. (2014). Renal resistive index 2014: A case of mistaken identity. *Hypertension, 64*(5), 914–917.

O'Shaughnessy, A. M., & Fitzgerald, D. E. (2001). The patterns and distribution of residual abnormalities between the individual proximal venous segments after an acute deep vein thrombosis. *Journal of Vascular Surgery, 33*(2), 379–384. https://doi.org/10.1067/mva.2001.111983.

Oates, C. P. (2008). *Cardiovascular haemodynamics and Doppler waveforms explained.* New York: Cambridge University Press.

Oates, C. P., Naylor, A. R., Hartshorne, T., Charles, S. M., Fail, T., Humphries, K., et al. (2009). Joint recommendations for reporting carotid ultrasound investigations in the United Kingdom. *European Journal of Vascular and Endovascular Surgery, 37*(3), 251–261. https://doi.org/10.1016/j.ejvs.2008.10.015.

Older, R. A., Gizieski, T. A., Wilcowski, M. J., Angle, J. F., & Cote, D. A. (1998). Hemodialysis access stenosis: Early detection with color Doppler US. *Radiology, 207*(1), 161–164. https://doi.org/10.1148/radiology.207.1.9530312..

Oliver-Williams, C., Sweeting, M. J., Jacomelli, J., Summers, L., Stevenson, A., Lees, T., et al. (2019). Safety of men with small and medium abdominal aortic aneurysms under surveillance in the NAAASP. *Circulation, 139*(11), 1371–1380. https://doi.org/10.1161/CIRCULATIONAHA.118.036966.

Orbell, J. H., Smith, A., Burnand, K. G., & Waltham, M. (2008). Imaging of deep vein thrombosis. *British Journal of Surgery, 95*(2), 137–146. https://doi.org/10.1002/bjs.6077.

Patel, R., Sweeting, M. J., Powell, J. T., Greenhalgh, R. M., & EVAR trial investigators. (2016). Endovascular versus open repair of abdominal aortic aneurysm in 15-years' follow-up of the UK endovascular aneurysm repair trial 1 (EVAR trial 1): A randomised controlled trial. *Lancet, 388*(10058), 2366–2374. https://doi.org/10.1016/S0140-6736(16)31135-7.

Pellerito, J. S., Revzin, M. V., Tsang, J. C., Greben, C. R., & Naidich, J. B. (2009). Doppler sonographic criteria for the diagnosis of inferior mesenteric artery stenosis. *Journal Ultrasound Medicine, 28*(5), 641–650. https://doi.org/10.7863/jum.2009.28.5.641.

Pemble, L. (2008). A study of the validity of performing carotid duplex ultrasound with the patient in a seated position. *Ultrasound, 16*(2), 80–82. https://doi.org/10.1179/174313408X291070.

Piazza, G. (2014). Varicose veins. *Circulation, 130*(7), 582–587. https://doi.org/10.1161/CIRCULATIONAHA.113.008331.

Platt, J. F., Rubin, J. M., & Ellis, J. H. (1994). Diabetic nephropathy: Evaluation with renal duplex Doppler u/s. *Radiology, 190*(2), 343–346. https://doi.org/10.1148/radiology.190.2.8284379.

Radermacher, J., Chacan, A., Bleck, J., Vitzthum, A., Stoess, B., Gebel, M. J., et al. (2001). Use of Doppler ultrasonography to predict the outcome of therapy for renal-artery stenosis. *New England Journal of Medicine, 344*(6), 410–417. https://doi.org/10.1056/NEJM200102083440603.

Radermacher, J., Ellis, S., & Haller, H. (2002). Renal resistance index and progression of renal disease. *Hypertension, 39*(2 Pt 2), 699–703. https://doi.org/10.1161/hy0202.103782.

Redgrave, J., & Rothwell, P. (2007). Asymptomatic carotid stenosis: What to do. *Current Opinion in Neurology, 20*(1), 58–64. https://doi.org/10.1097/WCO.0b013e328012da60.

Reneman, R. S., van Merode, T., Hick, P., & Hoeks, A. P. (1985). Flow velocity patterns in and distensibility of the carotid artery bulb in subjects of various ages. *Circulation, 71*(3), 500–509. https://doi.org/10.1161/01.CIR.71.3.500.

RESCAN Collaborators, Bown, M. J., Sweeting, M. J., Brown, L. C., Powell, J. T., & Thompson, S. G. (2013). Surveillance intervals for small abdominal aortic aneurysms: A meta-analysis. *Journal of American Medical Association, 309*(8), 806–813. https://doi.org/10.1001/jama.2013.950.

Robertson, V., Poli, F., Hobson, B., Saratzis, A., & Ross Naylor, A. (2019). A systematic review and meta-analysis of the presentation and surgical management of patients with carotid body tumours. *European Journal of Vascular and Endovascular Surgery, 57*(4), 477–486. https://doi:10.1016/j.ejvs.2018.10.038.

Rothwell, P. M., Eliasziw, M., & Gutnikov, S. A. (2004). Endarterectomy for symptomatic carotid stenosis in relation to clinical subgroups and timing of surgery. *Lancet, 363*(9413), 915–924. https://doi.org/10.1016/S0140-6736(04)15785-1.

Rothwell, P. M., Eliasziw, M., Gutnikov, S. A., Fox, A. J., Taylor, D. W., Mayberg, M. R., et al. (2003). Analysis of pooled data from the randomised controlled trials of endarterectomy for symptomatic carotid stenosis. *Lancet, 361*(9352), 107–116. https://doi.org/10.1016/s0140-6736(03)12228-3.

Ruckley, C. V., Evans, C. J., Allan, P. L., Lee, A. J., & Fowkes, F. G. (2002). Chronic venous insufficiency: Clinical and duplex correlations. The Edinburgh Vein Study of venous disorders in the general population. *Journal of Vascular Surgery, 36*(3), 520–525. https://doi.org/10.1067/mva.2002.126547.

Sandford, R. M., Bown, M. J., Fishwick, G., Murphy, F., Naylor, M., Sensier, Y., et al. (2006). Duplex ultrasound is reliable in the detection of endoleak following endovascular aneurysm repair. *European Journal of Vascular and Endovascular Surgery, 32*(5), 537–541. https://doi.org/10.1016/j.ejvs.2006.05.013.

Santilli, S. M., Wernsing, S. E., & Lee, E. S. (2000). Expansion rates and outcomes for iliac artery aneurysms. *Journal of Vascular Surgery, 31*(1 Pt 1), 114–121. https://doi.org/10.1016/s0741-5214(00)70073-5.

Saver, J. L., & Feldman, E. (1993). Basic transcranial Doppler examination: Technique and anatomy. In V. L. Babijan, &

L. R. Weschler (Eds.), *Transcranial Doppler sonography* (pp. 11–28). St. Louis, MO: Mosby.

Schäfer, V. S., Juche, A., Ramiro, S., Krause, A., & Schmidt, W. A. (2017). Ultrasound cut-off values for intima-media thickness of temporal, facial and axillary arteries in giant cell arteritis. *Rheumatology*, 56(9), 1479–1483. https://doi.org/10.1093/rheumatology/kex143.

Schlager, O., Francesconi, M., Haumer, M., Dick, P., Sabeti, S., Amighi, J., et al. (2007). Duplex sonography versus angiography for assessment of femoropopliteal arterial disease in a "real-world" setting. *Journal of Endovascular Therapy*, 14(4), 452–459. https://doi.org/10.1177/152660280701400404.

Schmidt, W. A., Kraft, H. E., Vorphal, K., Völker, L., & Gromnica-Ihle, E. J. (1997). Color duplex ultrasonography in the diagnosis of temporal arteritis. *The New England Journal of Medicine*, 337(19), 1336–1342. https://doi.org/10.1056/NEJM199711063371902.

Schmidt, W. A., Seifert, A., Grominica-Ihle, E., Krause, A., & Natusch, A. (2008). Ultrasound of proximal upper extremity arteries to increase the diagnostic yield in large-vessel giant cell arteritis. *Rheumatology*, 47(1), 96–101. https://doi.org/10.1093/rheumatology/kem322.

Sensier, Y., Bell, P. R., & London, N. J. (1998). The ability of qualitative assessment of the common femoral Doppler waveform to screen for significant aortoiliac disease. *European Journal of Vascular and Endovascular Surgery*, 15(4), 357–364. https://doi.org/10.1016/s1078-5884(98)80041-5.

Sensier, Y., Hartshorne, T., Thrush, A., Nydahl, S., Bolia, A., & London, N. J. (1996). A prospective comparison of lower limb colour-coded duplex scanning with arteriography. *European Journal of Vascular and Endovascular Surgery*, 11(2), 170–175. https://doi.org/10.1016/s1078-5884(96)80047-5.

Sinha, S., Houghton, J., Holt, P. J., Thompson, M. M., Loftus, I. M., & Hinchliffe, R. J. (2012). Popliteal entrapment syndrome. *Journal of Vascular Surgery*, 55(1), 252–262. https://doi.org/10.1016/j.jvs.2011.08.050.

Siracuse, J. J., Nandivada, P., Giles, K. A., Hamdan, A. D., Wyers, M. C., Chaikof, E. L., et al. (2013). Prosthetic graft infections involving the femoral artery. *Journal of Vascular Surgery*, 57(3), 700–705. https://doi.org/10.1016/j.jvs.2012.09.049.

Sloan, M. A., Alexandrov, A. V., Tegeler, C. H., Spencer, M. P., Caplan, L. R., Feldmann, E., & Therapeutics and Technology Assessment Subcommittee of the American Academy of Neurology., et al. (2004). Assessment: Transcranial Doppler ultrasonography. Report of the Therapeutics and Technology Assessment Subcommittee of the American Academy of Neurology. *Neurology*, 62(9), 1468–1481. https://doi.org/10.1212/wnl.62.9.1468.

Souza de Oliveira, I. R., Widman, A., Molnar, L. J., Fukushima, J. T., Praxedes, J. N., & Cerri, G. G. (2000). Colour Doppler ultrasound: A new index improves the diagnosis of renal artery stenosis. *Ultrasound in Medicine and Biology*, 26(1), 41–47. https://doi.org/10.1016/s0301-5629(99)00119-2.

Spencer, M. P., & Reid, J. M. (1979). Quantitation of carotid stenosis with continuous-wave (C-W) Doppler ultrasound. *Stroke*, 10(3), 326–330. https://doi.org/10.1161/01.STR.10.3.326.

Staub, D., Canevascini, R., Huegli, R. W., Aschwanden, M., Thalhammer, C., Imfeld, S., et al. (2007). Best duplex-sonographic criteria for the assessment of renal artery stenosis – correlation with intra-arterial pressure gradient. *Ultraschall in der Medizin*, 28(1), 45–51. https://doi.org/10.1055/s-2007-962881.

Stavros, A. T., & Harshfield, D. (1994). Renal Doppler, renal artery stenosis and renovascular hypertension: Direct and indirect duplex sonographic abnormalities in patients with renal artery stenosis. *Ultrasound Quarterly*, 12(4), 217–263. https://doi.org/10.1097/00013644-199412040-00003.

Stuart, W. P., Adam, D. J., Allan, P. L., Ruckley, C. V., & Bradbury, A. W. (2000). The relationship between the number, competence, and diameter of medial calf perforating veins and the clinical status in healthy subjects and patients with lower-limb venous disease. *Journal of Vascular Surgery*, 32(1), 138–143. https://doi.org/10.1067/mva.2000.105666.

Talbot, R. (2012). Duplex ultrasound assessment of upper extremity arterial occlusive disease. In J. S. Pellerito, & J. F. Polak (Eds.), *Introduction to vascular ultrasonography* (6th ed.) (262–280). Philadelphia: Elsevier Saunders.

Tessitore, N., & Poli, A. (2019). Pro: Vascular access surveillance in mature fistulas: Is it worthwhile? *Nephrology Dialysis Transplantation*, 34(7), 1102–1106. https://doi.org/10.1093/ndt/gfz003.

The National Institute for Health and Care Excellence (NICE). (Stroke and TIA in over 16s: Diagnosis and initial treatment: NG 128. (published: 1 May 2019) www.nice.org/guidance/ng128.

The UK Small Aneurysm Trial Participants. (1998). Mortality results for randomised controlled trial of early elective surgery or ultrasonographic surveillance for small abdominal aortic aneurysms. *Lancet*, 352, 1649–1655. https://doi.org/10.1016/S0140-6736(98)10137-X.

The UK Small Aneurysm Trial Participants. (2007). Final 12-year follow-up of surgery versus surveillance in the UK small aneurysm trial. *British Journal of Surgery*, 94(6), 702–708. https://doi.org/10.1002/bjs.5778.

Thompson, S. G., Ashton, H. A., Gao, L., Buxton, M. J., Scott, R. A. P., & Multicentre Aneurysm Screening Study (MASS) Group. (2012). Final follow-up of the multicentre aneurysm screening study (MASS) randomized trial of abdominal aortic aneurysm screening. *British Journal of Surgery*, 99(12), 1649–1656. https://doi.org/10.1002/bjs.8897.

Thrush, A. J., & Evans, D. H. (1995). Intrinsic spectral broadening: A potential cause of misdiagnosis of carotid artery disease. *Journal of Vascular Investigation, 1*, 187–192.

Tordoir, J., Canaud, B., Haage, P., Konner, K., Basci, A., Fouque, D., et al. (2007). EBPG on vascular access. *Nephrology Dialysis Transplantation, 22*(Suppl. 2), ii88–ii117. https://doi.org/10.1093/ndt/gfm021.

Tordoir, J. H. M., Rooyens, P., Dammers, R., van der Sande, F. M., de Haan, M., & Yo, T. I. (2003). Prospective evaluation of failure modes in autogenous radiocephalic wrist access for hemodialysis. *Nephrology Dialysis Transplantation, 18*(2), 378–383. https://doi.org/10.1093/ndt/18.2.378.

Tsivgoulis, G., Alexandrov, A. V., & Sloan, M. A. (2009). Advances in transcranial Doppler ultrasonography. *Current Neurology and Neuroscience Reports, 9*(1), 46–54. https://doi.org/10.1007/s11910-009-0008-7.

US Preventive Services Task Force Recommendation Statement, Owens, D. K., Davidson, K. W., Krist, A. H., Barry, M. J., Cabana, M., et al. (2019). Screening for abdominal aortic aneurysm: Recommendation statement. *Journal of American Medical Association, 322*(22), 2211–2218. https://doi.org/10.1001/jama.2019.18928.

Utter, G. H., Dhillon, T. S., Salcedo, E. S., Shouldice, D. J., Reynolds, C. L., Humphries, M. D., et al. (2016). Therapeutic anticoagulation for isolated calf deep vein thrombosis. *JAMA Surgery, 151*(9), e161770. https://doi.org/10.1001/jamasurg.2016.1770.

Van den Bos, R., Kockaert, M., Neumann, H., & Nijsten, T. (2008). Technical review of endovenous laser therapy for varicose veins. *European Journal of Vascular and Endovascular Surgery, 35*(1), 88–95. https://doi.org/10.1016/j.ejvs.2007.08.005.

van Marrewijk, C., Buth, J., Harris, P. L., Norgren, L., Nevelsteen, A., & Wyatt, M. G. (2002). Significance of endoleaks after endovascular repair of abdominal aortic aneurysms: The EUROSTAR experience. *Journal of Vascular Surgery, 35*(3), 461–473. https://doi.org/10.1067/mva.2002.118823.

Veith, F. J., Baum, R. A., Ohki, T., Amor, M., Adiseshiah, M., Blankensteijn, J. D., et al. (2002). Nature and significance of endoleaks and endotension: Summary of opinions expressed at an international conference. *Journal of Vascular Surgery, 35*(5), 1029–1035. https://doi.org/10.1067/mva.2002.123095.

Venous thromboembolism in over 16s: Reducing the risk of hospital-acquired deep vein thrombosis or pulmonary embolism. Retrieved September 21, 2020, from, www.nice.org.uk/guidance/ng89.

Virchow, R. (1846). Die Verstopfung den Lungenarterie und ihre Folgen. *Beitr Exp Pathol Physiol, 2*, 1.

von Reutern, G. M., & von Büdingen, H. J. (1993). *Ultrasound diagnosis of cerebrovascular disease*. Thieme Verlag.

Webber, G. W., Jang, J., Gustavason, S., & Olin, J. W. (2007). Contemporary management of postcatheterization pseudoaneurysms. *Circulation, 115*(20), 2666–2674. https://doi.org/10.1161/CIRCULATIONAHA.106.681973.

Wells, P. S. (2007). Integrated strategies for the diagnosis of venous thromboembolism. *Journal of Thrombosis and Haemostasis, 5*, 41–50. https://doi.org/10.1111/j.1538-7836.2007.02493.x.

Whittingham, T. A. (1999). Tissue harmonic imaging. *European Radiology, 9*(Suppl. 3), S323–S326. https://doi.org/10.1007/pl00014065.

Whittingham, T. A., & Martin, K. (2019). Transducers and beam-forming. In P. R. Hoskins, K. Martin, & A. Thrush (Eds.), *Diagnostic ultrasound: Physics and equipment* (pp. 37–71). Boca Raton, FL: CRC Press.

Williams, S. K., Campbell, W. B., & Earnshaw, J. J. (2014). Survey of management of common iliac artery aneurysms by members of the Vascular Society of Great Britain and Ireland. *Annals of the Royal College of Surgeons of England, 96*(2), 116–120. https://doi.org/10.1308/003588414X13814021676512.

Yusof, N. N. M., McCann, A., Little, P. J., & Ta, H. T. (2019). Non-invasive imaging techniques for the differentiation of acute and chronic thrombosis. *Thrombosis Research, 177*, 161–171. https://doi.org/10.1016/j.thromres.2019.03.009.

Zhou, W., Felkai, D., Evans, M., McCoy, S. A., Lin, P. H., Kougias, P., & et al (2008). Ultrasound criteria for severe in-stent restenosis following carotid artery stenting. *Journal of Vascular Surgery, 47*(1), 74–80. https://doi.org/10.1016/j.jvs.2007.09.031.

Zierler, R. E., Jordan, W. D., Lal, B. K., Mussa, F., Leers, S., Fulton, J., et al. (2018). The Society for Vascular Surgery practice guidelines on follow-up after vascular surgery arterial procedures. *Journal of Vascular Surgery, 68*(1), 256–284. https://doi.org/10.1016/j.jvs.2018.04.018.

Zitek, T., Baydoun, J., Yepez, S., Forred, W., & Slattery, D. E. (2016). Mistakes and pitfalls associated with two-point compression ultrasound for deep vein thrombosis. *Western Journal of Emergency Medicine, 17*(2), 201–208. https://doi.org/10.5811/westjem.2016.1.29335.

Zuker-Herman, R., Ayalon Dangur, I., Berant, R., Sitt, E. C., Baskin, L., & et al (2018). Comparison between two-point and three-point compression ultrasound for the diagnosis of deep vein thrombosis. *Journal of Thrombosis and Thrombolysis, 45*(1), 99–105. https://doi.org/10.1007/s11239-017-1595-9.

FURTHER READING

Anvari, A., Forsberg, F., & Samir, A. E. (2015). A primer on the physical principles of tissue harmonic imaging. *RadioGraphics*, *35*(7), 1955–1964. https://doi.org/10.1148/rg.2015140338.

Bland, M. (2015). *An introduction to medical statistics* (4th ed.). Oxford: Oxford University Press.

BMUS Safety Group. (2009). British medical ultrasound society. *Guidelines for the safe use of diagnostic ultrasound equipment*. Retrieved November 15, 2020, from https://www.bmus.org/static/uploads/resources/BMUS-Safety-Guidelines-2009-revision-FINAL-Nov-2009.pdf.

Evans, D. H., & McDicken, W. N. (2000). *Doppler ultrasound: Physics, instrumentation and signal processing*. Wiley.

Ferrara, K., & DeAngelis, G. (1997). Color flow mapping. *Ultrasound in Medicine and Biology*, *23*(3), 321–345. https://www.umbjournal.org/article/S0301-5629(96)00216-5/fulltext.

Guidance for Industry and Food and Drug Administration Staff. (2019). *Marketing clearance of diagnostic ultrasound systems and transducers*. Retrieved November 16, 2020, from https://www.fda.gov/media/71100/download.

Guidelines for Professional Ultrasound Practice. Society and College of Radiographers and British Medical Ultrasound Society Revision 4. December 2019. Retrieved September 3, 2020, from https://www.bmus.org/static/uploads/resources/Guidelines_for_Professional_Ultrasound_Practice_v3_OHoz76r.pdf

Hoskins, P. R., Martin, K., & Thrush, A. (Eds.). (2019). *Diagnostic ultrasound: Physics and equipment* (3rd ed.). Boca Raton, FL: CRC Press.

Industry standards for the prevention of work-related musculoskeletal disorders in sonography. (2017). Developed through a 2016 consensus conference hosted by the society of diagnostic medical sonography. *Journal of Diagnostic Medical Sonography*, *33*(5), 370–391.

Kim, E. S., Sharma, A. M., Scissons, R., Dawson, D., Eberhardt, R. T., Gerhard-Herman, M., et al. (2020).

Interpretation of peripheral arterial and venous Doppler waveforms: A consensus statement from the Society for Vascular Medicine and Society for Vascular Ultrasound. *Vascular Medicine*, *25*(5), 484–506. https://doi.org/10.1177/1358863X20937665.

Kremkau, F. W. (2019). *Sonography principles and instrumentation* (10th ed.). Philadelphia: WB Saunders.

Mahé, G., Boulon, C., Desormais, I., Lacroix, P., Bressollette, L., & Guilmot, J. L. (2017). A statement for Doppler waveforms analysis. *Vasa*, *46*(5), 337–345. https://econtent.hogrefe.com/doi/pdf/10.1024/0301-1526/a000638.

Pellerito, J., & Polak, J. F. (2019). *Introduction to vascular ultrasonography* (7th ed.). Elsevier.

Pozniak, M. A., & Allan, P. L. (2013). *Clinical Doppler ultrasound* (3rd ed.). London: Churchill Livingstone.

Quality Improvement Guidelines for Accuracy of Examinations in the Vascular Laboratory. (2018). *Society for vascular ultrasound*. Retrieved September 3, 2020, from https://higherlogicdownload.s3.amazonaws.com/SVUNET/c9a8d83b-2044-4a4e-b3ec-cd4b2f542939/UploadedImages/19__Quality_Assurance_Guidelines_for_Accuracy_of_Examinations_in_the_Vascular_Laboratory__Updated_2018_.pdf.

ter Haar, G. (2012). *The safe use of ultrasound in medical diagnosis* (3rd ed.). BIR publications. Retrieved November 15, 2020, from https://www.birpublications.org/pb/assets/raw/Books/SUoU_3rdEd/Safe_Use_of_Ultrasound.pdf.

Ultrasound Transducer Decontamination – Best Practice Summary 2020 The Society and College of Radiographers. Retrieved October 4, 2020, from https://www.sor.org/news/health-safety/effective-and-safe-decontamination-of-ultrasound-m.

Work Related Musculoskeletal Disorders (Sonographers). (2019). *The Society and College of Radiographers*. Retrieved October 3, 2020, from https://www.sor.org/getmedia/6698659d-2910-4bca-a826-ea942acaf80a/work_related_musculoskeletal_disorders_sonographers.pdf_2.

Note: Page numbers followed by "*f*", "t", or "b" refers to figures, tables or box respectively.